Towards Optimal Management of Diabetes in Surgery

Sanjeev Kelkar • Shubhangi Muley
Prakash Ambardekar

Towards Optimal Management of Diabetes in Surgery

Springer

Sanjeev Kelkar
Private Practice
Pune
Maharashtra
India

Shubhangi Muley
Senior Consultant Anesthesiologist
Central India Institute of Medical Science
Nagpur
Maharashtra
India

Prakash Ambardekar
Consultant, Anesthesioligist
Fortis S L Raheja Hospital
Mumbai
Maharashtra
India

ISBN 978-981-13-7707-5 ISBN 978-981-13-7705-1 (eBook)
https://doi.org/10.1007/978-981-13-7705-1

This Springer imprint is published by the registered company Springer Nature Singapore Pte Ltd.
The registered company address is: 152 Beach Road, #21-01/04 Gateway East, Singapore 189721, Singapore

Dedicated to the general, orthopedic, and plastic surgeons, anesthetists, and physicians and their understudies

To the faculty in Medical Colleges

To the resident doctors and the nurses of ICUs, operating theatres, and surgical, medical, and gynecology wards

To our students who, over the last 20 years, have practiced these ideas across India

And to anyone who has a need to understand these ideas for implementation

And to all agencies and individuals who have helped us to propagate these ideas for long.

Preface

Routine diabetes management itself has remained suboptimal in India. The mammoth effort put in by those who understood diabetes and willingly taught it over hundreds of continuing medical education programs, conferences, small booklets, and other forms of communication on diabetes has resulted in a large body of physicians in India with far better understanding of diabetes. The role of the various societies dedicated to diabetes as well as the pharmaceutical industry in this sphere must be gratefully acknowledged. Many of these efforts have looked into developing better understanding of the perioperative management of diabetes also as part of the overall teaching content. Even then, the perioperative situation of a patient with diabetes remains a large gray area in modern medicine till date. Despite many refined advancements of techniques in surgery, anesthesia, finer anesthetic drugs, and fairly widespread understanding of diabetes management, something extra was required to be done to make these matters also better.

The optimal management for best results in any complex situation needs an integrated, collaborative, proactive approach among the three specialties—surgery, anesthesia, and medicine. It is not only a question of their individual understanding of diabetes. In the practical management, issues of significance and of great importance are not the medical knowledge only. These relate to logistics for better coordination of them, understanding the contribution each one makes and limitations of each of these specialties. These issues neither get discussed in any forums and even in textbooks on diabetes nor are they addressed where these three specialists work or are expected to work together. This volume we believe will be of great help to make these matters also better.

Pune, Maharashtra, India — Sanjeev Kelkar
Nagpur, Maharashtra, India — Shubhangi Muley
Mumbai, Maharashtra, India — Prakash Ambardekar

Acknowledgments

In this long journey, we received support from many individuals and institutions. Ex-vice chair of the World Diabetes Foundation, Copenhagen, Dr. Anil Kapur, and former director of the Central India Institute of Medical Sciences, Late Dr. G.M. Taori, were the first. Dr. Ravi Bapat, ex-HOD Surgery KEM Hospital, Mumbai, and ex-vice chancellor of Maharashtra University of Health Sciences, has appreciated this effort many years ago. The Association of Surgeons of India and its various state branches, medical colleges across India, Bhilai Steel Plant, and AMRI Hospital Kolkata were some of the institutes where we held these programs. Later, the University of Newcastle, NSW, Australia, incorporated this program in their educational initiatives in India; particularly helpful were Dr. Jean McPherson and Dr. Judith Scott. The Diabetic Foot Society of India and its founder, President Dr. Arun Bal, and other members also supported this initiative. It gave us an opportunity to interact with the professional spectrum intended to be benefitted by. The feedback we received was valuable for us to continue to improve. We are grateful to them all. Three individuals, Mr. Mohan Naik, Mr. B.S.V. Naidu, and Mr. Aravind Kashyap, have exerted themselves for the success of this journey.

In preparation of this volume, we are thankful to Ms. Guneet Kaur, New Delhi, for the considerable work on transcription which made our work far easier. Mr. V.P.M.R. Prasad from Bengaluru has been of enormous help in reference work needed. It has lent depth to our writing. Dr. Shreerang Godbole, endocrinologist, Pune, and Dr. Ashu Rastogi, Asst. Professor, Department of Endocrinology, PGI, Chandigarh, have carefully gone through a few, rather intricate, chapters and corrected them. The idea that it should be published as a volume was initiated by Dr. Naren Agarwal of Springer Nature, New Delhi. We thank him for accepting the proposal and encouraging the development and publication of this volume. We also thank Ms. Teena Bedi and Mr. Ejaz Ahmad of Springer Nature for their assistance and follow-up. We are grateful to all of them.

About the Book

August 2019

We developed a teaching program on perioperative management of diabetes in 1995. From 1995 till 2005, we presented this in many forum and conferences, particularly to surgeons, in medical colleges across India which has continued till date albeit more sporadically. The principle these programs followed was to build the right perspective and establish the logic behind the themes related to the core ideas, rather than to cram the lectures with enormous details. One forum which trained nearly 700 medical consultants through a process of problem-based learning in India from 2001 to 2005 was found to be particularly rewarding in emphasizing the logic of this ill-understood area. Our efforts were highly acknowledged by all those who listened to it. The persistent suggestion from all of them was to bring this information in one book.

The later years witnessed an explosive growth in the much deeper understanding of diabetes due to extensive fundamental and therapeutic research, introduction of many newer surgical techniques which made the surgery itself quicker and safer, investigative modalities that helped the management of the critical care situation, and more elegant and finer equipment, techniques, and newer, safer anesthetic medication. All this became available in India on a widespread scale in a short period of time. The need to accommodate these details in a work only reinforced the desire of attempting to write a volume on this area.

We also realized that despite the explosion of these developments, the principles of management, and the logic behind how these new facilities should be incorporated in practice have remained the same. This has shaped the structure and the contents of this volume. The volume thus attempts to achieve the following:

The first half of the book purposely focuses on the critical care aspects of diabetes management in surgical setting. In doing that, we have emphasized the need to shift the focus of control of diabetes and other abnormalities arising there from to the residents and the ICU or the ward nurses. Thus, the first chapter addresses to empower these doctors to manage these situations primarily. For that, we have used most of the situations they routinely confront, the reasoning behind why they develop, and, as a fallout, the measures, monitoring, and precautions they should take. We have also pointed out the huge practical benefits that result out of this. It also addresses the consultants in all the above branches and how to support the management from behind without getting in to minute-to-minute management.

The critical surgical (and medical) care in diabetes is invariably accompanied by diabetic ketoacidosis and hyperosmolar states, the most difficult to control. This chapter extends the glucose management in more complete management of all other abnormalities. It also indicates the fundamental relation of the surgical state, giving rise to these two states and the intriguing aspects related to it.

The third chapter builds upon this understanding in emergency major situations and its management. The emphasis now changes from practical management to the understanding of the more fundamental pathological dysfunctions of all the organ systems which are potentially dangerous to survival. It also discusses the barriers in taking such a patient up for surgery early, the most crucial issue in this area.

Logically, the fourth and fifth chapters enter in the discussion of intra- and post-operative management, followed by the discussion of the single factor of hypoglycemia and how it keeps the routine or critical surgical and diabetes management suboptimal in perioperative situations.

The next chapter gives a detailed expose of the numerous issues that arise in the elective, routine surgical situations.

The number of surgical options to rectify different disorders has increased. Even if they are elective in nature, there is a need to have a better understanding of the pathophysiology, organ effects, and its perioperative and longer term risks, we have grouped all of them in two chapters of Special Surgical Situations. This chapter thus goes in greater depth of theory but much greater degree of management as well. Two areas have been given special importance since these are generally not covered in detail in discourses or in the textbooks. The first is the gestational diabetes. The professional attention in diagnosis and good management needs a boost since it is related also to the primordial and primary prevention of diabetes in the future generations. The numbers are also rising, and a different specialty of gynecology now works with the physicians and anesthetists.

The second emphasis is on the regional anesthesia in diabetic foot and such other local surgical procedures. We believe that its importance lies in its sheer high prevalence, highly suboptimal conditions in which the patients present, difficulties in taking them up for surgery and devastating consequences both on life and economy as no other condition in diabetes does.

The other need we felt strongly was to give an in-depth knowledge of the diabetes as such. Without that, the discussions on practical management with its reasoning, we felt, would not be complete. Secondly, the later stages of perioperative management, at discharge and beyond also, must see the optimal understanding of it. Hence, we have written detailed chapters on insulin physiology with its actions, its pharmacodynamics, and its pharmacokinetics. The same has been applied to other drugs used in diabetes, comorbid conditions, and their drug-to-drug interactions.

The knowledge of the deeper understanding of the pathological basis of diabetes was scattered throughout the volume. There were many aspects which was essential to elaborate. In order not to disturb the flow of the discussion, we did not include them but decided to present them as a separate chapter titled Metabolic Havoc of Uncontrolled Diabetes, which is profound in theory.

The same difficulty arose in including several aspects of care. Many of them are smaller areas. Some are areas where a conflict is apparent. In other places, the historical understanding of some of the changes that have occurred was required to build the full care perspective. The Commonly Asked Questions collected together in the last chapter fall in these categories. They are as instructive as the metabolic havoc. On the whole, there might be a miniscule minority of issues we may not have touched.

The authors have a combined clinical and teaching experience of nearly 100 years. We have some insight in the exact needs of the doctors. Therefore, lastly, our endeavor is geared to improve the in-depth understanding by identifying the learning gaps and attempts to develop the habit of critical clinical reasoning which presently is rather dim. We sincerely hope the volume will be of help and will be welcomed by the medical fraternity.

Sanjeev Kelkar
Shubhangi Muley
Prakash Ambardekar

Contents

About the Authors

Sanjeev Kelkar an MD in Internal Medicine has worked in many fields of health care, but diabetes has remained his focus for the last three decades. A key figure in India, he has successfully conducted innovative teaching programs for postgraduate doctors in collaboration with the Australian University in Newcastle. He was awarded for this work by the Australian Government and Australian Industry. With a few other doctors, he founded the Diabetic Foot Society of India, which has since become recognized throughout the Diabetes World. Improving the understanding of Diabetes and Diabetic Foot among allopaths, paramedics, and doctors from traditional systems of medicine in India through numerous interactive workshops is another of his achievements. He has written and edited many books on Diabetic Foot Management.

Shubhangi Muley holds an MD in Anesthesia from AIIMS, New Delhi. After working at AIIMS, she became a Senior Consultant in Neuro and Cardiac Anesthesia and was the chief of critical care for nearly 8 years at the CIIMS, Nagpur. During this time, she worked to develop and adapt many methods for smoothly managing these heavy burdens in simple, straightforward ways, making their management more efficient. Many of these ideas can be found in this volume.

Prakash Ambardekar is a veteran anesthetist who has pioneered, developed, and refined the techniques of regional anesthesia particularly in infected diabetic foot surgery in hemodynamically unstable patients with grossly altered vital parameters, as well as other infected lesions elsewhere in the body—innovations that have made these surgeries far safer than under general anesthesia. He has performed thousands of these surgeries with successful outcomes.

Role of Residents and Nurses in Perioperative Diabetes Management

1

Contents

S. Kelkar et al., *Towards Optimal Management of Diabetes in Surgery*,
https://doi.org/10.1007/978-981-13-7705-1_1

1.1 The Present Culture of Indoor Medical Management

Managing diabetes optimally in emergency or routine surgery is still a gray area. In patients who are critically ill, it is much more complex. Optimal control within limitations of surgical setting is rarely achieved in most places. Excessive or too frequent monitoring without dynamically changing plans for controlling the blood glucose to its optimal level is common. Optimal/tight blood glucose control leads to far better outcomes in all types of surgical settings [1].[1] The primary reason for not undertaking aggressive management is the illogical fear of hypoglycemia and its consequences. The second is the inability to understand the relation between hyperglycemia in surgical setting and the causes leading to it. This in its turn leads to further indecisiveness about continuously altering the insulin administration to the dynamically changing causes. The third is the lack of knowledge of the pharmacokinetics and pharmacodynamics of administered insulin. Fourth is the high levels of insulin resistance that is obtained in these situations and how to break the resistance to achieve normoglycemia. Insulin resistance increases by seven- to eightfold in patients undergoing surgical procedures [2]. All of these factors with many more lead to a state of continuous hyperglycemia.

1.1.1 The Indoor Management Culture

Currently, in most places, particularly the private setups, glucose control is consultant centric. For every smallest decision, the residents and the nurses are expected to inform the consultant and get the advice. For example, if a particular intravenous infusion or the pumps used routinely nowadays are coming to an end, or a latest of the blood glucose result or any other report has been communicated to the nurses, they have to inform the residents, the residents then contact the consultant, and the change in the orders goes back in the reverse direction to be executed. The situation

[1] In this landmark study in 2001, Van den Berghe et al. controlled hyperglycemia with or without a history of diabetes. The setting was critical surgical ICU. Majority were critical postcardiac surgery patients. It was a large, prospective, randomized controlled trial with a treatment group that was tightly controlled for glucose levels. The other control group was treated conventionally. All other management modalities were the same for both groups. It reported a dramatic 42% decrease in mortality in tightly controlled group. It had several other collateral benefits like reduced patients' needs for antibiotics, blood transfusions, and kidney failures, and support for ventilation was much shorter. The polyneuropathy as a result of critical illness was also reduced in the treatment group.

will and does get complicated when more than one consultant are managing the case since the same dialogue has to take place again with the remaining ones.

It is not uncommon that the original order passed by the A consultant here is reversed or modified by the main or some other consultant, ensuing the same chain of communication immediately or later in the evening or late night rounds of all these consultants. The result is highly suboptimal and leading to haphazard management which does not have any planned and consistent approach for the day or the next few days. It becomes an unintelligent and mechanical exercise which is so completely boring for the nurses as well as the residents and is demeaning to them. More disastrous is the outcome that most important human agencies, the residents, and the nurses experience a completely meaningless existence while managing the cases for blood glucose control. We need not go in the reasons for this type of management at this place. It has been discussed in extensive detail in my volumes on health policy in public and private health care in India. All we need to find out is if there is a simpler way to solve the problem. The answer is to make the residents and the nurses *primarily* responsible to optimize the blood glucose control and take decisions during the day and in the night, and consultants should play a different role during the routine rounds which will be explained later in detail. Delegating not just serious but highly complex issues like optimization of glucose during the surgical setting to nurses and residents may look either ridiculous or too dangerous an approach to most consultants. The authors of this volume have not only advocated but practiced this approach since 20 years that have gone by. These objections were there then, as they are now. Some of the issues related to this positional and perspective change will be discussed later in this chapter.

The authors also refuse to accept that this is a highly complex and serious issue. It is extremely important yes, but it is neither complex nor serious. In diabetes management, in any setting only three things can happen. The blood glucose will go either high or very high, low or very low, or remain in a desirable range. All that one needs to know is what the causes are behind any of the three situations, the logic to manage these three situations, and the iatrogenic effects of the treatment given in its totality which includes surgical, anesthesia, and critical care. Before we introduce to the professional reading these pages the magic formulae that make the management easy, we would like to talk about a few more ideas.

The management at resident and nurse level should be a reflection of the joint decisions taken over the fluid, electrolytes, calorie management, and antibiotic regimes by the three specialists. Unless these basic agreements are reached, no method of glucose control will ever work. Fluctuations of fluid, electrolyte, and acid base balance could also be as much or more troublesome than any other problem created by hyperglycemia.

The types of residents/nurses involved usually are:

1. Newly operative medical residents at junior most levels.
2. Medical residents of intermediate level of experience.
3. Surgical or anesthesia residents of the above categories.
4. Newly graduating nurses who are facing complex situations.

The first job that any one of them is expected to do is to follow the instructions related to surgery per se and the "metabolic management." The second job expected of them to do is to undertake to intently watch any variations or abnormalities that may develop in the course and report them. They are not allowed to think about the reasons behind the transgression of physiological or acceptable limits of parameters—clinical, radiological, and, more importantly, biochemical and hematological. For them to be able to do that in the initial periods of their service, they need a considerable input of logic and reason as to why the matters are out of control as well as the meaning and logic behind what management steps are being taken and what they will do to the situation. This will give them an insight to solve these issues while faithfully reporting the same to the senior consultants.

Unfortunately, no such empowering exercise is undertaken by today's consultants, anywhere in India. The alertness and ability to see a parameter in the total perspective of the surgical/diabetic situation can be developed only by such teaching. They will be then able to act upon the knowledge by themselves or follow the instructions more intelligently with greater understanding, reasoning, and logic and see the effects of these instructions, on the situation, for even better understanding. It will help the specialists even more if they undertake this exercise.

Now let us start from the beginning where this saga begins.

1.2 Interpreting the First Glucose Value in Perioperative Setting

This value could be the one the patient has come to the treating facility with. It could be a few days or weeks old when the surgical setting was not fully set, especially the emergency surgery. Or it could be the one done immediately before or after admission. This is the value we need to consider to unravel the entire mystique of glucose control in pre-operative settings. To make matters easier to understand, we will make another assumption that the patient has got admitted in an acute or critical surgical condition. It will however hold true for nonsurgical acute or critical cases as well. The same logic presented below also holds for all glucose readings the residents or the consultants are faced later with, throughout the management from the outpatient, emergency room, surgery, and the discharge.

The most important thing to understand is that any glucose reading is the result of:

(a) The native insulin resistance that has got enhanced due to the surgical condition.
(b) The rate at which calories are being supplemented, its variability or nonsupplementation.
(c) The plasma levels of insulin at the point of monitoring for which the surrogate marker could be taken as insulin infusion rate—U/min.

Therefore if the blood glucose is high as will be the case in most majority of the cases, it has to be managed by taking steps to reduce the intensity of the causes or elimination of it which has led to enhanced insulin resistance as in a. above. That done—the next and the crucial step are to increase the blood level of insulin in whichever way one wants to do (and there are several ways of doing it which will be discussed in the volume at different places.) *This is the main domain of the residents and the nurses to manage, without a necessary recourse to consultants all the time.* The third is the rate at which calories are being supplemented. At the resident level, some attempts should be made to change the management strategies in short term and getting it confirmed with the consultants later.

1.2.1 The Converse of This Logic

(a) If the factors which raised the insulin resistance start getting treated effectively, it will lead to the reduction of the insulin resistance which continues to decline at steady speed initially and when under control, rapidly. It is a dynamic reduction, and the only way to understand it is to observe the patient's condition, his vitals, well-spaced blood glucose values, and laboratory results.
(b) Once the situation in a, has got set, the blood or the plasma level of insulin should be brought down *proportionate* to the blood glucose reading, by well-spaced out monitoring. If this is not done, it will either not control hyperglycemia or may lead albeit rarely to hypoglycemia.
(c) As the blood glucose readings lower or tend to normal, calorie supplementation comes in for detailed understanding leading to a plan of administration of calories. The basic principle is to *administer calories at a uniform rate* in the days to follow. We will discuss that at appropriate places.
(d) The course of the management then is to titrate the blood glucose levels with the rate of insulin infusions for the next few days to maintain glucose at desirable, optimum level (see below and later).
(e) If the cause of insulin resistance is not controllable except via surgery, the insulin resistance will remain high, and blood glucose and some other vital parameters will rarely reach normal pre-operatively. More about these aspects will follow.

We will elaborate on the components due to or arising out of the surgical condition shortly below creating the insulin resistance and briefly the treatment initiation.

1.3 Monitoring Blood Glucose

The various avenues open for the blood glucose monitoring are:

(a) Biochemistry laboratory of the indoor care facility.
(b) Testing by rapid glucose assay meters.
(c) Testing without rapid glucose assay meters—though outdated—could still be useful in remotely located facilities at times.

Any good functioning laboratory, doing venous plasma glucose by glucose oxidase method and doing electrolytes, could be considered as the prevailing gold standard of that local area. In a perioperative situation, laboratory testing has several disadvantages for a variety of reasons especially when a patient needs to be monitored repeatedly, at odd hours.

(a) A good laboratory may not be at one's disposal at odd hours.
(b) It involves delay of at least an hour before the result can be learnt. This delay is inevitable. Laboratories have their own problems, and further delay in getting the result is expected normally. During this period, dangerous hypoglycemia may persist, or severe hyperglycemia will continue to be operative.
(c) It involves a venous puncture. In any person with diabetes, preservation of veins must get priority.

The singular advantage of a standard laboratory is to check the rapid glucose assay meter reading against a highly reliable gold standard. How and when to utilize such a laboratory is discussed below.

1.3.1 Common Errors in Monitoring Glucose and Other Laboratory Parameters

1. One should be careful not to draw blood from central lines running with glucose or any other fluids. It is highly debatable whether right readings can be assured even after aspirating and rejecting 5–10 mL of blood initially, which anyway is a waste.
2. One should also be careful over *not* drawing blood, preferably from the same arm on which glucose infusions are running. This is not proven but is precautionary. Both these readings are likely to be on a much higher side than blood drawn from sites away from this, will lead to increase in the insulin infusion rate (i.e., concentration of or the rate of insulin infused), and could lead to dangerous hypoglycemia. One could also question the staff when an abnormally high reading is obtained in a patient otherwise coming well under control to ascertain that the above two precautions were take nor not. If not, then it is advisable to get an assured sample of freely mixed venous blood, by drawing blood from the opposite arm (obviously without any glucose infusions going).

The glucose monitoring described below is framed the context of an acutely ill/critical surgical patient. This setting calls for the most careful monitoring and its precise interpretation each time over days. It is, on the other hand, a useful setting to illustrate all the variations that a glucose monitoring can have.

The logic of control of blood glucose in hemodynamically stable, uninfected patients who have to be controlled for routine surgery is much different than an acute surgical case. This part will be discussed much later in this volume in Chap. 6.

1.3.2 The Second First Reading of Glucose

After the initial capillary blood glucose reading (as is the case nowaday in most places) is read, the step necessary is to take a venous blood sample to get the glucose done once again, along with electrolytes, renal and hepatic parameters, and hemogram. The management especially with fluids should start after this. The fluid running already could be glucose- or nonglucose-containing fluid. The decision is whether to continue the same fluid based on the first reading of the rapid glucose assay meter or change it to another type before subsequent glucose testing and other parametric management is undertaken. There could be further changes in the fluid composition as laboratory readings become known later.

1.4 Testing by Rapid Glucose Assay Meters

This is a useful, dependable, and extremely rapid way of assessing blood glucose which has now become quasi universal. One should encourage use of it in the perioperative period and in wards, in all situations where frequent daily monitoring is required for several days. By frequent monitoring, we mean blood glucose testing more than 3–4 times a day; hourly/2/4/6 hourly. It is not worthwhile for occasional monitoring of a sick patient where it can be left to be collected with other blood samples.

The rapid glucose assay meters in the nineties were rather unreliable, error prone, failing in reading the sample, highly susceptible to ambient temperature and humidity. In the initial stages of new technology, the human errors were also frequent. Now it is an extensively used technology which has controlled the adverse factors, and the reading has become much more reliable. On all counts by 2003, it was a well-established technology. However a meticulous and extensive study challenged the technical accuracy. It alleged that it has not become more accurate even after its use in 1993–2003 [3]. That certainly is not the situation today in 2018 in standard assay meters. Meters not able to attain such accuracy are also there in India. They do give erroneous readings.

Towards the turn to the twenty-first century, their reliability was established when its use was sanctioned even in epidemiological studies. A little knowledge about which company is selling this product and personal experience should decide which the reliable ones are. It is not uncommon to get rapid glucose assay meters ordered by hospital management which does not know much about them, and the purchase depends upon many other factors related to cost, etc. Such meters should be discarded by the professionals if found unreliable.

1.4.1 Choice of Rapid Glucose Assay Meter and Its Placement in Wards, ICUs

Today's rapid assay meters by default should come with automatic spring needles. Care should be taken to see that these needles are neither stolen nor lost. If an admitted patient has his assay meter and needles, it should be put to use. Initially it is wise to calibrate it with the laboratory with a technique given below in this chapter. The needle of the patient's assay meter can be used for a number of readings. It reduces cost and utilizes his resources well.

Using rapid glucose assay meters by the bedside for inpatients with diabetes is quite common now. The accuracy has improved to an extent that variations in the PCV or the packed cell volume can be corrected [4, 5].

1.4.2 Method of Testing

The method of testing blood glucose by rapid glucose assay meter needs a mention. The needle puncture is done usually on the pulp of the third finger after it is cleaned and is dry without any residue of the cleaning agent left. This finger does not connect to the other palmer spaces; hence if on a rare event it gets infected, the infection will not spread to the palmer spaces. The method nowaday preferred is to prick the side of the fingertip as it is somewhat less painful. This is of help in those who monitor their glucose more frequently as in gestational diabetes.

First the assay meter has to be put on. The finger is then cleaned and allowed to dry. Then the needle is to be fitted in a casement to the spring lock and then covered with a top portion. A small lever loads the spring needle. The slightly concave tip from which the needle projects out in spring action should be released by pressing the button. The concave surface has to be snugly fitted to the skin. These needles give a small prick which is hardly painful. It is a regulated prick force unlike injection needles where there is no control over the force used, hence on the depth of needle going in, and it is far more painful. In using the automatic needle, the needle may go for a very minimum depth of barely 1–1.5 mm to get an adequate drop of blood.

With this technology instead of pricking the pulp of a finger, one may prick to the side of a finger to escape the synovial sheath and avoid spread of infection upwards. Another advantage of pricking sides of fingers not the pulp is - it makes available radial side of index finger, second and third finger on both sides of these fingers, and the ulnar side of little finger on one hand. It makes six sites on one hand to prick, making it 12 sites on two hands.

The pulp of the finger is then gently compressed at the base of the first metacarpal joint so that the pricking site becomes a little turgid. It is then best to do the puncture with an automated spring needle while holding the pulp so that a small drop of blood is formed. That drop is then placed on the testing pad squarely so that at the first touch, the pad gets evenly soaked. Nowaday the readings are obtainable in 5–15 s.

It is very commonly seen that those who do this capillary glucose testing squeeze the pulp hard and repeatedly before puncturing. This actually causes dilution of the capillary blood and gives a lower reading. There is hardly ever any need to do this.

The strips supplied by the meter company with it only should be used; else it may give inaccurate readings.

The glucose values of the rapid glucose assay meters are higher than the venous blood/plasma glucose values by about 8%. This testing is done on the capillary blood glucose which is passing through the tissue bed which absorbs the glucose it needs, before this blood proceeds in the small venules and then the bigger veins. This is the reason why the venous blood is lower in its glucose value. The difference between venous and capillary values and therefore the reliability and accuracy even now come for discussions with the relatives of acutely sick people; the residents and the nurses should be well versed with this knowledge.

In one ward or one ICU, only one meter should be used. Using more numbers even of the same type will have variations resulting in variability of treatment within the same or different patient. That is not acceptable. Going further there should be only *one type of meter and its corresponding strips for any testing throughout a hospital, health-care facility, or service.* The experience of laboratory, ward nurses, and diabetes educators (if they are a part of the treatment group) should be taken to make a choice of the rapid assay meter [6].

1.4.3 How Do the Rapid Glucose Assay Meters Work?

The newer type of the rapid glucose assay meter that has been in the market for many years now is used in the same manner as far as placing a drop of blood on the strip is concerned. But these meters work on the principle of reflectance photometry or generating a current after the capillary blood glucose reacts. The strength of the current gives the reading in digital display. These meters are claimed to be unaffected by a large temperature moisture range.

1.4.4 Calibration of the Rapid Glucose Assay Meter

There is no reliability of any laboratory testing unless the instruments are calibrated against an invariant standard. Reproducibility under the same initial conditions is the *hallmark* of modern science, and calibration is the first step to it. Hence it is important to calibrate which unfortunately is not done routinely or hardly ever. In addition are the human errors which should be eliminated or minimized by good training and practice.

Calibration can be done by using calibration strip or a calibrating solution which gives a particular result mentioned in the accompanying literature. This should remain constant. The calibration strip or the solution is supplied with each box of strips which show a reading that gives standard reading for that glucometer on insertion. If the calibration strip reading mentioned in the literature is not the same as the one shown on the digital display window of the glucometer, the calibration and other strips are likely to have been damaged by exposure to light heat or moisture. This happens if in the hurry of doing a test, the box is not capped immediately after the calibration or after the testing strip is removed from the box. Such readings from the strips are not to be relied upon.

In most instances the calibration strips are missing or lost in wards and ICUs. In such situations also, the calibration must be carried out once every day. It can be done by using venous blood once a day. This is not the most accurate way but is reliable enough. The first author has tried this numerous times in his career and can vouch for undertaking this method. It is done as follows:

(a) In a perioperative situation, electrolytes, urea, and creatinine have to be done frequently. All of these cannot be done in the bedside meters. When blood is drawn as a venous sample for any such testing, additional random blood glucose may be ordered even if a glucose testing has been done a little while ago.
(b) When the laboratory bulbs are filled up, the rapid glucose assay meter may be set ticking, and a small drop of the same venous blood is put on the square pad of the glucometer strip covering it fully, and the rapid glucose assay meter reading is then noted on the indoor paper.
(c) When the laboratory results come back, the random blood glucose reading can be compared with the test carried out on the rapid glucose assay meter strip and compared. In most instances the variation will be minor which indicates a well-functioning meter and considered as standard and well calibrated.
(d) This is the nearest that one can come if there is no other way to calibrate a meter. The technical requirement this method satisfies is that the blood for both testing modalities comes from the same sample without any time delay.

An uncalibrated glucometer is like a boat without a compass and cannot be expected to reach one to the safety of control blood glucose with any efficiency.

A somewhat surprising argument has come up in 2012. It cites studies to recommend glucose measurement during the perioperative period by central-laboratory-device (CLD) and not by point-of-care (POC) devices. This would be difficult to accept even in 2012, much more now in 2018. Whatever the reasons given, the learning probably should be to do the estimations at point of care more carefully. We have also shown above how the point of care devices can be checked for accuracy with the central laboratory devices [7, 8].

One of the important precautions that one must take is to clean the optical chamber of the rapid glucose assay meter. The blood on the pad or any part of the soaked pad can stick to the optical window and reduce the area through which the light is passed. If that is narrowed due to clotted blood, the readings will be low or error may be shown. The cleaning has to be done frequently depending upon the use of the glucometer. The matters should not be allowed to reach clogging levels [9].

1.4.5 Limitations of the Rapid Glucose Assay Meter Readings

If the venous plasma glucose is beyond 400 mg/dL or below 30 mg/dL, the rapid assay meter readings are represented as Hi, but not quantified or undetectable. Here the venous sample blood glucose mentioned above will be helpful. The authors at times have seen blood glucose readings so low that there is no reaction on the strip visible, the patients improving rapidly with rapid infusions of glucose.

1.4.6 Blood Glucose Estimation in Remote Area Settings

In the days long gone by, it was done without rapid glucose assay meters. This was the then principle of self-home blood glucose monitoring. The same strips that we use for rapid glucose assay meters had to be used, in the same manner instilling a drop of blood on the reactive pad. These strips came from a bottle of the hemoglucotest. The time for which one has to wait after soaking the pad with blood is mentioned on the bottle. The bottle also has a line of squares with different colors indicating a somewhat broad range of glucose reading. At the exact time, the color the strip pad develops has to be matched with the colors on these squares to get the range. If the procedure has been followed properly, it is a dependable method even in relatively complex or serious ward situations in areas where better means are not available.

1.5 Principles of Calorie Management

Any acute illness, surgical even more so, is a highly catabolic state. In diabetes, it is worsened by two pathological abnormalities. One is the high insulin resistance which does not allow the available insulin to act effectively to metabolize glucose for the calories needed by the sick body. The immediate effect is the protein breakdown from the muscles since there is no storage of proteins in the body. The breakdown results in glutamine and alanine as the principle of three carbon amino acids which are then deaminated and enter the Kreb's cycle as acyl CoA. The second is the release of fatty acids as a substitute fuel for glucose. However due to the insulin resistance, the fatty acids do not proceed to full combustion, and a process called beta-oxidation takes place. These are the precursors of the ketonemia and then ketoacidosis.

It therefore follows that to metabolize these fuels fully and to prevent protein catabolism, adequate calorie supplementation as glucose under accentuated supply of insulin becomes necessary. In critical settings high levels of plasma insulin are necessary. Effectively high levels will achieve:

(a) Full glucose disposal and consumption intracellularly.
(b) Prevent protein loss.
(c) Halt the beta-oxidation process and prevent ketoacidosis by normal free fatty acids metabolism.
(d) The only way to maintain high insulin values in plasma consistently is continuous insulin infusions.

It is not always possible to start supplementing the calories in acutely ill patients mainly due to high or very high levels of plasma glucose. It is a matter of skill to bring plasma glucose to an initial level of 250 mg in diabetic ketoacidosis (DKA) or to 300 mg in other conditions like hyperosmolar hyperglycemic state (HHS) in 6–8 and 24 h, respectively, in a gradual manner. It is a matter of judgment as well as art to decide when to start supplying adequate calories. As a general principle, it must start as soon as can be. But in the practice of acute or critical illness, both surgical and nonsurgical, this supplementation gets delayed, and/or when started it may be inadequate, particularly in case of diabetes (see below).

The reasons for this are many:

(a) The clinicians are overcautious for fear of hypoglycemia in not allowing the blood glucose brought under tight control with aggressive effort.
(b) The reluctance to substantial calorie supplementation is with idea of not allowing the blood glucose to rise again. This is bound to happen if extra calories are supplied. But the catabolic state demands that it must be done to prevent catabolism.
(c) There is certain reluctance or apprehension due to which the clinicians are often unwilling to step up aggressively the insulin infusion to what may look to them as abnormally high rate.
(d) The effects of calorie deprivation or insufficient insulin supplementation or both become manifest if the illness is prolonged and recovery is not rapid. It finally leads to hypoalbuminimia which is one of the strong indicators of fatality.

The first principle behind calorie management is *adequacy, quality, particularly protein, and using insulin, even in high quantities* to restore the fuel metabolic homeostasis.

The second principle of calorie management in diabetes is that severe hyperglycemia in acute illness is the only state, from whatever cause, where calorie supplementation is withheld and insulin is administered. In severe hypoglycemia calories are administered without insulin. In all other situations, calories and insulin go hand in hand. Calories without insulin will lead to quick hyperglycemia, and insulin without calories will result in severe hypoglycemia.

The plasma insulin levels and rate of glucose or non glucose-containing infusions determine blood glucose level. By varying one of the two any desired blood glucose level can be maintained as in HHS, around 300 mg/dL in initial control. To achieve this, it is worldwide practice now to use the calorie supplementation and the insulin infusion *only intravenously*, till the patient is able to take food orally or at times by nasogastric tube. After the desired level of blood glucose is obtained during Intravenous calorie and insulin administration, these two infusions should be constant. *Any mismatch even in short periods causes wide glucose fluctuations*. This is the main principle of calorie management.

In other words, neither insulin nor glucose can be interrupted at any given point of time unless hyper- and hypoglycemia develops when the calories and insulin have to be reduced or stopped, as the case may be.

The second offshoot is that both these supplies should be uniform in their rate of supplementation and rate of disposal resulting in balancing glucose concentration after a certain point when the acute surgical problem can be or is resolved satisfactorily. Resolution of such a problem reduces insulin resistance in the immediate short term and continues to do so for long after.

The reversal of all the pathological and biological aberrations the illness had created takes a few days, especially in acute emergency cases before the patient heads towards normalcy through the recuperative processes. The road to achieve this is higher calorie and higher insulin.

Significant reduction (nearly 50% or more) in insulin concentration may be called for in situations in which postoperatively the insulin requirements may drop and suddenly at the end of a drip blood glucose of say 80 mg/dL. This generally indicates that the cause of illness which has resulted in such high insulin resistance and high insulin requirements has been removed now effectively. Again, such reductions should not be done by the sliding scale method but by percentage reductions of the rate of reduction of insulin (see below).

1.5.1 The Instability of Control at the Beginning of Glucose Transfusion

This stage starts when the cutely elevated blood glucose has been brought to a reasonable level mentioned above. It is at this stage the diabetes control starts fluctuating widely. The first is the transition phase from purely intravenous administration of the calorie insulin combination to starting and increasing the oral intake and continuous reduction in the intravenous calories. A mixed model of long-acting basal insulin with much lowered concentration of intravenous insulin may be brought in. Or a fully subcutaneous insulin administration with short as well as intermediate/long-acting insulin could be employed once the patient is on full and only oral intake. These two routes and types of insulins used are not as uniform in their effects as intravenous route is. That makes the management difficult resulting in widely fluctuating glucose levels, at least in the initial stages till controls are achieved.

The answer to improve this situation will lie in the understanding of:

(a) Insulin pharmacokinetics.
(b) Insulin pharmacodynamics.
(c) The qualities of the calories, its glycemic index, absorption rates given orally or via nasogastric tube.
(d) The need to anticipate the likely blood glucose. This dilemma is not as complicated as it may look. Some of these matters will be explained again below.

1.5.2 Glucose Control in Acutely Sick Patient, Surgical or Nonsurgical

The principles are the same for both types. The stages faced at the time of admission by a resident or the ICU nurses are:

(a) In the emergency room (ER) where the initial clinical assessments are often done and laboratory specimens are sent.
(b) Immediately after the admission from the ER room to ICU.
(c) After the blood glucose is done by a rapid blood glucose assay meter if not done in the ER room.
(d) When all the laboratory parameters are available and the initial management is started in full.
(e) When the need for glucose infusions arises, to be backed by the insulin infusion already going on, which have to be now recalibrated. In this section we will be talking *only about glucose monitoring* before going in to the management of all other abnormal parameters.

1.6 The Syringe Pump with Insulin, the Best Tool for Glucose Control

1.6.1 When the Blood Glucose Is High

In most patients the blood glucose is shown to be high, i.e., 400+ mg/dL, or higher, 600–700 mg/dL. The ruling principle here is of intravenous use of insulin without any infusion of the calories. The safest route is to start a normal saline infusion with A concentration of insulin from the syringe pump.[2] If a syringe pump is not available, then the best way to manage is to place adequate easily measurable quantity of insulin in a steadily running nonglucose infusion.

There are two other alternatives if the syringe pump is not available. One can easily use a microinfusion set used in pediatric practice which gives 60 microdrops/mL. It should run as a separate infusion as is the case with syringe pump so that the fluid rates of other infusions do not alter the speed of microinfusions It is a chamber of 100 mL, in which one can add 50 U of crystalline insulin which gives 0.5 U of insulin every 60 microdrops. If 1 U is to be given, the drip rate can be adjusted to 120 and so on. But it would be more desirable to add 100 U of insulin to minimize the flow rate. Then it is 1 U of insulin for every 60 drops. This can be fine-tuned to a fraction of a unit. For example, 1.5 U will translate to 90 microdrops.

Such a micro-chamber infusion set is connected to 500 mL infusion bottle, preferably normal saline or 0.45% saline. It should also run as a separate infusion as is

[2] Twenty years back when the authors presented the comprehensive vision of optimal glucose control in surgery, the syringe pumps was a rarity. Nowaday it is a common accompaniment in most places, probably in the government medical colleges as well, except in remote areas.

the case with syringe pump so that the fluid rates of other infusions do not alter the speed of microinfusions. In this 100 mL chamber, one can take whatever required volume and add necessary dose of insulin which can be administered by a microphone with 60 drops/mL. If we take just 20 mL and add 50 U of insulin, each 60 drops will translate to 2.5 U. This has two advantages. If the glucose goes well beyond the 400 mg limit, then all glucose can be stopped for an hour or so, and 3–5 U could be given for an hour or 2 to bring the blood glucose down and restart the other infusions with dose calculation as explained in this chapter below. The second advantage would be that it will also help in, if required, reducing the infusion volume.

In the absence of syringe pump, 50 U of insulin can be injected in a 500 mL normal saline where the insulin concentration will be 10 U/100 mL of normal saline, or in a 100 mL normal saline unit with 50 U of insulin, the concentration for which will be 0.5 U of insulin in every mL of saline. Either of them should be infused by a separate line initially at least. The reason for separating the two is that initially the rehydration fluids flow at a much faster rate. The 100 mL preparation facilitates the change in insulin concentration by upscaling or downscaling the flow rate, as frequently without having to change the 100 mL infusion.

Whichever way the insulin is infused, there has to be a dual intravenous route—one that is for rapid rehydration, almost always with nonglucose-containing fluids, and the other with insulin going at a steady rate, which is varied per the glucose reading. The mid drip techniques that we have described below are far more useful in this situation.

1.6.2 Preparing a Syringe Pump with Insulin

These pumps have a 50 mL syringe with thin tubing attached to an intravenous line, by a two-way adopter fitted in a contraption, which under pressure delivers a fixed volume of the syringe contents irrespective of the speed of the infusion to which it is attached.

The easiest way to operate this is to take 50 U of regular, crystalline human insulin and draw normal saline in it reaching 50 mL and mix the two thoroughly by tilting slowly a few times and attach it to the infusion (which at this stage will be a nonglucose-containing fluid).

In simple terms—the 50 mL of insulin syringe with 50 U of regular crystalline insulin charged and put in a syringe pump could be started at 1–5 or even 7 U/h. The syringe pump has a concentration of 1 U of insulin/mL. It means that the pump speed is to be set at 1–5 or even 7 mL/h. The common experience is that this connection – one unit is equal to one mL is not quickly recognized by the ICU nurses or the ICU or duty doctors. If the insulin flow rate has to be changed it is just altering the mL flow is also not done immediately.

Insulin infusion rate depends upon the level of blood glucose. Higher the glucose greater is the insulin infusion unit rate per hour, lowered proportionately as the glucose level drops.

There are at least six different regimens described in literature in extremely well-planned trials, all coming from the USA or Europe. All of them are algorithmical, designed with the primary purpose of being nurse driven (the purpose of this chapter is to delegate care to the lower levels.) Over the last 25 years the authors have come across its use in various settings in many places in India. It has lead only to wide fluctuations and not a steady, acceptable level of glucose.

These regimens popularly known as the sliding scale always result in wide fluctuations if we continue to use them once the blood glucose has come to a reasonable level on nonglucose infusions under insulin effect. There are reasons for it which will be described later. The authors then shifted the entire management with intravenous insulin administration by abandoning the sliding scales 25 years ago. We have used other methods regularly in the management of even DKA or HHS. In the many lecture tours and teaching programs, the authors have taught these aspects. We have been getting exceptionally good and stable results to *any* desired level one wants to maintain the blood glucose by using these methods.

Over the years our departure from the sliding scales was rewarded by the dissatisfaction voiced by many authorities who discarded these scales, often denouncing them in harsh words. Over years we have come to call these regimes of ours as the common sense regimes or individual regimes as may be seen fit.

The typical scenarios one encounters under any of these insulin infusions are:

(a) The initial reading on the display panel shows the word "Hi." It appears if the blood glucose level is 400 mg/dL or above that. After an hour or two after starting insulin infusions, it may still remain high. In practical terms it means that the present rate of insulin infusion has not affected the blood glucose levels in any way. The reason for the glucose not getting lowered described above is that of high insulin resistance due to the surgical condition, in which the insulin levels achieved through the infusion are not able to dispose the glucose in to the cells and tissues thereby unable to lower the blood glucose.
(b) The second scenario is that of a blood glucose reading on the rapid blood glucose assay meter as a figure, 400 mg or less, confirmed by the regular standardized venous plasma glucose sent to the laboratory for other investigations. An insulin infusion is established and the blood glucose is done again after an hour or two. This may not drop to a level more than 10% of the initial reading.

The action in both these scenarios is the same—double the rate of insulin infusion and repeat the exercise of blood glucose estimation after one more hour. If the second hour blood glucose also turns out to be less than 10% of the reading prior to doubling the insulin infusion, the next step is to once again double the insulin infusion rate and repeat the estimation of blood glucose after one more hour and see what difference it has caused.

The more common experience of these two doublings will be that the blood glucose drops down to a level between 300 and 200 mg/dL. The number of doubling however depends on the initial level of insulin infusion, whether it is low, just 1 or, 2U/mL of insulin/h or higher at 5 to 7 units/h. In such cases it will need at least two or more often three more doubling, generally speaking. Hence the common and commonsense advice well supported by the Alberti regime[3] is to start the infusion at 5 mL or 5 U of insulin/h [9].

In acute surgical cases, the stress levels are high and are the ones with sepsis among other stresses. In such cases the high rates of insulin infusions also will not produce hypoglycemia which is a concern to all. In fact in all acute perioperative cases, it is extremely difficult to produce hypoglycemia unless heroically high doses are indiscriminately administered without bothering about the glucose monitoring. That makes insulin even in high infusion rates a safe drug while becoming effective cumulatively over time.

The second aspect is that of easy and quick reversal of hypoglycemia if it ever occurs in such a situation. It is common clinical experience for hypoglycemia to occur in routine or non-acute conditions in patients who are on insulin many more times in terms of patient-years than those who are on OHAs. It can be often severer, but it is quickly reversible hence much safer than any cohort which is on the oral drugs. The latter is more difficult to reverse, takes a long time before it is done, causes severe glucose excursions in either direction, and is likely to be more damaging than insulin-induced ones. The third aspect is the likelihood of cerebral and/or myocardial damage in hypoglycemia under insulin compared to one on oral drugs. The brain matter changes that are seen in cases of frequent hypoglycemia are confined to patchy gliosis of the cortical white fibers for which no functional significance has been attributable [10].

1.7 Coming Back to the Further Management: A Picture in Practice

It is a common practice to stop insulin and recheck the blood glucose and then restart the infusion which rises invariably after that. As an example, suppose the blood glucose reading from "Hi" has now come down to 300 or 250 mg under the insulin infusion rate of 10 U/h. These are the recommended levels to shift from the non glucose-containing to glucose infusions with insulin. A new and often arbitrary rate of insulin infusion is set up leading to one more or hourly monitoring. The wide fluctuations in glucose levels continue. As was succinctly put by one of my friends and colleague, Dr. Uday Phadke, DM endocrinology, "it is here the period of chasing glucose starts." A simple and convincing alternative strategy would be found in the blood glucose control usually in the OPD practice. It is to fix the fasting first, without which no

[3] High-dose insulin infusion was the practice in the initial periods long ago before low-dose insulin regime was invented and standardized by KGMM Alberti in 1970s with much better efficiency. This method still holds. To conclude as the authors will reiterate in this volume, intravenous insulin administration under monitoring is one of the safest drug modern medicine has invented.

control can ever be achieved. Here we vary the operational terms by fixing a value to which we want the blood glucose to be brought and fixed by changing dosing without following any algorithm.

We go back to the continuing example of 10 U of insulin/h with normal saline flowing. This rate of insulin infusion has brought blood glucose to 250 or 300 mg. What would be the next step?

1.7.1 Scenario 1

One of the recommended practices is to lower the insulin infusion rate by half, that is, 5 U/h in the above example, but not to stop it. If stopped then all the insulin we have infused will be reduced to half its concentration in about 7 min, and there will be no trace of it in 30–60 min or even earlier. In less than an hour, the supraphysiological level required to act effectively to save all proximate principles will rapidly decline, utilizing glucose and free fatty acids, and prevent protein breakdown. The blood glucose then starts rising rapidly [11].

The management should then continue as follows:

(a) In another hour the blood glucose estimation should be repeated. This is the fifth blood glucose in 5 h that will be done.
(b) The blood glucose continues to remain between 300 or 250 mg. It indicates that 5 U of insulin/h will not be able to lower it further.
(c) If (and as will be the case) the clinical decision-making for taking up a patient for surgery demands that a lower glucose level be achieved, the reasonable way to achieve it is to raise the infusion rate back to 10 U/h and see how the glucose level drops.
(d) Depending upon the glucose level thus obtained, the insulin infusion rate could then be adjusted between 7, 10, and 15 U/h.

1.7.2 Scenario 2

If the blood glucose falls further on 5 U/h, then there is every reason to lower the 5 U/h to 2–3 U/h but not to stop and watch the glucose levels. By simple titration in a couple of more hours from the point of view of taking the patient for surgery, the patient will be in safe conditions.

1.7.3 Scenario 3

At this time the non glucose-containing fluids may continue depending upon the hydration and electrolyte needs, but glucose-containing fluid could/should now be added and the insulin infusion rate readjusted, in the theater or intraoperatively. A number of variations encountered practically are described below under the situation of need to start infusing glucose.

(a) If a miraculously normal level on *X* U rate of insulin infusion is achieved and if the blood glucose drops to a narrow level between say 140 and 180 mg/dL, what should be done?

Some of the many studies quoted below suggest that the insulin infusion rate at this level then should drop to 1–2 U and the dextrose normal saline should be started. The blood glucose estimations should again be done, and the insulin infusion rate rescaled up or down. We perused at least nine studies over the years. There is overall consensus on the optimal perioperative glucose level between 140 and 170 mg/dL. But the methodologies differ. One general principle which has emerged from all these trials is that whatever scale or protocol one may use, it should be manageable at the level of nurses and medical officers [9, 12–18].

We reiterate that starting with 1 U with added glucose infusion will not work. The result would be a rise of glucose well beyond the level of 250 mg or so. The reason is that the blood glucose has got lowered at *X* U of insulin since there was no glucose being infused. Now glucose is being introduced. The stress levels have not dropped so significantly since the cause of destabilization has not been removed as yet. These two together logically lead to the conclusion that if glucose has to be introduced, there is no need to change the prevailing insulin rate immediately but will have to be done subsequently to a likely higher level.

The practice we have suggested above is to continue the same rate of insulin infusion when the glucose level reaches well below 200 or between 140 and 180 mg but add glucose containing fluids. It differs from all other regimens. Whether the glucose will rise or not will have to be monitored, but certainly such a patient is not going to go hypoglycemic.

The next step would be to check the blood glucose after 1 h. Suppose *X* U/h were the insulin infusion rate and the glucose tested now continues to be in the above range of less than 200 or 140–170 mg/dL range as in this example. Then it demonstrates that the balance between the calorie supplies from glucose is equal to the disposal of glucose.

In addition the stress levels (not psychological but due to physical factors) develop in to insulin resistance. Insulin resistance means the inability of insulin at a plasma concentration that works in normal care. The same level cannot lower the blood glucose in acute illnesses. If the blood glucose remains well within the normal range as above, it indicates various clinical phenomena. The rate of insulin infusion is able to counter the insulin resistance due to the stress factors effectively. In addition it is able to dispose the blood glucose from the blood to tissues and cells and keep blood glucose in normal range. This situation will continue as long as the stress level induced resistance continues to remain the same. The concomitant care also helps in reducing the stress levels like antibiotics, fluids. If it comes down, the rate of insulin infusion also will have to be lowered. The most dependable and steady range is between 140 and 180 mg to which reference will be repeatedly made in the text in other chapters as well.

(b) On the contrary, if after starting the glucose drip without lowering the insulin rate the blood glucose goes well above 200 mg dL, what should be the next step then?

It is obvious that the insulin rate of X from the hypothetical one assumed here should go to $X + 2$ or $X + 4$ or 6 or more units of insulin would be required per hour. Equally obvious would be the impossibility that 1–2 U of insulin as advised by most, mentioned above, would have maintained the glucose level between 140 and 180 mg.

(c) In the above examples, the blood glucose will never come down to hypoglycemic range. There is no need to consider lowering of insulin infusion rates unless the blood glucose on glucose insulin drip drops to a level below 100 mg. In such situations the insulin infusion rate could be halved or reduced by 25%, 75%, or lower as required but *should never be stopped* unless the patient is shifted to oral intake and subcutaneous insulin regime. The fatal error is to stop insulin at this juncture as it will immediately cause a destabilization of the blood glucose.

1.7.4 Proof of Concept

If blood glucose is kept in a narrow range of 80–110 mg/dL, the outcomes in critical surgical care are far better. The evidence from trial has reported reduction in mortality by over 42%. In Chaps. 7 and 13, we will discuss many more trials in this respect [1].

1.7.5 The Additional Mechanisms of How the Blood Glucose May Actually Get Lowered

Depending on the kind of surgical emergency, the surgeon and the anesthetist will have instituted other measures like hydration, antibiotics, and correction of electrolyte imbalance in these hours. As the first reports of all the investigations sent at admission are at hand, these measures will be modified or intensified. Each of these steps helps and facilitates the blood glucose control by finally reducing insulin resistance and intracellular transport of glucose.

The high levels of infusion of insulin aided by the abovementioned interventions result in breaking down the insulin resistance caused by or arising from the surgical condition itself or the counter regulatory hormones discussed in detail in later chapters. As soon as this happens, the level of insulin in plasma required to further lower the blood glucose also drops.

Up till now we have not discussed anything about the factors needing corrections other than the glucose which will be done in later chapter. At present what is being clarified is the single factor which is the most intriguing and unsatisfactorily controlled in acute surgical (and for that matter any critical illness). Steady desirable glucose control is all about monitoring-action-monitoring. We discuss this aspect in considerable detail here on the backdrop of what is commonly found in the wards and ICUs.

1.7.6 About Monitoring Itself: Myths, Misconceptions, Errors, Frequencies, and Interpretations

Myth: Monitoring is more important; it does not or need not necessarily be followed by action for change. This is the situation that obtains in the wards and the ICUs and is widely prevalent but not acceptable.

(a) A change in the approach is needed. If the result of a monitoring is not going to change the management in either direction, i.e., increasing or decreasing the insulin infusion rate, then (especially) the hourly monitoring is in no way justified. In such case the monitoring interval should continue to be doubled each time, if no action is called for. In practice action is always required but never taken.
(b) On the contrary, if an action is taken, then a reasonable time interval should be fixed for the next monitoring. And this will not be 1 h unless other actions have resulted in drastic alteration of the condition.

Myth: That unless monitored frequently hypoglycemia will escape attention with serious consequences, when the patient is under insulin infusions. The answers given above indicate that this myth does not seem to be correct.

(c) Once a reasonably stable state of blood glucose is achieved and the doses of insulin administered have been decided to maintain the same as discussed above, the reasonable intervals should be 4 h or even more since the level remains stable for 4–8 h, before further changes are needed (see below).
(d) The "reasonable" level could vary from 110 to 250 mg/dL. It depends upon the experience and the expectation of the anesthetist and the physician; the lower the level of blood glucose considered as safe for anesthesia or surgery the lesser is the experience level. The agreement between these two which is an outcome of working together over a period of time in managing such critical cases jointly in the pre-operative scenario will result in controlling the glucose at a much lower level before handing the patient over to surgery. Collaboration and the strength of the stand to help each other out in critical situations and their ability to convince the surgeon together for taking up a case will be then enhanced.

1.8 The Mid Drip Monitoring Technique

This is a technique devised by the authors and experimented with over long years. This helps in reducing the frequency of monitoring considerably without increasing the risk of undetected hypoglycemia and saving resources as discussed below. Let us continue with the commonly met situation, assumed to be operating here as discussed above. Let us carry the example further.

The patient is on some nonglucose-containing fluid administration at 100 mils/h with an insulin infusion pump running at X mL/U/h, as in the example from above continuing. The blood glucose monitored before the current fluid is started stands at 250 mg/dL as above. We change the insulin infusion rate upwards by a $X + 4$ more units trying to reach the goal of glucose level of 140–170 mg/dL.

Suppose instead of monitoring this patient hourly we do glucose estimation again when the fluid is half finished ie two and a half hours after. If we obtain the same level of 250 mg/dL, we could easily raise the insulin infusion rate to $X + 8$ or $X + 10$ U/h without any fear of precipitous hypoglycemia as should be obvious from the above discussions.

Supposing further that we monitor the blood glucose again, when the fluid is about to end, i.e., after another two and a half hour, and get a level of 170 mg, we need not change the insulin infusion rate at all and avoid one more monitoring immediately after starting a new infusion. This is the essence of the mid drip monitoring technique.

Do a mid drip glucose with the insulin infusion rate of $X + Y$ U/h, that is, X plus 4, 8, or 10 U. If we find that the blood glucose is still around 150 mg/dL, we need not change the rate. In that case one more end drip result say 100 or 90 mg, not dangerous but more satisfactory, immediately tells us that the infusion rate should be set somewhere between $X + 4$ and $X + 10$ that is (W) units for all the glucose-containing infusions as long as the rate of glucose infusion does not change. This will also lead now to a monitoring schedule of 5 h or more about which we have to say something more, later.

1.8.1 Interpretation

In about 5 h with minimal monitoring, we have brought the patient to a stage when insulin even with the backing of caloric infusion has given us an eminently acceptable value in the pre-operative setting by a calculated but substantial increase in the insulin infusion rate. The matter that needs further interpretation is with the next 4 U of glucose-containing fluid; what level of insulin should we continue? If we continue with a value W units per hour, most certainly the blood glucose will drop to 120 or 130 or 100 mg/dL. The possibility that it may go even lower is also genuine. If this is the expected outcome, given the overall improvement in the clinical situation, the next infusion would be W—2, 4, or 6 U. Such equilibrium lasts for about 12 h before the insulin requirement starts dropping on account of surgical intervention and removal of the cause of hyperglycemia.

As the experience grows, the rate of change of insulin infusions can be with fractions like 12.5 or 15.7 U. The change does not have to be in full integers. In places where these kind of situations have not been faced for long, where the staff is new or changing, a range of 140–170 mg can be suggested where the apprehension of hypos will be minimal and yet a measure of aggressive blood glucose control could be practiced.

The absurdity of the sliding scale will now become quite clear. What would happen if the rate of insulin infusion at 250 mg level is reduced from X to 2.5 U where an increase is necessary? Or if the level of 135 at the rate of $X + 4$ U was reduced to 1.4 as the sliding scale demands, when the dynamic balance between the glucose/insulin level required has been such high levels of insulin? It should therefore be clear that in no circumstances the sliding scale should feature in the management of blood glucose in the acute perioperative setting.

There is no need to repeat that it will be a series of widely fluctuating high-level results, not at all satisfactory if the sliding scale is used. That will necessitate finding out a new scale to control glucose since calorie supplementation has become mandatory now. This is waste of time, and deregulation of the desirable blood glucose level will continue for many more hours, in fact for days together as is the experience. The control will never be achieved, and one of the two parties either the anesthetists or the surgeons will decline to take the case up creating further delays and gross deterioration of the patient's condition soon making it irremediable, leading to death.

1.8.2 Maintenance

Once an appropriate level of steady glucose infusion rates and counterbalancing insulin infusion rates are found as mentioned above, such a situation will last in equilibrium for about 8–12 h with minor variations in blood glucose causing minor changes in the insulin infusion rates. In the interim surgery could have taken place since the glucose levels were highly satisfactory. The subsequent management will be discussed under the postoperative care in a separate chapter. The golden rule in this kind of management is the higher the quantum of reduction of blood glucose, the greater will be the reduction in insulin concentration, i.e., the infusion rates. The lesser the quantum of blood glucose reduction much higher will be the level of the quantum and concentration of insulin infusion.

1.8.3 Other Advantages of the Mid Drip Glucose Monitoring

(a) A mid drip glucose reduces the number of estimations from 5 to 2 or even 1 every 5 h.
(b) It avoids hourly blood glucose when changes expected to occur may not be substantial.
(c) A mid drip glucose can detect impending hypoglycemia as well as hyperglycemia reasonably early.
(d) In case of impending hypoglycemia without throwing the infusion away or reusing it later, it can be continued to be used by changing glucose concentration in the drip. In a mid drip reading, the remaining volume in the fluid is 250 mils, be it glucose-containing or nonglucose-containing one. This is how the variation can be undertaken.

    In case of impending hypoglycemia, a quantum of 10% glucose, 50–100 mils could then be safely added to the running drip without disturbing the insulin infusion rate or the insulin rate can be reduced by a few units. The addition of 10% glucose to the fluid results in dilution of the hypertonic 10% dextrose and lessens the chances of thrombophlebitis. It has an added advantage of pulling the blood glucose away from hypoglycemic ranges but not allowing it to escape in the hyperglycemic range. It happens due to both dilution and slower infusion rate and since it is administered not as a bolus but as infusion over the next 150 min. His helps in maintaining the near euglycemic state till the next fluid is introduced.

(e) Alternatively if the glucose levels are in the hypoglycemic range, the insulin infusion rate could be reduced considerably but not switched off, to allow for the glucose to rise.

In the older days, when syringe pumps were not as universal as they are today, it was common practice to add insulin to the 500 mils standard infusions with or without glucose if the blood glucose tended to hyperglycemic range. In a situation where a mid drip reading showed a substantial hyperglycemic range, an appropriate quantity of insulin can be added to the remaining 250 mils instead of glucose.

(f) The idea behind both these situations, d and e, is the same—it is the interplay between the glucose insulin ratio on the background state of insulin resistance described above.
(g) The logic thus emerges is in hypo states the glucose concentration or rate of infusion will go up and in hyperglycemic states the insulin concentration (in the plasma) will have to be pushed up.
(h) The situation has changed for better after the universal availability of syringe pumps; the rate of insulin can then be stepped up for the next 150 min without changing the infusion starting another and wasting resources.
(i) These reductions or increases change the situation within minutes since the glucose insulin dynamics of adjustments works in minutes. This eliminates the need for an immediate monitoring and could wait till the 2½–3 h when the intravenous infusion is about to be over. The requirements of both glucose and insulin can then be recalibrated more readily and easily for the next infusion.

1.9 Precautions About the Insulin Infusion Pumps

In theory the insulin pumps will push the desired mils set on it with a steady rate. But it would be wise to check that it is so once in a while. It can be done by checking the volume delivered since it started till the time of observation against the rate. At times when the other intravenous fluids are going at a fast rate of 200–500 mils/h especially in the initial period (as will be discussed later), the pump may slow down perceptibly but not always. In such a situation or even otherwise, the technique of dual intravenous infusion will have to be employed, as is routinely done nowaday.

It is also mandatory that the insulin infusion rate should be checked as frequently as possible or necessary even in steady state where the infusion rates of other fluids are fixed. It is extremely common for these infusion rates to vary and must then be set again. For example, if the patient is shifted for any reason, bed to bed, for CT MRI, or if some other injection is to be given, the intravenous infusion is stopped and then restarted without again setting the rate of the infusion properly or while changing the intravenous fluid once empty and so on.

The reason for avoiding this at all costs is described in detail in the principles of calorie supplementation. It is clearly stated there that this rate should be constant; it can be 100 mils/h or 200 or 150 or whatever, but any variations thereof will disturb the continuous dynamic equilibrium of the insulin glucose concentrations aimed to be maintained to get reliable results of glucose levels.

1.10 Conflict of Fluid Administration

Till such time the insulin-backed glucose infusions are not started, i.e., only nonglucose-containing fluids are being administered, there is no conflict of fluids. Here the only responsibility of the residents and the ICU nurses is to see that the prescribed rates are maintained while watching for signs of fluid overload. In the initial periods for about 24–36 h, these fluids are given a rapid rate.

Once acceptable glycemia is attained and the management cannot go further without calorie supplementation, the glucose-containing fluids generally at a fixed rate are then added. The management of dehydration may not yet be over, and non glucose-containing are also running. Giving both these fluids through a single line *is absolutely inadvisable*, since neither will go according to the prescribed rates. Hence the practice that must be followed is of two intravenous lines—one for the nonglucose-containing fluids and one for the glucose-containing fluids with the syringe insulin pump attached to it. This arrangement helps to segregate all orders coming from various consultants involved.

In either category there are various fluids with different compositions the use of which will be decided by the clinical and more importantly the laboratory parameters. The consideration is about those which have been made with glucose 5% as the base with different electrolytes, with saline in varying concentration. Even if such of them are chosen, *the rate of their infusion should not change to compensate for other elements or electrolytes* in a more urgent manner. In such cases the elements needing hasty correction (as in case of say severe hypokalemia which is common) should be added to the nonglucose-containing fluids since the rate of these fluids can be increased to very high levels. These matters will be discussed in the appropriate chapter with many theoretical inputs without which it is not easy to obtain the homeostasis. It is also desirable that all other intravenous administration of drugs should be through the nonglucose-containing line.

1.11 The Second Stage of Pre-operative Glucose Level Maintenance

Another way one can look at the blood glucose level at the end of a glucose insulin drip as described above is to consider it as the cumulative way in which it overcomes the insulin resistance, over the initial few hours of intensive treatment. What we mean by that is the signs of improvement, the most important being the reduced rate of insulin requirement, at times even going down significantly. Also, as the blood glucose lowers, the efficiency of glucose disposal by insulin may go up, and the sensitivity returns resulting in lower insulin concentration, in next infusions. The higher the quantum of reduction in blood glucose levels, the lower will be the subsequent insulin requirements.

1.11.1 Fitness for Surgery

This is the next issue to arise when encouraging blood glucose levels as in the example carried from the beginning are achieved. Here are a few variations on the theme here:

(a) If the blood glucose levels after all such heroic measures do not drop below 250 or 300 mg, what is the next alternative?

The greatest and the most important realizations at this point and this scenario are that unless the surgical cause is removed, it will be impossible to expect the blood glucose to normalize. Seen otherwise it means that the surgical condition is the cause for recalcitrant hyperglycemia. Hence surgical intervention takes the primacy to be attacked than infinitely waiting for the "safe" blood glucose levels to be reached. It will never be reached. The only outcome of not intervening at this point is the continued worsening of the patients which makes them even more risky, soon making them irremediable under the very nose of all these specialists, resulting in untoward outcome.

(b) This sort of a situation or a deadlock between the demands of the anesthetists, the impatience of surgeons to act, and the physician getting squeezed in between for better control are not at all uncommon. In fact this is the scenario that obtains in a very large majority of acute surgical cases all over the country.

(c) That makes the alternative criteria mentioned below useful to break this deadlock and get optimal results. Three biochemical and three clinical criteria are considered necessary to be fulfilled to consider a patient reasonably fit for surgery, even if there would be some increased risk for surgery. These criteria need to be explained in context somewhat more complex and will be described later.

The role of residents as well as the consultants during the intraoperative and postoperative phases from ICU to wards and at the time of discharge as well as follow-up is described in detail in Chap. 4. A technique of minimum most monitoring is also elaborated in a later chapter which can be applied to any situation, especially once the glucose insulin balance is established.

1.12 Concluding Remarks

While this chapter is aimed at improving the understanding of residents, all the consultants may find it is useful in some way or the other in clarifying and crystallizing their ideas about the perioperative management of diabetes especially in emergency major surgery and as an extension critical care medicine as well.

Perioperative control of glucose is primarily a science of understanding the physiology of insulin and of practicing it. Yet, it is as much as an art that it is a science.

References

1. Van den Berghe G, Wouters P, Weekers F, Verwaest C, Bruyninckx F, Schetz M, Vlasselaers D, Ferdinande P, Lauwers P, Bouillon R. Intensive insulin therapy in critically ill patients. N Engl J Med. 2001;345:1359–67.
2. Ljungqvist O, Jonathan E. Rhoads lecture 2011: insulin resistance and enhanced recovery after surgery. J Parenter Enter Nutr. 2012;36(4):389–98.
3. Böhme P, Floriot M, Sirveaux M-A, Durain D, Ziegler O, Drouin P, Guerci B. Evolution of analytical performance in portable glucose meters in the last decade (1989 to 1990). Diabetes Care. 2003;26:1170–5.
4. National Diabetes Service Scheme. Use of blood glucose meters March 2015, Diabetes Australia.
5. Van den Berghe GH. Role of intravenous insulin therapy in critically ill patients. Endocr Pract. 2004;10(Suppl. 2):17–20.
6. Roche. user_manual_active_infinity, by Accu Check.
7. Rice MJ, Pitkin AD, Coursin DB. Glucose measurement in the operating room: more complicated than it seems. Anesth Analg. 2010;110(4):1056–65.
8. Mraovic B, Schwenk ES, Epstein RH. Intraoperative accuracy of a point-of-care glucose meter comparedwith simultaneous central laboratory measurements. J Diabet Sci Technol. 2012;6(3):541–6.
9. Alberti KGMM, Gill GV, Elliott MJ. Insulin delivery during surgery in the diabetic patient. Diabetes Care. 1982;5(1):65–77.
10. Kelkar SK. CIIMS bulletin, 1994.
11. Gavin LA. Perioperative management of the diabetic patient. Endocrinol Metab Clin N Am. 1992;21(2):457–75.
12. Hirsch IB, McGill JB. Role of insulin in management of surgical patients with diabetes mellitus. Diabetes Care. 1990;13(9):980–91.
13. Reynolds C. Management of the diabetic surgical patient. A systematic but flexible plan is the key. Postgrad Med. 1985;77(1):265–79.
14. Peters A, Kerner W. Perioperative management of the diabetic patient. Exp Clin Endocrinol Diabet. 1995;103(4):213–8.
15. Fetchick DA, Fischer JS. Perioperative management of the patient with diabetes mellitus undergoing outpatient or elective surgery. Clin Podiatr Med Surg. 1987;4(2):439–43.
16. Smail PJ. Children with diabetes who need surgery. Arch Dis Child. 1986;61(4):413–4.
17. Marks JB. Perioperative management of diabetes. Am Fam Phys. 2003;67(1):93–100.
18. Gill GV, Alberti KGMM. The care of the diabetic patient during surgery. In: Edwards CMB, editor. International textbook of diabetes mellitus, vol. 2004. New York, NY: John Wiley & Sons.

Additional Reading

Böhme P, Floriot M, Sirveaux M-A, Durain D, Ziegler O, Drouin P, Guerci B. Evolution of analytical performance in portable glucose meters in the last decade (1989 to 1990). Diabetes Care. 2003;26:1170–5.

Ginsberg BH. Factors affecting blood glucose monitoring: sources of errors in measurement. J Diabet Sci Technol. 2009;3(4):903–13. © Diabetes Technology Society.

Goldberg PA, Inzucchi SE. Selling root canals: lessons learned from implementing a hospital insulin infusion protocol. Diabetes Spectr. 2005;18(1):28–33.

National Diabetes Service Scheme. Use of blood glucose meters March 2015, Diabetes Australia.

Roche. user_manual_active_infinity, by Accu Check.

Sudhakaran S, Surani SR. Guidelines for perioperative management of the diabetic patient. Review article. Surg Res Pract. 2015;2015:Article ID 284063. https://doi.org/10.1155/2015/284063.

Van den Berghe GH. Role of intravenous insulin therapy in critically ill patients. Endocr Pract. 2004;10(Suppl. 2):17–20.

Van den Berghe G, Wouters P, Weekers F, Verwaest C, Bruyninckx F, Schetz M, Vlasselaers D, Ferdinande P, Lauwers P, Bouillon R. Intensive insulin therapy in critically ill patients. N Engl J Med. 2001;345:1359–67.

Perioperative Diabetic Emergencies

2

Contents

S. Kelkar et al., *Towards Optimal Management of Diabetes in Surgery*,
https://doi.org/10.1007/978-981-13-7705-1_2

2.1 Preamble

Diabetes in surgical setting, in all the complex aspects of both, has not been covered as a separate chapter in major textbooks on diabetes [1]. The information on the concomitantly present myriad aspects have remained scattered in the textbooks on surgery, anesthesia, or ICU protocols. All major textbooks on medicine have provided less than meager space for diabetes. As a result, the plethora of issues arising for the three major contributors, surgeons, physicians, and anesthetists have not been satisfactorily answered to conduct safe surgery and splendid recovery. A cohesive, comprehensive, and not ad hoc approach towards resolution of these difficulties has not been available. The iatrogenic issues that arise when multiple specialties must collaborate, agree upon certain matters, and take joint responsibility have never been discussed. This has led to fragmentation of care which cannot be more detrimental than in managing patients with diabetes undergoing major, acute, or critical surgical situations than in any other. This volume is one such effort to ease the situation.

Any acute surgical condition in a person with diabetes will be accompanied by diabetic ketoacidosis (DKA) most of the times and hyperosmolar hyperglycemic state (HHS) with lesser frequency. The challenge here is to correct these conditions conservatively and treat surgical condition and its aftermath together. It should be done as early as possible so that the patient is brought to a reasonable level of safety, not at all optimal, just reasonable, for the surgeon anesthetist team to be able to take him/her for surgery. There are many issues associated with these twin dangers which also have to be discussed to reach a common understanding and aim to take such patients up for surgery. The intraoperative and postoperative issues are no less important. They will be discussed separately. Here the discussion is limited to preparing the patient for surgery in presence of these two presenting conditions related to diabetes.

In the preceding chapter, we have discussed glucose control in emergency surgery, considered to be by far the most difficult clinical situation to manage. Glucose control however needs concomitant management of several other parameters, without which the patient cannot be considered as adequately, if not fully, fit for anesthesia and surgery. The risk for anesthesia and surgery is heightened, and the outcome may be suboptimal or poor, even after these efforts. There are only a few absolute contraindications for general anesthesia, like extreme hyperkalemia of 10 meq/L or a sodium level of less than 120 mmol/L where the patient is likely to go into cardiac arrest, while intubation is done. In most other situations, we should be able to take the patient up for surgery. However the safety criteria and the understanding thereof between the surgeons and the anesthetists are the biggest barriers. In emergency surgery and with or without the diabetic emergencies, we will, in most situations, not be able to reach these so-called safe limits since it is the surgical situation at its bottom which prevents it from reaching. If surgery in such circumstances is denied, then mortality in such cases will be extremely high, an outcome which is far too unacceptable than the risks of surgery itself.

This chapter will elaborate on what these serious risk factors are and how should they be corrected, the various intricacies of it, and some simple rules which guide us to accomplish this job of preparing the patient for surgery in as short a time as possible, even if not in the safe limits.

Acute or critical surgical or nonsurgical illness accompanies a state of diabetic ketoacidosis (DKA) in its full-blown spectrum or on its way to it. DKA is characterized by significant ketonemia, 3+, presence of ketones in urine, metabolic acidosis, and hyperglycemia. The blood glucose level should be 250 mg/dL or higher for diagnosis of DKA. Arterial blood pH is less than 7.3, and bicarbonates less than 15 meq/L are the additional diagnostic criteria. It is also accompanied by significant dehydration to complete the DKA picture. Early clinical signs and symptoms also suggest the impending nature of this development. Diabetic ketoacidosis is not restricted to patients of type 1 diabetes. It occurs in type 2 patients of diabetes also and quite frequently. Hence the diagnosis and the definition of the severity of all parameters must be looked for in the initial assessment to ascertain the degree of DKA in type 2 as well. Aggressive treatment should be followed by monitoring to see whether these factors are improving or deteriorating and at what speed.

Overall DKA occurs at 4.6–8 cases per 100 patient-years. Nowaday type 2 diabetes is found in adolescents, teenagers, and morbidly obese children also. Twenty-five percent of this group of patients, at the time of diagnosis, present in the state of DKA with or without an accompanying severe illness. Up to 20% of newly diagnosed people with diabetes and 1.6% of general population of people with diabetes may develop DKA. In 100 diabetic years, 3–8 episodes of DKA may occur. This statistics will vary depending upon the competence for treating diabetes as would be available in any locale. Among diabetes-related admissions, DKA is seen in nearly 30% as primary or presenting problem. Six percent DKA is diagnosed as a secondary or associated diagnosis [2, 3]. What is more important—DKA as compared to hyperosmolar hyperglycemic nonketotic syndrome, HHNS—is far more common but has much less mortality between 1% and 5% as compared to the latter, which stands at around 50–70% [2].

2.2 DKA as It Presents in Clinical Situations

In clinical emergency practice, a DKA patient may be received de novo. Many children and teenagers get detected as having type 1diabetes during the first admission in DKA. They may or may not have any other illnesses. The presentation in DKA is merely the rapid culmination of undiagnosed onset of type 1 diabetes. At times a child may be taken off insulin for an alternate therapy, but the results are disastrous. In the absence of any other precipitating cause, this development can occur within a matter of few weeks or days, deteriorating into DKA.

In type 2 diabetes, a major illness, usually sepsis of a severe degree, could push the patient in DKA. In spite of an explosive appearance, DKA however is more easily and much more quickly reversible even in these situations. Needless to say, it is mandatory to look for any other illnesses which could have precipitated DKA and manage accordingly.

The other set of situation is slightly more complex when a patient diagnosed elsewhere, not necessarily a teenager, is partially treated and is referred. For example, a full-blown DKA may present with a blood glucose level less than the definitive level of 250 mg or more. Here the higher level of care facility should strive to identify where possible the agent(s) of intervention, their quantum, and the time of the pre-referral intervention. The treating team should look at in particular the insulin administration details. An especially large subcutaneous dose of regular-, intermediate-, or even long-acting variety may have been delivered in the previous treatment facility. All of them form a depot, keep getting released in the bloodstream during the transfer, and will continue to act. The patient in such situations may present with blood glucose less than that diagnostic of DKA. Such insulin administration with high levels of plasma insulin results in some decrease in glucagon. Consequently these patients may have lower levels of acidemia as well as glucose.

Such subcutaneous doses should also be considered because it will dictate the moderation instead of aggressive glucose and DKA management for the initial 12–24 h. By then the depot will have exhausted and only the intravenous insulin would be the insulin acting.

Patients could also be taking oral hypoglycemic drugs, the effect of which will last for the first 24 h at least as the management proceeds. There may be intravenous coadministration of fluids with or without glucose which must be identified as the patient is admitted. In rare situations such patients may actually present in hypoglycemia. Neither this nor lower blood glucose nor lower levels of ketonemia should deter the diagnosis of DKA if other features, both clinical and laboratory, are

Box 2.1 DKA Precipitating Causes

DKA precipitated by infections like pneumonia, meningitis, gastroenteritis, viral infection, peritonitis, carbuncles, polytrauma, acute myocardial infarction, and strokes, i.e., all varieties of severe illnesses significant surgical stress; DKA status many a times is altered by the administration of insulin in other facilities, elsewhere

Box 2.2 Clinical Presentation of DKA

20% patients are comatose
14% patients are stuporous
40% patients are drowsy
Osmotic symptoms, i.e., polyuria, polydipsia and polyphagia, are weight loss, are common before DKA, vomiting, at times severe abdominal pain, weakness, S/o dehydration, shock, Kussmaul's breathing, and evidence of obvious infection

indicative of DKA. In persons with long-standing diabetes and catecholamines, glucagon secretion may also be reduced, lessening the effects of counter-regulatory hormones and producing less severe DKA.

In surgical practice, carbuncles, peritonitis, polytrauma, and surgical stress may precipitate DKA. In an already uncontrolled state of diabetes, the precipitation may be quicker.

2.3 Etiology and Pathogenesis

Three factors make important contributions to the development of DKA. These are the level of insulin deficiency, excess of other hormones, and dehydration. These hormones antagonize the insulin actions. In literature they are called as counter-regulatory hormones, a term which will be retained in this volume all along. These are released due to many conditions listed in Table 2.1 and many more. Degree of dehydration plays a substantial part in worsening the situation and should take precedence in the earliest management, at times, even over insulin administration. More details about this will be found below. To ascribe sole importance to any one aspect might cause us to lose perspective of the totality of DKA. In this context it will be useful to understand in more detail the physiology of the insulin actions in the body discussed in detail elsewhere.

Insulin deficiency is the primary and the most powerful cause to develop DKA. Hence the plasma levels of insulin become the determinant of DKA, HHS, or other hyperglycemic states. Different levels of plasma insulin have different effects

Table 2.1 DKA and HHS—clinical and laboratory features in a 60 kg person

Clinical features	Mild DKA	Moderate DKA	Severe DKA	HHS
Thirst	Moderate to severe	Severe	Severe	Severe but could be stuporous to report
Vomiting	Significant	Significant	Significant	Not likely
Severe abdominal pain	Present	Present	Present	If HHS precipitated by abdominal catastrophe
Polyuria	Striking	Striking	May not be striking due to severe dehydration	History of, may be oliguric at presentation
Consciousness status	Alert	Alert/drowsy	Stupor/coma	Stupor/coma
S/o dehydration	Significant	Significant	Severe	Sever
Pulse	Rapid, thready	Rapid thready	Rapid thready	Rapid thready
Blood pressure	Low normal	Low normal/ hypotension	Hypotension	Hypotension
Breathing	Slow deep	Slow deep		
Infective foci/ surgical causes/ insulin withdrawal	Very likely	Very likely		Very likely, typically elderly type 2 diabetics not type 1
Laboratory values				
Plasma glucose (mg/dL)	>250	>250	>250	>600
Water deficit (mL/ kg body weight)	100, 6–8 L			100–200, 6–12 L total
Sodium deficit (meq/kg body weight)	7–10, 420–600 meq total deficit			5–13, 300–780 meq total deficit
Chloride deficit (meq/kg body weight)	3–5, 200–300 meq total deficit			5–15, 300–900 meq total deficit
Potassium deficit (meq/kg body weight)	3–5; 200–300 meq total deficit			4–6; 240–30 meq total deficit
Phosphate deficit (meq/kg body weight)	5–7; 300–20 meq total deficit			3–7; 180–420 meq total deficit
Magnesium deficit (meq/kg body weight)	1–2			1–2
Calcium deficit (meq/kg body weight)	1–2			1–2
Urine ketone	+	++	+++	Small

Table 2.1 (continued)

Clinical features	Mild DKA	Moderate DKA	Severe DKA	HHS
Serum ketone	+	+	+	Small
Serum osmolality	Variable	Variable	Variable	>320 mosm/kg
Anion gap	>10	>12	>12	<12
Arterial pH	7.25–7.35	7.0 to <7.25	<7.0	>7.3
Serum bicarbonate (meq/L)	15–18	10 to <15	<10	>15

on the principal organs of insulin resistance, glucose storage, and glucose release, that is, the liver, muscles, and substitute fuel sources like adipose tissues. These actions are described in detail elsewhere. Lipolysis in DKA, not proceeding through the normal metabolism in the absence of insulin, goes through beta-oxidation process which is the cause of ketosis.

2.3.1 Hyperglycemia and Its Central Role in Genesis of HHS and DKA

The mechanisms described below have been elaborated later and in much greater detail in Chap. 10. At concentrations less than 15 μU/mL, ketosis will develop since none of the physiological processes maintaining the milieu interior can work effectively at this level. In addition to that, any acute illness both surgical and nonsurgical results in raised levels of cortisol, catecholamines, tumor necrosis factor alpha, cytokines, and growth hormone. Pyrogens and tissue trauma also cause release of counter-regulatory hormones. Each has a different mechanism of action, but the net effect of all of them is the rise in insulin resistance. They have an additive effect in presence of high levels of glucagon. These dynamical changes set, with low insulin levels, the stage for development of DKA.

On the contrary if the insulin level remains higher than 15 μU/mL, the lipolysis does not take place, and free fatty acids do not take the path of beta-oxidation. But this level is not sufficient to facilitate intracellular glucose disposal. Glucose continues to rise, causing continued further osmotic diuresis; with it the electrolyte losses resulting in severe dehydration, hypotension, and cerebral dysfunction, which finally lead to HHS. Any other factors described later below in the discussion of HHS which may increase insulin resistance will cause further elevation of glucose levels resulting in extreme levels of hyperglycemia.

2.4 Metabolic Alterations in DKA

The clinical signs have been described in Box 2.2. The metabolic alterations are seen in the laboratory reports in a quantified manner. Hyperglycemia, ketonemia, lipolysis leading to increased free fatty acids, osmotic diuresis causing dehydration and electrolyte losses, proteolysis, and phosphate and magnesium losses are the principal metabolic alterations and will be dealt with one by one.

2.4.1 Hyperglycemia

By definition a blood glucose level above 250 mg/dL is enough to diagnose DKA. DKA usually precipitates rapidly and does not unfold over days like HHS. Therefore extreme hyperglycemia like HHS above 600 mg of glucose is not a definitive requirement.

2.4.2 Ketonemia

This is the second most essential factor. Serum ketone levels 2+ or urinary ketones 3+ indicate substantial ketosis. This is an essential element to diagnose DKA. As the intervention proceeds intensively, the clinical condition improves rapidly, generally within 4–8 h, but ketone levels may not decrease but may actually rise. This is not a cause for alarm, nor one to decline the patient from taking up surgery. The reason behind this paradox is simple. Under the beta-oxidation process mentioned above, beta-hydroxybutyrate levels in blood rise. These are not detectable as ketones, though they represent the penultimate state of ketone bodies. The ketones are oxidized under the rising levels of insulin and decline of glucagon and other measures taken to correct other abnormalities. The ketonemia reduces. But the beta-hydroxybutyrate in blood then starts getting converted to ketones before being oxidized completely under insulin administration. As ketones they become detectable which in the improved clinical setting should be understood as a natural biochemical process and not as a sign of alarm.

An attitude of alarm towards ketonuria should be given up. It should not be used as a convenient excuse to refuse to take the patient up for surgery. There is no need to do ketones every few hours and especially when the clinical signs are improving. Ketonuria persists for at least 24–36 h even when the diabetic ketoacidosis is well controlled, other parameters have been restored, for a patient to be taken up for surgery or who is in a position to resume oral intake.

If ketonuria is mild, it could be correctible in the next 8–12 h. If not, then of course, the matter must be tested further. In mild ketonuria, the same urine sample which detects ketones should be double diluted. If the test becomes negative, it is an indication that these ketones are due to starvation and feeding would resolve the ketonemia. In strongly positive ketonuria testing after dilution is not necessary. Ketones may reappear during the course of treatment. If the urine is tested for ketones after double dilution and if it is negative for ketones it again indicates the need of feeding. Reappearance without clinical or biochemical worsening should cause no worry.

2.4.3 Acidosis

Acidosis and electrolyte imbalance are intimately connected in DKA. The correction of both is equally intimately connected with glucose control. The detailed theory and practice of correcting acid base and electrolyte balance will be described here without always differentiating between the two. A few remarks at this stage would be sufficient. Correction of acidosis in DKA separately is almost never required. Even if it is given for such low pH as 6.9, it has not shown any benefits. When used it has to be in a diluted form; 100 mils may be diluted to 400 mils and infused at 200 mils/h.[1] Other measures necessary to correct DKA are all that is necessary.

Acidosis is the hallmark of DKA. To add to the clarity, acidosis is either metabolic or respiratory. Clinically they present differently. The respiratory acidosis is more likely to be of shallow rapid or slow breathing. Almost always it will have inflammatory involvement of lungs which in its most fully developed form usually is acute respiratory distress syndrome with extensive bilateral inflammatory changes in lungs. It could be due to severe compromise of gas exchange in the lungs due to obstructive pulmonary disease.

The acidosis is metabolic in DKA or in uremia. Even at early stages, it will be detectable as slow rate of and deepening of respiration, with a long pause between the inspiration and expiration, with or without sighing ([1] p. 3). This is the Kussmaul's breathing. One must train oneself to detect and see the changes in respiratory pattern as the intervention proceeds. The respiratory acidosis will usually require ventilator support which DKA rarely does as it starts improving rapidly within hours and if it does not have compromised lung capacity.

When available, blood gas analysis gives a clear picture of what kind of acidosis is present. The respiratory acidosis typically will have hypercapnea, i.e., a very high arterial PCO_2 and much lower than normal PO_2 which at times is unlikely to be corrected even adequately on ventilator support. In DKA typically the PO_2 will be high normal, and the PCO_2 will be low since the diffusion capacity of lungs is intact and even if slow, the respiration is deep, which with unaffected alveolar capillary bed surfaces allow full gas exchange. Significant pulmonary disease may alter this.

An arterial pH and bicarbonate levels of less than 7.3 and 15 meq/L, respectively, are diagnostic of DKA. Acidosis is the excess of hydrogen ions in the plasma. It is neutralized in two ways. One is through stepped-up production of bicarbonate anion by kidneys. It combines with excess hydrogen to form H_2CO_3. It will dissociate in H_2O and CO_2 in alveoli by carbonic anhydrase. The CO_2 diffuses across the alveolar surface and is lost to the atmosphere during expiration. H_2O returns to circulation. When this response becomes inadequate, the second largest buffer against acidosis available is that of intracellular potassium which comes into the circulation (see below). Ketones however cannot be neutralized in this way.

[1] Potential adverse effects of bicarbonate infusions are – overshoot alkalosis, paradoxical cerebrospinal fluid acidosis, hypokalemia, volume overload alteration in tissue oxygenation and overproduction of ketoacids.

2.4.4 Fatty Acid Metabolism

It is grossly disturbed. Free fatty acids, VLDL, and chylomicron levels would be high. Total cholesterol, LDL cholesterol, and IDL cholesterol do not show any change. Their estimation under the altered plasma component conditions is neither necessary nor would be accurate. It is the chylomicrons that give a lipemic or milky appearance to the serum in extreme cases. The presence of high levels of fatty acids and VLDL also has some other impacts with reference to electrolytes in particular and creatinine levels which will be discussed with dehydration below. The resultant plasma composition also has some important bearings on intravenous administration of electrolytes. LDL, IDL, decreases and HDL improves under prolonged insulin therapy.

2.4.5 Dehydration

Dehydration is always a significant accompaniment of DKA. It is generally as severe as 100 mL/kg body weight, in fully developed DKA. As the blood glucose rises beyond the renal threshold, it starts appearing in urine. It is theoretically assumed that in normal kidneys, blood glucose up to 180 mg in glomerular filtrate is completely reabsorbed. Beyond that the renal capacity is overwhelmed and glucose cannot be absorbed fully. As the glucose continues to increase, so does the osmotic diuresis and dehydration and becomes more dangerous. Increased glucose in plasma may draw water from extracellular compartment to the intravascular compartment from which it is lost to osmotic diuresis.

2.4.6 More About the Process of Dehydration

The total body water in person weighing 70 kg will be 0.6 × 70 kg = 42 kg. Roughly 3.5 L are present in intravascular, 11 L of fluid in the extracellular compartment, and the remaining 28 L in the intracellular compartment. The osmotic diuresis originates in the intravascular volume in the non-cell compartment. The subtle changes in the osmolarity and specific gravity result in some fluid shift, water, absorbed from the extracellular compartment in the intravascular tree. It maintains as near normal an intravascular volume which is essential for homeostasis via blood pressure maintenance, tissue perfusion under adequate pressure, and preventing tissue hypoxia.

Later the extracellular compartment fluid is osmotically absorbed in intravascular compartment and lost in osmotic diuresis; the intracellular compartment of fluid is then drawn in the extracellular and from there to the intravascular compartment osmotically and lost the same way in urine. At the beginning of this stage, the acidosis, dehydration, and hypotension will have become very prominent.

2.4.7 The Process of Rehydration

When the rehydration starts, the hydrating fluid to be chosen should first normalize the intravascular fluid compartment. It has a few consequences. The capacitance vessels which are severely constricted to accommodate for the reduced intravascular volume dilate and the intravascular volume need to be readjusted to normal. As more fluid is pumped in, an osmotic gradient is established between the intravascular and extracellular compartment causing a fluid shift in the opposite direction towards the extracellular compartment which regains the fluid it has lost. Once the fluid escapes into the extracellular compartment and gets diluted, the intracellular compartment starts getting hydrated causing the third major shift of fluids.

Thus rehydration occurs in the reverse direction compared to the dehydration. These fluid shifts are massive. They can lead to transient hypotension reversing back to a normotensive stage as the rehydration continues. The swift as well as massive fluid shifts also cause wide fluctuations in plasma levels of sodium, potassium, and glucose. That is why, be it HHS or DKA, in the initial management, 4-hourly monitoring of these parameters and rate of rehydration should be judged by frequent clinical monitoring also. For fluid shifts leading to normalization of all three compartments, it takes about 24 h at its minimum. That is why rehydration process should be prolonged with energetic fluid replacements.

2.4.8 The Fourth Compartment Losses

Many a surgical condition can and do cause a large fluid, electrolyte, and blood loss in what is called the fourth compartment. Intra-abdominal surgical sepsis, obstruction, and massive gangrenes could be sited as a few. Here the fluid is lost in the organs affected as well as in the peritoneal cavity. Posttraumatic blood losses or transfemoral fractures also cause massive losses. Unlike the other three compartments, this fluid or blood is lost to the body as it does not participate in the fluid shifts described so far. Thus, estimating these losses at appropriate stages becomes an additional measure that needs to be undertaken while the dehydration is computed and corrected. In abdominal surgery with long incisions, as much as 10–15 mils/kg could be lost under the blazing lights of the operation theater.

The fluid that chronically collects in the abdomen or elsewhere is seen in chronic congestive heart failure or in hepatic cirrhosis or in full-blown SIADH—syndrome of inappropriate antidiuretic hormone. Such fluids are in equilibrium with the other compartments of the body. If such fluids are drained rapidly, it could at times cause circulatory collapse due to massive fluid shifts. This is mentioned here although not related to the topic to complete the understanding of fluid dynamics.

2.5 Evaluation of Fluid Status of Patient in the Emergency Surgical Situation

Fluid loss is an integral and vital part of the emergency surgical situation, whatever may be the nature of the emergency. It may be trauma entailing blood loss or an abdominal emergency like perforation of bowel with peritonitis, or even with significant sepsis requiring an emergency intervention, fluid loss of a significant nature has to be expected. Concomitant water losses due to osmotic diabetic diuresis get added to the fluid deficit. The picture is at its worst for emergency abdomen presenting with established DKA. This fluid loss will be further compounded once the abdomen is opened and surgical loss sets in. So, assessment of fluid status and correction *has* to start pre-operatively in an aggressive and anticipatory manner.

While the clinical parameters of heart rate, blood pressure, pulse volume, moistness of tongue, urine output, and nature of skin and its temperature are the primary assessment criteria, these often do not suffice to judge the extent of fluid deficit. Correction of these clinical parameters with fluid administration does help to assess the improvement of patient's condition, but more objective parameters are required especially if the patient with diabetes also has cardiac disease.

To optimize fluid therapy, therefore, invasive monitoring methods will have to be instituted. The commonest and easiest invasive monitoring tools employed are the CVP monitoring and intra-arterial pressure monitoring. This approach is mandatory especially in those patients who remain hypotensive in spite of initial aggressive fluid resuscitation.

2.5.1 Central Venous Pressure (CVP)

The CVP is an index of preload of the heart. Preload is the volume of venous return which includes the lymphatics pouring their contents in the venous system. However, CVP is influenced by a few more factors. If the myocardial contractility is poor, venous return coming from the right heart to the left cannot be pumped out. The failing heart dilates and myocardial fibers get stretched beyond the optimum. It makes the Starling's Law ineffective. The excess volume results in increase of both the end diastolic volume and pressure within the heart. This gets reflected in the rise of the CVP.

The heart pumps blood also against the systemic arterial or peripheral vascular resistance, also called the afterload. Afterload, the arterial resistance depends upon the contractile status of arteries. If the contractility of the left heart is poor, it cannot pump out the blood fully, even if the peripheral vascular resistance is normal. It will also result in increased CVP due to damming effect. Poor contractility against higher peripheral vascular resistance will result in even higher CVP as the blood continues to accumulate the ventricles and atria.

Additionally if the intrathoracic and intraabdominal pressures are high, the venous return will be obstructed, and the heart will not get the full venous return. Full venous return optimally stretches the heart muscle fibers for a full contractibility. It does not happen if the venous return is low. That will engorge the vena cavas and the recorded CVP will be higher than normal. Hence, single values of CVP cannot be relied upon; rather the rising or not rising trend of the CVP value in response to fluid administration is more relevant.

Absolute CVP values are expected to be low in a patient with fluid deficit, and as fluid resuscitation proceeds, this value will start improving.

The aim optimal for CVP value is of 8–10 cm of water, always remembering that to achieve this value would be a matter of massive fluid administration in a patient with diabetes especially with established DKA or HHS in the emergency surgical situation. Here lies the importance of an improving trend of CVP.

A higher CVP value (10–12 mmHg) is recommended in situations like mechanically ventilated patients as it results in obstruction to the venous return which could be partially overcome for better filling of the right heart. Diastolic dysfunction, the characteristic feature of diabetic cardiomyopathy, is found in people with diabetes quite frequently. It is the inability of the heart to adequately relax to accommodate the full volume of venous return. Lowe than normal or normal CVP will not achieve the filling fully where a higher VP could be of help. In chronic obstructive pulmonary disease (COPD) leading to higher intrathoracic pressure or/and in case of increased intra-abdominal pressures, the inflow obstruction will be overcome by higher level of CVP.

The CVP catheter also gives us access measure of the central venous oxygen saturation or $SCVO_2$. The $SCVO_2$ level is lower than the arterial oxygen saturation level which supplies the oxygen to the tissues. After the tissues have utilized the oxygen, the returning venous blood will be desaturated. Measuring $SCVO_2$ thus is actually a measure of the balance between oxygen demand (VO_2) and supply (DO_2) to the tissues. Alternatively it is a measure of tissue perfusion and its adequacy. An $SCVO_2$ of 70% and above indicates an adequate tissue perfusion. Achieving this balance between oxygen demand and supply has been shown to be associated with reduced complication rates in high-risk patients. This can be monitored continuously with the help of specialized CVP catheters or intermittently by venous blood gas measurement as a cheaper alternative. It is of major relevance in septic shock.

2.5.2 Intra-arterial Blood Pressure Monitoring

In addition to continuous values of arterial pressure, the intra-arterial waveform can be an important guide to the fluid status of a patient. Hemodynamic interpretations that can be made from the wave forms are:

(a) Systolic blood pressure variations (swing in wave form) can be seen with hypovolemia.
(b) Steep slope of upstroke means good contractility and vice versa.
(c) Area under the curve represents stroke volume.
(d) Slope of the descent if steep indicates low systemic vascular resistance (SVR).

2.5.3 Pulmonary Artery Occlusion Pressure (PAOP)

We would like to mention PAOP only in order to complete the issue of hemodynamic monitoring. We have hardly used this monitoring method in routine clinical practice, even in the very worst clinical situations. The reason, obviously being the fact that it is a difficult monitoring to establish, requires skill and is expensive.

Besides we have been managing adequately with the other invasive monitoring methods available to us. However the value of PAOP monitoring in cardiac surgeries, definitely, cannot be denied.

2.5.4 Preload Responsiveness in Intra-arterial Monitoring

Fluid resuscitation is essential to treat hypovolemia and restore organ perfusion. However excessive fluid administration will contribute to tissue and pulmonary edema and right ventricular dysfunction. Therefore, in a hypotensive patient, whether further fluid administration is warranted or not may sometimes be a tricky issue.

An important tool in the armamentarium is provided by the intra-arterial monitoring method in the form of two parameters, pulse pressure and stroke volume variation, explained below. These parameters are of use *only* in mechanically ventilated patient. As such these are more useful for the anesthesiologist intraoperatively, rather than in ICU setting perioperatively. During the phase of pumping air in the lungs and the phase in which the passive exhalation takes place, the volume the heart receives for pumping will vary. That will reflect and result in the pulse pressure variation (PPV) and stroke volume variation (SVV). Depending upon the extent of variation, the various measures of fluid infusion or factors of mechanical ventilation and other ones can be adjusted intraoperatively.

2.5.5 Pulse Pressure Variation and Stroke Volume Variation

Static measures are single point of time and not real-time continuous measures of preload, that is, CVP or PAOP. Decisions to give a fluid challenge are often tricky. In a given number of fluid challenges, half the times CVP or PAOP may fail to predict fluid responsiveness. That means these many times these two do not predict whether fluid loading will result in an increase in cardiac output. In addition, fluid has to be given before the response to fluid challenge can be evaluated. This is potentially hazardous in some patients since it can lead to fluid overload, dangerous to a compromised heart or renal insufficiency.

Dynamic parameters of pulse pressure variation and stroke volume variation in such situations predict the response to fluid loading without having to give a fluid challenge. Hence, they may reduce the number of situations where a fluid challenge will not work and avoid the potential hazards of fluid loading. The principles behind these parameters are outlined below.

1. Transmural pressure is the difference between the pressure inside the aorta and the (pleural) pressure outside. During inspiration in a fully controlled mechanically ventilated patient, afterload to the left ventricle decreases. It happens because the transmural pressure decreases.

2. The preload to the left ventricle increases due to squeezing of pulmonary capillary blood to the left side of the heart. It will then stretch the myocardial fiber length according to Starling's law where up to a point stretching increases the myocardial contractility. This causes increase in the left ventricle output the stroke volume during inspiration. This will lead to increased systolic pressure as well. Pulse pressure is the difference between the systolic and diastolic blood pressure. As the systolic pressure goes up, the pulse pressure also widens or increases.
3. During inspiration, due to less venous return to the right ventricle, its preload decreases. At the same time due to lung inflation and higher alveolar pressure, the pulmonary arterial pressure, that is, the afterload, increases. It results in decreased right ventricular stroke volume or the beat-to-beat output. Then there is a transit time for the blood volume to shift from the right- to the left-sided heart. All these changes lead to decrease in systolic pressure, pulse pressure, and stroke volume which is reflected during expiration due to transit time.
3. During expiration, this phenomenon is reversed.
4. Thus there is a respiratory cycle during which these changes and variations occur. The stroke volume variation (SVV), systolic pressure variation (SPV), and pulse pressure variation (PPV) increase during inspiration. These parameters will decrease during expiration. These changes are called as dynamic indicators of how responsive the system will be to preload.
5. In hypovolemic patients, these changes are exaggerated. Values more than 13% are indicative of fluid responsiveness.
6. The physiology behind the volume responsiveness or pressure variation with respiration can be explained in simple terms. Both the ventricles of healthy subject have a preload-stroke volume relationship. The stroke volume response is with preload rising steeply. During respiratory cycle there is a normal preload reserve. Therefore detecting the volume responsiveness must not systematically lead to the decision to infuse fluid. The presence of signs of cardiovascular compromise must be taken into consideration since it will have a potential risk of pulmonary edema formation. In that case the gas exchange may worsen. Such a decision must be balanced and be based on these factors.
7. There are a few limitations of SPV, PPV, and SVV. These cannot be used in patients with spontaneous breathing activity. These are not reliable in patients ventilated with low tidal volume either, and in those patients with increased intra-abdominal pressure in case of arrhythmias, the ventricles are particularly liable for fluctuating preload due to a loss of sequential atrioventricular function. Hence these parameters are not reliable during arrhythmias.
8. There is also a much simpler way to do it. In these cases, raising the leg passively is an alternative choice. Passive leg-raising maneuver is an endogenous fluid challenge. A continuous monitor of stroke volume, SVV, PPV, or aortic blood flow by esophageal Doppler is required. Increase in stroke volume of more than 10% and aortic blood flow of more than 10% or decrease in SVV/PPV after passive leg raising indicates a good response to fluid loading.

The next important parameters are those of fluid, electrolyte, and acid base deficits to be corrected in DKA. Below a tabulated depiction for the deficits is given. These figures will be mentioned repeatedly in this volume about perioperative diabetes management. Suffice to say that the importance of fluid and electrolyte assessment cannot be emphasized enough in the management of an emergency surgical diabetic patient.

2.6 Electrolyte Abnormalities

The schedule for electrolytes and acid base assessment is— to be sent from the ER; if it is not sent, then as soon a patient is admitted, then after 4 h once the resuscitative measures have begun and then 8–12 hourly in the first 2 or 3 days. If the free urine flow is established in 24 to 48 hours is adequate. If severe chronic kidney disease is also present, then it depends on dialysis schedules.

With sodium and potassium, it is highly desirable that chlorides also be done. It should be in the protocol of the laboratories to include it when electrolytes are asked for. Again for some uncanny reason, testing of chlorides has disappeared from the practice. They are particularly important in diabetes since hypochloremia is often present with acidosis. The blood gas analysis with electrolytes gives values of calcium which are worth noting to decide if any action is needed on that count. The most important electrolyte is potassium and should be *adequately monitored and courageously replaced*. Intracellular actions which include insulin secretion also cannot be initiated unless potassium rises inside the cells and its efflux channels are closed.

2.6.1 Sodium

With glucose lost in the urine is also lost sodium. These two solutes (substances which dissolve completely in water) always go together. When the kidneys are absorbing glucose till its maximum capacity, it also absorbs sodium with what is called as the sodium glucose cotransporter. When greater quantities of sodium continue to be lost in urine, the cellular mechanisms of urinary tubules let out the potassium in exchange of absorbing sodium to maintain the osmolarity. Thus the situation leads along with dehydration to a stage of significant to serious hypokalemia and an uncertain sodium level, about which more will be discussed below. Sodium is an extremely important plasma ingredient which keeps the plasma osmolarity as near to normal as possible. A near-normal osmolality is essential for the maintenance of milieu interior or the homeostasis and the preservation of organs.

2.6.2 Sodium Values in DKA and How to Interpret Them

Sodium estimation is dependent on the actual volume of water in plasma. Therefore anything that alters physically the water content of plasma will also alter the sodium levels in three directions. The direction is decided by the ratio of volume of water lost with the quantum of sodium lost. If water is lost in excess over sodium in osmotic diuresis, the plasma will show either a high or a normal level. If sodium is lost in excess of water, it will give a lower reading of sodium. In the face of volume contraction in plasma, all three values could be false. Vigorous efforts for rehydration with iso-osmolar fluids within hours can change the water content of plasma to give much more reliable readings.

The other confounding factor in this respect is the lipid abnormalities. In micro terms, the effective volume of water in plasma is displaced by the lipids, over and above that lost in osmotic diuresis. This volume contraction may also lead to either high or low or normal levels of sodium and high levels of creatinine in particular. That also contributes to the different values of sodium mentioned above, more suitably called as pseudohyponatremia, pseudonormonatremia, and pseudohypernatremia.

Sodium values have a direct bearing on the rehydration process. None of the above values can be believed to be correct in the first estimation. In hyponatremia or (pseudo) hyponatremia or (pseudo) normonatremia, the choice of rehydration fluid will be normal saline. If the sodium is found to be normal or high, it is common practice to start hydration with either a 0.45% saline or in pediatrics even a 0.33% saline, at rates dictated by the level of dehydration, discussed in more details in the treatment/management section.

In gross dehydration 0.45% or normal saline can be infused at 500–1000 mils in the first hour or two. Infused saline stays much longer in the blood than 5% dextrose alone does. With a liter or two of saline, the water level in the plasma expands over 4 h. A repeat reading of sodium (with potassium and chlorides) is taken. It may throw up quite a different level of sodium, and the concentration of saline will have to change accordingly. If the sodium reading is high normal or higher, 0.45% saline will suffice. Therefore while replacing sodium, it is better to re-evaluate these values intermittently as dehydration is corrected and after DKA has been reversed long enough to reach the level of homeostasis. It is necessary to watch the patient carefully in these 4 h to see if formation of urine is on the rise and to detect signs of fluid overload, to moderate the speed of rehydration. Once urine starts flowing freely, more aggressive rehydration can be undertaken.

2.6.3 Hyponatremia

Hyponatremia results in cerebral dysfunction and emotional lability, and severe hyponatremia can lead to irreversible brain damage or coma. Hyponatremia caused by SIADH is not as dangerous but difficult to treat. One of the most frequent side effects of high-concentration mannitol given rapidly is hyponatremia with other electrolyte disturbances. Mannitol as it is has been discontinued from the practice of neurology over decades and should not be used except under dire neurosurgical emergencies. The management of persistent or gross hyponatremia if revealed is quite different. One of the frequent causes of hyponatremia is the use of 5% or 10% glucose without 0.9% saline since it causes dilutional hyponatremia fairly quickly.

Suffice it to say that discontinuation of intravenous dextrose alone without sodium should be the first step. This could be the single most important cause for hyponatremia. Instead it should then be replaced by normal saline with or glucose depending upon the glucose level. Plain glucose with potassium alone is also no longer recommended for the same reasons. This is a common practice which should be given up.

Hyponatremia per se does not call for hypertonic saline infusions of 1.8% or 3%. If the need to use 1.8% or 3% saline arises, it should be infused at the rate of 100 mils over 4–6 h intermittently or continuously at the same rate. It depends upon the comfort and the experience of the ICU in charge with the choice of either method. The correction of hyponatremia should always be more gradual. Rapid correction may lead to acute central pontine myelinolysis leaving the patient quadriplegic, severely and permanently disabled.

If hyponatremia persists even after these measures, the diagnosis of either SIADH or salt-losing nephropathy must be considered. The latter is rare. We have time and again tried to diagnose it by estimating urinary losses of sodium and have not come across this entity. The common situations that lead to SIADH are prolonged use of diuretics with dietary sodium restriction as is common with hypertensive patients. It is also caused by massive infusions of solutions like dextrose not backed by sodium.

2.6.4 The Mechanism of the Development of SIADH

In severe hypovolemia the consideration of maintaining volume overrides the consideration of maintaining osmolarity, and water in excess of sodium is retained. This is accomplished by inappropriate secretion of ADH or antidiuretic hormone which acts on the V2 receptors of distal renal tubules and reabsorbs large volumes of water. The key to treatment is the severe or serious restriction of hypotonic fluids, i.e., mainly water or glucose solutions without electrolytes in sufficient quantities. Added to the fluid restriction where possible, excess salt, as much as can be tolerated, helps resolve SIADH. Oral salt intake may not be possible in severe hyponatremia as it frequently causes severe cognitive dysfunction and coma. In general Hyponatremia severely affects the higher cortical cognitive functions. Hypokalemia causes cardiac rhythm disturbances.

Hypernatremia is extremely dangerous as it causes extensive diffuse cerebral white matter damage leading to brain death. Such levels of hypernatremia are seen in diabetes insipidus due to complete absence of ADH, complicating the situation if it goes unrecognized. This is more likely to happen in pituitary surgeries or hypothalamic damage in skull base trauma. Vasopressin is the drug of choice which should be aggressively administered in such dangerous hypernatremia. It is discussed in more detail in Sect. 7.10. High normal or higher than normal sodium levels during rehydration and other treatments will necessitate introducing a unit of plain glucose and withdraw all electrolyte containing fluids to normalize the situation, if detected early.

2.6.5 Potassium in DKA/HHS

Loss of potassium is a given in DKA and HHS with or without an acute surgical condition accompanying. In places where these emergencies are managed, ICUs or a lesser intensive care unit like HDU or the high-dependency unit, continuous EKG monitoring is available. Even before the first value of potassium is at hand, the monitor can give indication of the potassium levels.

2.6.6 EKG Changes in Altered Potassium Levels

The T wave height decreases as the hypokalemia continues to get lowered. It may become flat or even inverted as the hypokalemia progresses. It would be proportionate to the degree of hypokalemia. The U wave is the second positive deflection after the T wave. As the T wave flattens, U wave makes its appearance. It is seen most easily in the leads V_2 and V_3 on EKG. Appearance of U wave results in the QT interval getting longer. The T and the U waves may fuse. It gives rise to a giant T wave. This happens in severe hypokalemia. When the U wave exceeds the T-wave amplitude, the serum potassium level is <3 meq/L (for that to happen, an earlier record of EKG may be required because in an already presenting hypokalemic state, it may be absent). Severe hypokalemia can also cause ventricular tachycardia/fibrillation and rarely atrioventricular block. In hypokalemia the PR interval can be prolonged and the P waves will become taller than before [4, 5].

In hyperkalemia, first the P wave starts flattening and then disappears, the QRS complex starts widening, and the T wave starts becoming taller. Bradycardia ensues. These changes will lead to cardiac asystole if not corrected.

2.6.7 Potassium Kinetics

Potassium is mainly found inside the cells of the body. Sodium is an extracellular cation. In case of potassium, it should always be remembered that the serum values are not indicative of either intracellular or total body potassium status. There are three mechanisms in DKA or HHS causing loss of potassium from within the cells first to the extracellular compartment. It is then lost via kidneys once it enters the vascular compartment. As the sodium is lost in osmotic diuresis, maintaining a cationic balance is necessary. Acidosis develops which requires a basic cation to counter it. Sodium is continuously lost after the maximum renal tubular absorption in DKA or HHS. To maximize sodium retention, a cation is needed to be exchanged in the renal tubules by a mechanism known as Na^+ K^+ ATPase. To correct all three deficiencies, the only other cation which is immediately available in adequate quantities that can be mobilized is potassium. Under these conditions potassium effluxes from the intracellular compartment and is taken up by the intravascular compartment.

Potassium is also in dynamic equilibrium with intracellular shift of glucose which takes place under adequate levels of insulin. If glucose is lowered rapidly in states like HHS in particular, it will, among other effects, result in massive and sudden lowering of plasma potassium values resulting in severe hypokalemia. Both severe hypo- and hyperkalemia are dangerous life-threatening situations. Secondly, the serum potassium levels do not reflect the adequacy or deficiency or the true status of potassium requirements. Thus a serum level of potassium of 5.5 meq/L in DKA or HHS still indicates lowering of the total body potassium. A potassium level of 3.5 meq/L merely indicates a far more serious total body potassium deficiency state. Suffice it to say that raising intracellular potassium is the first and the final target and not just normalizing the serum values.

The few rules of management that emerge from this discussion are that the potassium deficiency is a given in states like DKA or HHS. Hence even if the potassium levels are high or normal, the potassium replacement should start with hydration and insulin infusions. In higher potassium levels, initial replacement of potassium should be more gradual. Only about 20 meq of it may be added in a liter of saline to be infused in an hour. The caution is necessary before the urine flow is established. In lower levels higher concentration of potassium up to 40 meq or more can be given in a liter of saline in an hour. In extremely low levels of potassium, it is *recommended to first correct potassium* with rehydration and *start insulin infusion later* by a couple of hours to avoid fatal hypokalemia (see below).

The need for higher quanta of potassium is reflected in the common experience that even after aggressive replacement, the serum potassium values keep sliding down, as the glucose lowers. The lesson is to keep the potassium supplements high. It follows that repeated estimation of sodium potassium and chlorides as therapy progresses and improvement occurs is absolutely necessary. Initially 4- and later 8- to 12-hourly or once-daily estimation of electrolytes in the first couple of days is sufficient.

Potassium and glucose are interconnected by a different mechanism. With hydration and insulin administration, the glucose in the plasma starts entering the cells for the purpose of producing energy. This glucose influx is concomitant with potassium influx as that is where most potassium physiologically is located. This last fact has some bearing on the difficulties of potassium correction in both DKA and HHS. Proper level of intracellular potassium is essential for cellular functions. The greater the glucose lowering, i.e., its shift intracellularly, the more rapid will be the reduction of serum potassium levels, creating a state of hypokalemia of significant to serious degrees which is also detrimental to cardiac rhythm and causes excessive muscle weakness, especially in pediatric age group. Hence it is a dictum to first load the rehydrating infusions with potassium if the serum values are low, during which time there is no need to enthusiastically start insulin also since the effects of severe serum hypokalemia will be equally dangerous. Vice versa with high potassium levels, serum insulin will take precedence over potassium replacement which should be started with smaller doses ([1], p. 896–897). It also follows that there is no apprehension in infusing large quanta of potassium once urine flow of 1 mL/min or more is established except in a few conditions discussed below.

2.6.8 Hyperkalemia and Antihypertensive Medication

Hypertension is far more common in diabetes than in nondiabetic state. The choice of antihypertensive medication is the class of drugs called angiotensin-converting enzyme (ACE) inhibitors and angiotensin receptor blockers (ARBs). Both these drugs retain potassium; hence the serum levels may be higher even in DKA. Clinically one may have to be cautious in replacing potassium in such situations.

ACE inhibitors and ARBs are discontinued at serum creatinine levels of 3 mg/dL or low GFR of less than 30 mL/min. This represents an ESRD, i.e., end-stage renal disease, which adds to the metabolic acidosis and may develop hyperkalemia under potassium infusions. Here the potassium replacement will have to be gradual and more frequently monitored.[2] Once urine flow is established, aggressive potassium replacement becomes safer. An accidental load of potassium is not absorbed by the kidneys and is allowed to pass off.

2.6.9 Chlorides, Phosphates, and Magnesium Deficiencies

Chloride estimations are essential since the anion gap can then be calculated. Hyperchloremic acidosis is common in diabetes. It gives rise to headache, difficulty in concentrating, drowsiness, stupor, rapid and deep breathing, and muscle weakness. To avoid that, intravenous potassium phosphates are recommended. In DKA there is a simultaneous phosphate deficiency also which condition can be corrected by potassium phosphates. This preparation however is not available easily in India. Magnesium deficiency like phosphates is common in both DKA and HHS. Parenteral replacement is not particularly needed in DKA since the patient starts taking nutrition orally within a few hours. In HHS it can be done by intramuscular two or three injections of 2 g each of magnesium sulfate, or the same could be added to the drip. The latter option adds to fluid load and makes therapy a little more complex. If it is given in a fresh glucose drip, it will alter the caloric supplementation rate.

2.6.10 Creatinine Levels

For the same alterations in plasma composition in DKA, described above as well as the possibility of continuing ACEI or ARBs, the initial creatinine level could also come as higher and becomes a cause of worry, especially from the point of view of rehydration. ACE inhibitors and ARBs do cause a dose-dependent elevation of

---

[2] Under outpatient care if potassium and creatinine levels are estimated when the patient is on ACEI or ARBs, it is not uncommon to find potassium levels as high as 6 mmol or more. However it does not seem to cause much discomfort, notwithstanding that these levels must be lowered to acceptable levels like 4.5 mmol. Potassium-sparing diuretics must be discontinued first, with fruit juices and other potassium-containing fluids or food (e.g., urinary alkalinizers) and putting these patients on loop diuretics in high doses or urgent dialysis as necessary.

creatinine. As much as 30% of the value could reduce if these agents are discontinued and other antihypertensives are used.

Creatinine and amylase are usually abnormal because keto acids interfere with their estimation. The apprehension is that fast rates of rehydration will produce overload and congestive cardiac failure, if urine output does not improve quickly. On further dilution of plasma on hydration as the water compartment expands, the creatinine levels will come down, more so if the urinary output increases.

The other unseen contributions of the grossly dehydrated state are that it increases the concentration of all the counter-regulatory hormones, further contributes to acidosis, and increases the viscosity of blood, thereby increasing the risk of intravascular thrombosis, which may cause hypoxia, bleeding, and hypotension.

2.6.11 Abnormalities of Protein Metabolism

A negative nitrogen balance up to 9–12 g/day gets established in DKA. Non-lysosomal proteolysis and decreased protein synthesis are noted. Aminoacidemia occurs. Alanine after the initial release declines and is low because it gets converted to pyruvate for gluconeogenesis. Ketogenic amino acids, leucine, isoleucine, and valine increase.

In India protein content of the diets in general is low. In acute illness nutritionally balanced intake cannot be established early. That results in further lowering the protein content of the body. Insulin levels in such situations may be high as the patient comes under treatment, but the plasma levels of amino acids would be low; adequate to high plasma value of amino acids is a prerequisite for protein synthesis. The protein synthesis, an energy-costing process, therefore will be slowed. If the acute illnesses get prolonged, it takes just a couple of weeks to develop hypoalbuminemia, if not adequately supplied with proteins, a serious indicator of mortality.

Renal function should not be equated with normal ranges of creatinine, since it is partially a reflection of muscle mass also which in thin persons may be low. For complete Renal evaluation in diabetes test for microalbuminuria in early stages and when frank proteinuria develops, urinary albumin creatinine ratio is a must. Renal function oftentimes can be upset easily since even in pre-complication days it would be without reserves. It further alters in DKA and progressively worsens. Initially renal excretion of glucose, ketone, and nitrogen compounds increases. As dehydration, insulin deficiency, rising cortisol, and impaired tissue utilization develops, ketone clearance declines. Kidneys cannot absorb three beta-hydroxybutyrate and acetoacetate which cause large losses of electrolytes as these compounds are lost.

Kidneys normally reabsorb small proteins which in full-blown DKA become inefficient and may take many days to correct even after DKA is corrected. The body proteins are acidic, basic, or neutral in nature and have different rates of degradation in an insulin-sufficient state. This keeps the cyclical protein synthesis and its degradation in balance. In insulin-deficient states, all the proteins start degrading at the same rate disturbing the balance between synthesis and degradation and the cell function. While new protein synthesis may not be efficient, the high levels of insulin attained at least effectively reduce the catabolism of proteins.

Presence of infection in DKA is indicated by a leukocyte count beyond 25,000 mm^3. Such high counts up to 25,000 mm^3 without infection are not uncommon. Liver function test may be abnormal because of increased lipids.

2.6.12 Other Contributors

The serious plethora of disturbances of DKA or HHS are the serious pathological changes the acute illness itself adds. Those changes can specifically target an organ or many organs, setting the stage for multiorgan failure. The DKA or HHS is a state in which the immune function is ineffective, leading to endotoxemia and septicemia, leading to DIC, i.e., disseminated intravascular coagulation, which causes further tissue ischemia and could result in serious coagulopathy and life-threatening hemorrhage. It needs many more inputs to effectively manage DIC other than the packed red blood cells, like FFPs and PRPs which makes the management of the DKA even more complex.

The difficulty primarily is to maintain a steady level of glucose infusion and corresponding insulin level and manage rehydration and electrolyte acid-base correction while accommodating these fluids. The matter gets much simplified if the principle of one IV line for glucose-containing fluids with insulin pump at steady rate and one more for all the remaining fluids is maintained. We will discuss this at other places as well. It must be remembered that the glucose control does not always result in full correction of electrolytes and hydration. Thus it becomes mandatory that there should be two intravenous lines, what is now routinely called as the separate line infusions, one for a steady rate of glucose infusion supported by insulin pump in which the per hour insulin rate can be easily calibrated as discussed in the previous chapter. It is easy and highly effective. There are situations where two or more glucose-containing fluids may have to be run. Syringe insulin pumps are ideally suited for temporary variation of rate till the steady-state calorie supplementation is resumed.

This brings us to the actual deficits and excesses in DKA of the normal body parameters that needs correction while the causes of the acute illness are treated as the cause may be.

2.7 DKA Deficits and Excesses

In an adult weighing 70 kg, dehydration is to the tune of 5–8 L of water. Roughly it is about 100 mL/kg body weight. Average sodium loss is 400–700 or 3–10 meq/kg body weight. Average potassium loss is between 3 and 5 meq/kg body weight, which translates to about 210–350 meq. There is excess water loss over sodium loss. Anion gap is increased due to chloride losses up to 5–7 meq/kg and presence of ketones. Anion gap is the difference between sum of the sodium and potassium levels and the chloride levels. Hyperchloremic acidosis is sometimes present when dehydration starts, causing chloride retention as urine output falls. Phosphates are lost about 1 mmol/kg and magnesium 0.5–0.8 meq/kg. A table depicting the deficits and excesses in DKA and HHS is given below under the discussion of HHS.

2.8 Clinical Profile in DKA

Only 20% or less number of patients, who arrive in the hospital with DKA, are in coma. The usual clinical picture is that of a sick individual, retching, vomiting, and complaining of moderate or severe abdominal pain. At times it would be so severe that laparotomy has been performed which turn out to be negative. Thirst is very common. Drowsiness is present in nearly 40%. Fourteen percent of them may be stuporous. Fever may or may not be present. Dehydration and its signs are obvious. Kussmaul's breathing may or may not be present but should be spotted early. It is one of the early signs to start recovering. There may be evidence of pneumonia, peritonitis, sepsis, carbuncles, acute myocardial infarction, gastroenteritis, and viral infection which constitute common causes for precipitation of DKA.

In history of the patient, the most important single factor however *is the withholding of insulin*, under the belief that since the patient is unable to eat properly and vomits, his insulin requirement goes down. On the contrary, infection or the stress being the most common cause of small doses of short-acting insulin even with little intake as possible could still avert major DKA. A total 20% increase over the regular dose is assumed. That dose is divided in smaller rapid-acting insulin injections with whatever possible intake and can be repeated 3–4 hourly. By keeping good hydration, one can avert full-blown picture of DKA. This aspect is covered further under the sick day rules in Chap. 13.

2.9 Treatment of DKA

2.9.1 Rehydration Measures

The most important is to correct dehydration first. It can be done by infusing normal saline or 1/2 NS if available at the rate of 200–1000 mL/h depending upon the severity of dehydration. If it can be done under central venous pressure monitoring, the better it will be for the safety. For initial quick rehydration, measures can be undertaken while awaiting results of investigation. Rehydration in DKA should be done with non-glucose-containing fluids, an error commonly met within wards. 1/2 NS is the best initial fluid to start with till the sodium values are obtained. Ringer's lactate is not indicated till DKA is reversed and surgery is performed. In postoperative state it can be used liberally (see below) as a rehydration fluid. Roughly half of the estimated loss is to be restored in the first 12 h without causing fluid overload. The remaining volume is to be replaced in the next 24 h.

Rehydration decreases the concentration of counter-regulatory hormones in plasma, thereby decreasing intensity of some of the abnormalities of DKA. An insulin bolus is often administrated at 0.4 U of crystalline insulin/kg body weight. It alters the insulin/glucagon ratio, an important consideration in ketogenesis, and will further block glucagon release and effectively reverse continued ketogenesis. Not all follow the bolus injections, and not giving bolus does not materially affect the situation since insulin levels in plasma are achieved rapidly under IV infusion.

Rehydration should be under close observation. It can be best described as controlled aggression in "a hurry under leash." There is no substitute to frequently checking the patient's sensorium, hydration status, vital signs, central venous pressure, basal rales, breathing, and hourly urinary output. From the beginning of treatment, watching for cerebral edema is a must. The level of stupor, drowsiness, bradycardia, depth of respiration at presentation may deepen or may develop newly, indicating raised intracranial tension.

Box 2.3 Treatment of DKA 1

DKA—Treatment—1

Most important

Correct dehydration first, potassium next, and watch for fluid overload

Begin and establish reversal of high blood glucose and electrolyte abnormalities

Reversal need not be complete

Watch for cerebral edema

Box 2.4 Treatment of DKA 2

DKA—Treatment—2

Rehydration under CVP monitoring with 1/2 NS 200–1000 mL/h depending on dehydration

Bolus insulin 0.4 U/kg body wt, 1/2 the dose IV, or full-dose IV or not at all

Insulin infusion at 5 U/h

Bladder catheterization

Hourly urine output, >50 mils/h

2.9.2 Other Immediate Measures

While biochemistry results are awaited, urinary catheter is passed. It is mandatory to monitor *urine output hourly* and to decide on the speed and quantum of hydration against urine output. Every hour the bag must be emptied into a measure and the quantum noted. Fluid losses in sweating and in breathing are physiological losses which may be increased in febrile conditions. These losses should also be compensated by increasing the quantum of rehydration. Catheter enables to decide on the quantity of urine passed per hour comparing hour-to-hour increases. This helps to decide rapidity of fluid and potassium administration. Once the free dilute urine flow is established, more aggressive potassium administration without danger of creating hyperkalemia is possible. Ryle's tube should be passed and stomach fully and repeatedly aspirated if required so that retching and nausea do not lead to vomiting and it does not become a threat for aspiration with the serious consequences of ARDS.

What is important is to begin and establish reversal of dehydration and acidosis by insulin administration and fluids. Wherever required, antibiotics may have to be used or surgical correction undertaken. While the reversal may not be complete, the patients are able to start taking small feeds orally in a matter of 6–8 h, if not contraindicated by the surgical illness. *One pitfall of the reversal is to slacken over these energetic measures*. After the initial intensive management and once the illness seem to be coming under control, sudden deceleration of all measures may happen for many reasons. This may at times cause the DKA to reappear. This particular condition has to be distinguished from reappearance or elevation of ketones in spite of the visible clinical recovery with the patient taking orally as explained above.

2.9.3 Correction of Potassium: In Addition to What Has Already Been Discussed

Each time potassium is to be replaced, a formula serves as a useful indicator for amount of potassium to be added in fluids and the rate at which it is to be given. The formula $(4\text{-}K^{+}) \times 0.3 \times$ kg body weight gives the net potassium needed at that point. Generally half of it is replaced over 3–4 h, and the rest more gradually by adding 10 or 20 meq of potassium in each of the running intravenous infusion.

2.10 Insulin: The Mainstay of DKA Treatment

Insulin administration is best carried out by a syringe pump. It has evolved to this method after having undergone many variations historically. In the early era, small doses are used to be administered. Later in the 1970s, dogmatic use of large doses ranging up to 263 ± 45 U was used intravenously or subcutaneously. It was found to be of no extra benefits with respect to normalization of blood glucose or reaching the biochemical endpoints, as with low-dose insulin. On the other hand, hypoglycemia was common. Hypokalemia was seven times commoner than low-dose insulin, both being dangerous in a high glucose state.

The real breakthrough came with low-dose continuous intravenous insulin therapy or the Alberti regime mentioned in the earlier chapter. The total number of units of insulin required was much smaller, 46 ± 5 U. There were no episodes of hypoglycemia and hypokalemia was many times less. Nowaday the standard insulin infusion is through syringe pump. Further discussion on Alberti regime will be found in Chap. 13.

Two suggestions are frequently made about using syringe pump. One—the pump once charged should be run through the intravenous tubing to saturate the sites with insulin so that all subsequent insulin infusions will be delivered with the full concentration intended. More often than not, it is forgotten. However once the insulin infusion has started, it need not be undertaken. The authors however have not found in their long practice any lag in reaching the desired insulin effects delivered without running the fluid first. For the same reasons, the suggestion frequently made earlier to mix the first insulin infusion with albumin may not be particularly useful and add to the logistical difficulties of procuring albumin, much of which will be anyway wasted and the added considerable costs.

To repeat, the IV route is the preferred route in these situations over the subcutaneous one. In a state of hypoperfusion of tissues due either to hypotension or frank shock, the absorption of subcutaneous insulin would be highly unpredictable to build the plasma levels. Two—once given, the quantum of insulin cannot be withdrawn or stopped from acting, which makes glucose fluxes more erratic and would call for more watchfulness, anxiety, and more monitoring. In case of intravenous insulin, it can be stopped for short intervals, its speed can be reduced or increased, or the glucose insulin ratio can be changed easily as many times as needed as discussed in the previous chapter.

Rapid lowering or high-speed reduction of glucose additionally gives rise to hypoglycemic symptoms which are quite alarming without reaching anywhere near the true hypoglycemic values. It will also lead to a disequilibrium within the cerebral fluid content Needless to say, all actions of whichever nature should always be followed by well-calibrated schedules of clinical and laboratory monitoring.

Box 2.5 Treatment of DKA 3

DKA—Treatment—3
IV insulin route far better than IM/SC route, not recommended
Low-dose insulin infusion in saline
5–10 U/h IV by syringe pump, results in immediate attainment of pharmacologic insulin levels
At least 10% reduction of blood glucose in first hour expected
If not, double the insulin rate
More rapid reduction in ketones
Repeat loading dose unnecessary

Box 2.6 Treatment of DKA 4

DKA—Treatment—4
Low-dose insulin rarely causes hypoglycemia, hypokalemia is much less frequent
50 U of crystalline insulin in 50 mils of normal saline in a syringe pump
Lower blood glucose to 200 or 150 mg before starting glucose with saline
Insulin pump rate to be adjusted per glucose monitoring

2.10.1 DKA and Major Surgical Causes: Nutrient Management and Calorie Supplementation

The nutrition supplementing second stage usually starts by giving intravenous glucose once the DKA abnormalities are under control. The recommended calorie supplementation is of 180–200 g/day of glucose infusion for a major surgery. Two considerations arise. If 5% dextrose has to be used, then it should be backed by the saline component within it. The required infusion rate then will be 150 mils/h, that is, 3.6 L of glucose infusion, i.e., 7 U of 500 mils of glucose-containing fluid. This could be difficult to maintain, when many other fluids may also have to be given mentioned earlier. It could lead to overhydration and excess sodium levels and is more likely to disturb the electrolyte milieu.

If 10% dextrose is used, the volume may be half, about 3.5 U, but the insulin infusion rate goes much higher than just the double in our experience. The frequency of thrombophlebitis increases considerably. One more difficulty is to find 10% dextrose with 0.9% saline concentration in most places. Its general nonavailability will lead to hyponatremic consequences. The authors therefore recommend using 5% dextrose saline initially and in cases where the oral intake is going to be delayed by many days institute total parenteral nutrition (TPN). All the issues related to the TPN are discussed in Chap. 13, in order not to distract this narrative from the more important other considerations at this stage.

It is also essential at resident level to know which fluids have or do not have glucose, in the set up and in the city. Plasma expanders like Haemaccel or dextrans do not alter glucose homeostasis. Newer, complex polysaccharides, excreted unchanged, do not cause glucose disturbances. Blood units—the acid citrate dextrose anticoagulant solution contains 2.45 g of dextrose monohydrate, anhydrous sodium citrate 2.2 g, and anhydrous citric acid 0.73 g (composition of Albert David Co). In an era of stored blood without the plasma, the glucose and gluconeogenic substrates will further reduce. Some glucose will be anaerobically oxidized during storage by the RBCs. Hence overall multiple transfusions of packed cell RBCs will not alter glucose homeostasis much.

The mixed intravenous electrolyte solutions come mostly with a glucose component with an electrolyte mix and sodium salts. They are hypertonic. If the situation requires that no intravenous glucose is to be administered, the residents should point out the glucose content. The fluid is then changed to nonglucose-containing one adding the needed electrolytes. In all other situations where 5% dextrose is used, these fluids can be used as multiple electrolyte solutions. The disadvantage of such infusions is that one may not have the adequate quantities of sodium potassium or any other electrolytes if present to meet the situation. The general advice therefore is to constitute the solutions as required rather than going for readymade mixes. In neonatal pediatric groups however, their use may be decided by the neonatologist and pediatricians.

2.10.2 Ringer's Lactate as a Rehydrating Fluid

It is a more physiological fluid which surgeons use liberally with saline. It is better avoided in DKA or HHS. In the recovery phase or postoperative stage when the primary pathology is removed, it can be used liberally in people with diabetes. It is most unlikely to adversely affect glycemic control as shown below. It will be infused over a few hours. Since the hypoperfusion and hypotension is corrected, the lactate in it will be oxidized to pyruvate. Since the insulin levels would be high, the pyruvate will enter the Krebs cycle to produce ATP.

Alternately, assuming that the 29 mmol of lactates per liter get converted to glucose, it would yield 14.5 mmol of glucose over 4–5 h. It comes to 3 mmol of glucose per hour which will be diluted in 5 L of plasma. Thus, the maximum increase in glucose concentration with 1 L of Ringer's lactate would therefore be much less than 1 mmol/L. It does not affect the glucose levels in any significant manner. Ringer's lactate also contains isotonic saline component. There has been an unnecessary as well as incorrect fear to use Ringer's in people with diabetes for long time. For development of hyponatremia in patients with diabetes, not using Ringer's Lactate could be an important reason [6].

It is contraindicated, to due to the lactates in it, in severe hyperglycemia with hypotension. In stable, well-hydrated, near euglycemic patients, with good oxygenation, without sepsis, we have not found lactates to create any problems.

Box 2.7 Treatment of DKA 5

DKA—Treatment—5

On saline insulin drip

- Hourly blood glucose
- Double insulin dose every hour if blood glucose level drops less than 10%
- Potassium monitoring every 2–4 initially; 8–12 hourly as the situation improves, creatinine checked every day for first few days

Box 2.8 Treatment of DKA 6

DKA—Treatment—6

- K^+ replacement if urine output is adequate
- Begin K^+ administration if K^+ level is less than 5.5 meq/L
- K^+ 3.3 meq/L indicates severe deficit—40 meq of $K^+ L^{-1}$ in hydrating fluid in an hour or two; repeat same if needed

Box 2.9 Treatment of DKA 7

DKA—Treatment—7

Switch over to glucose insulin

- Glucose<200 mg/dL
- D5 in NS 100–250 mL with 5–7 U rapid-acting insulin per hour

K+ correction by formula

- 0.3 × kg body wt. × (4-K^+)

Box 2.10 Treatment of DKA 8

DKA—Treatment—8

Ryle's tube aspiration

Watch for cerebral edema, basal rales

Watch for adequate urine output

Once patient is well and alert

- Gradually resume oral intake
- Reduce drips gradually

Treat the other causes of DKA

Switch to SC insulin

2.11 Hyperosmolar Hyperglycemic State (HHS): ADA Nomenclature

Extreme hyperglycemia, no ketosis, raised serum osmolarity, and extreme dehydration with hypotension and drowsiness form the basis of diagnosis of HHS. This is not a more severe, preceding, or sequential stage deteriorating in DKA but differs from it in many ways, in its genesis, clinical profile, and mortality statistics. In fact these two conditions represent in many ways opposite ends of the spectrum of hyperglycemic syndromes. HHS is more insidious, develops over many days, and is peculiar only to elderly, not optimally attended by type 2 diabetic patients, where thirst is blunted and high-glucose-containing solutions are consumed. Clinically, extremely severe dehydration and disorientation are more in HHS than in DKA. Dehydration is almost always has some degree of hypotension. The level of coma is proportional to the level of blood glucose and osmolarity as well as the duration and any new immediate surgical cause mentioned below. In DKA the primary defect is insulin deficiency. In HHS such extreme degrees of glycemia can result in high-degree insulin resistance which interferes with lowering of glucose. The kind of hyperosmolarity found in HHS is not found in DKA. A state of extreme hyperglycemia but mild ketosis is also found not infrequently—a mixed ketotic state.

If one goes by the strict criteria of blood glucose of 600 mg/dL or more without ketosis, one may find a much less diagnosable incidence of HHS in medicine and much less so in surgical practice. But a lesser blown picture with high but not as high blood glucose and absence of ketonemia, hypotension, or obtundation or severe dehydration should probably be managed in the same way one may manage HHS. Such situations are more frequent, and the discussion below includes any near HHS states also, e.g., blood glucose approaching or exceeding 500 mg/dL. Newly detected diabetes may occasionally have a near hyperosmolar state.

2.11.1 Precipitating Factors

The surgical conditions associated with HHS are mesenteric thrombosis, intestinal obstruction, GI bleeds, trauma, any major surgery postoperatively, gram-negative sepsis from surgical or medical conditions, acute pancreatitis, and burns. The medical conditions associated with HHS are cerebrovascular accidents and cardiovascular events, pulmonary embolism, heat illness and hypothermia, thyrotoxicosis, kidney failure, endocrine diseases like acromegaly Cushing's disease, steroid use, alcohol or cocaine abuse, pneumonia, or peritoneal dialysis. It is not uncommon to diagnose a patient with extremely high sugar levels who had no history of diabetes or was not diagnosed previously as having diabetes. Elderly, female, demented patients, and nursing home residents are more likely to develop it; delayed medical attention seeking may be a cause. The HHS may come to fore when surgery is contemplated and patient investigated prior to that. Near hyperosmolar blood glucose without other features of HHS is encountered in medicine frequently.

Some of the commonly used drugs associated with HHS are beta-blockers, carbamazepine, chlorpromazine, immunosuppressants, neuroleptics, lithium, phenytoin, thiazides and loop diuretics, and total parenteral nutrition [7].

2.11.2 HHS Differential Diagnosis

Stupor or coma due to HHS is more likely to be seen if the effective serum osmolarity crosses 340 mOsm and certainly if it crosses 350 mOsm/L. (Normal serum osmolarity is 275–295.) It represents very severe dehydration. Hypernatremia is a more prominent and effective contributor to such high levels of osmolarity than severe hyperglycemia is [2]. The neurological changes that may occur in HHS are unilateral or bilateral paralysis of movements and sensory deficits, aphasia, myoclonic jerks, chorea, nystagmus, and upgoing plantar reflex, seizures in about 15% cases, focal, intermittent, or continuous. If due to HHS these changes are completely reversible. These changes may lead to finding a neurological causation and may delay the diagnosis of HHS. These changes are likely to be due to intracerebral dehydration, microischemia, and changes in neurotransmitter levels [2].

The other common causes of altered levels of consciousness are hypoglycemia, hyponatremia, severe dehydration uremia, hyperammonemia (found in liver cirrhosis), drug overdose, sepsis, severe poisoning, head injuries, and massive ischemic/hemorrhagic cerebral strokes.

Diagnostic criteria of HHS [8]: laboratory findings that clinch the diagnosis of HHS and DKA are given below [9].

Blood glucose—600 mg/dL or more

Serum osmolarity more than 320 mOsm/kg or greater

Profound dehydration to the tune of 8–12 L with increased levels of BUN and a high BUN to creatinine ratio indicating prerenal nitrogen retention or azotemia

Small ketonuria, absent or low ketonemia

Bicarbonate levels are 15 mmol/L or more, blood pH 7.3 or higher

Some alteration in the consciousness

BUN to creatinine ratio could be as high as 30:1, indicating prerenal azotemia

The formula for calculating osmolarity is −2 [Na + K] + (Glucose in mmol). This level of osmolarity cannot be reached unless the glucose is 600 mg or more or there is significant hypernatremia due to excessive dehydration. Mmols for glucose is obtained by dividing glucose in mg/dL by 18.

2.11.3 Pathogenesis

The primary abnormality of high blood glucose develops as a result of low plasma insulin levels which are higher than those found in DKA as discussed above. Such levels as are found prevent ketosis but cannot control blood glucose since it cannot effectively cause glycogenesis in the liver or muscle. As a result the blood glucose rises further. The higher the levels of glucose, the insulin resistance increases due to that alone or other surgical/medical precipitating conditions mentioned above. The medication may not be taken properly or adequate care not given, as is known to happen in old age homes that the blood glucose continues to spiral up and osmotic diuresis sets in with all the abnormalities of DKA except ketosis develop in far greater degrees of seriousness. Levels of counter-regulatory hormones and free fatty acids in HHS are lower than DKA [10]. The insulin glucagon ratio is higher than in DKA. There may be inhibition of lipolysis, but hepatic glucose output cannot be inhibited, and inadequate glucose utilization may continue resulting in continued elevation of blood glucose leading to extremes of hyperglycemia, dehydration, and cognitive deficiencies. Infections, surgical or nonsurgical, as discussed above may accelerate the process.

Due to dehydration and hyperglycemia, the sodium level obtained in the laboratory parameters may not reflect the correct value. To get the correct sodium level, one of the two formulas can be used.

- Corrected Sodium = 1.6 × (glucose − 100)/100 or
- 2.4 meq of Sodium to be added for every 100 mg of glucose

For example, if the glucose is 600 mg, 14.4 meq should be added to the sodium level obtained. This formula is more suitable for extreme hyperglycemia. The correct levels guide better in the management of water and electrolyte abnormalities [11, 12].

2.12 Treatment of HHS

Treatment of infections first if present, as is appropriate:

- A liter of normal saline in first hour.
- To start on 1/2 normal saline till blood pressure improves or normalizes.
- One-half normal saline should be continued till the laboratory parameters are at hand.
- Depending upon the sodium level, half normal saline or normal saline with potassium as per the lab reports should continue at such rates till 12% of body weight is replaced by fluid in 24 h. Higher volume fluid rates are much more likely to cause cerebral edema if given too quickly which could be fatal.

- Intravenous bolus insulin 0.15 U/kg body weight.
- Intravenous insulin 5–7 U/h in normal saline; in HHS such high blood glucose levels cause high insulin resistance which may become hard to overcome.
- In that case if the blood glucose does not drop below 10% of the original reading, doubling the insulin dose every hourly or two hourly becomes necessary.
- The blood glucose is brought to 300 mg/dL and is maintained at that level for 24 h by changing to 5% dextrose in normal or half normal saline (if available) with insulin, as required. The rehydration continues apace.

- Potassium Replacement is directed by the adequacy of and improving urine output as the hydration improves.
- Replacement should begin at potassium level of 5.5 meq/L.
- Add 30 meq K^+ in 1 L of saline to be administered next, to keep K^+ level at 4–5 mmol/L.
- Monitor K^+ as required—4 hourly or less.
- Cautious K^+ administration if urine flow is less.
- If the CVP is low, rehydration will take precedence.

The real risk of HHS therapy is that cerebral edema may develop if rehydration is too rapid or blood glucose is lowered too rapidly in HHS. The corrections should be gradual. The mainstay of whatever treatment is given is clinically monitoring fluid overload and, to watch for signs of cerebral edema, as many times as possible, monitoring and appropriate decision-making. It is important to inform the relatives about the high mortality and record it on the case papers.

Further stages of management—preoperative evaluation, criteria for fitness for surgery, and intraoperative management will be discussed after further discussion on Chap. 3.

References

1. Joslin EP. Joslin's textbook of diabetes mellitus. 14th ed. Boston, MA: Lippincott, Williams & Wilkins; 2005, Indian edition.
2. Trence DL, Hirsch IB. Hyperglycemic crisis in diabetes mellitus type 2. Endocrinol Metabol Clin North Am. 2001;30(4):817.
3. Morales AE, Rosenbloom AI. Deaths caused by hyperglycemic hyperosmolar state at the onset of type 2 diabetes. J Pediatr. 2004;144:270–3.
4. Diercks DB, Shumaik GM, Harrigan RA, Brady WJ, Chan TC. Electrocardiographic manifestations: electrolyte abnormalities. J Emerg Med. 2004;27(2):153–60.
5. El-Sherif N, Turitto G. Electrolyte disorders and arrhythmogenesis. Cardiol J. 2011;18(3):233–45.
6. Milaskiewicz RM, Hall GM. Diabetes and anesthesia: the past decade. Br J Anesth. 1992;68:198–206.
7. Nugent BW. Hyperosmolar hyperglycemic state. Emerg Med Clin North Am. 2005;23:629–48.
8. American Diabetes Association. Hyperglycemic crisis in diabetes. Diabetes Care. 2004;27(Suppl 1):S94–102.
9. Chiasson J, Aris Jilwan N, Belanger R, et al. Diagnosis and treatment of diabetic ketoacidosis and hyperglycemic hyperosmolar state. Can Med Assoc J. 2003;168(7):859–66.
10. Umipierrez GE, Khajavi M, Kitabchi AE. Review: diabetic ketoacidosis and hyperglycemic hyperosmolar non ketotic syndrome. Am J Med Sci. 1996;311:225–33.
11. Launder M, Hammer D, Kelen GD.. Fluid and electrolyte problems In: Tintaneli JE, editor. Emergency medicine a comprehensive study guide. New York, NY: McGraw-Hill; 2004. p. 167–79.
12. Hitler TA, Abbott D, Barret EJ. Hyponatremia: evaluating the correction factor for hyperglycemia. Am J Med. 1299;106:399–403.

Emergency Surgery and Diabetes Management

3

Contents

S. Kelkar et al., *Towards Optimal Management of Diabetes in Surgery*,
https://doi.org/10.1007/978-981-13-7705-1_3

The perioperative period, especially the preoperative stage, is of such supreme importance. It is because of the "surgical stress" that really upsets the normal hemodynamic and metabolic state maximally and more seriously in this stage. In diabetes, it is all the more complicated because of its comorbidities than any other concomitant disorder in the emergent surgical situation. Any surgery in itself is a "stress." The stress to the patient is not only limited to the surgical procedure but also the anxiety to the patient and her relatives shared by the team of the professionals on account of the strong possibility of the patient being taken up for the surgical work, in a suboptimal condition of fitness and the dangers associated with it.

Severe hyperglycemia and glycemic fluctuations are detrimental to the outcome of the surgery in all three stages of surgery. Anesthetists have always experienced hyperglycemia around 200 mg/dL even in people without diabetes, even when they are not administered intravenous solutions with glucose (Ambardekar P., Personal communication, 2018). This is the critical level during perioperative period of any surgery. Beyond this threshold point, the chances of postoperative infection increase. General surgical wards showed an 18-fold increase in death during hospitalization in the perioperative period. This happened with even a moderate increase in blood glucose. Such moderate increases in glucose levels were associated with a longer hospital stay and a greater risk for infection [1]. The literature is replete with the association of hypo and hyperglycemia with above and many other serious or fatal outcomes all of which need not be cited. In particular, it may sometimes expose the patient to sudden and/or severe hypoglycemia which may go undetected. There is poor tolerance of hypoglycemia in the elderly [2]. Strokes are frequent and mortality increased with relatively low blood glucose levels [3].

Naturally, the better the control of all these factors before taking a patient for surgery, the less are the intra- and postoperative problems, costs, duration of stay in the hospital, and so on. The safety of anesthesia increases with as near-normal blood glucose. As mentioned in the first chapter of this book, blood glucose level in the range of 140–170 mg/dL appears to the authors the best level to achieve and maintain during all stages of surgery. It should be achieved by keeping the glucose level in this range by an appropriate dose of insulin infused on a per hour basis. It avoids the tight control levels, for which there is abundant evidence in literature in favor and against [4–7]. Similarly, there is abundant evidence for increased mortality when the average blood glucose rises above 200 mg/dL. The range 140–170 mg/dL avoids by more than fair distance the hypo-/hyperglycemic range for worse outcomes.

It is not always possible to reach these levels preoperatively. More often than not, they will not be reached, in spite of aggressive preoperative management. Hyperglycemia occurs due to high stress levels induced by surgical condition. Blood glucose therefore cannot be lowered beyond a point unless the surgical condition is effectively treated. This puts the situation on the horns of dilemma of whether the patient is safe to be taken up for surgery or can the blood glucose be lowered further to a safer limit. The latter cannot be achieved without surgical intervention.

The blood glucose levels before taking the patient up for surgery, as is emphasized here, are *not the sole criterion to accept or reject* a patient for surgery. The degree of metabolic improvement and hemodynamic stability are as important. Both these conditions may not be, like blood glucose, optimal, but there are criteria which dictate the patient to be taken up. Such a patient will have higher risk but could also be reasonably safe. Not accepting patient at all will lead to death, the professionals will commit an act of omission and refuse a reasonable chance for recovery. Such refusals are not acceptable both morally and from the professional view point, especially in the age of modern medicine with so many advances available in large majority of places. These preliminary remarks bring us to the pathophysiology of surgical stress.

Surgical stress is not just a figure of speech, nor the psychological stress. It comprises, in reality, a hormonal and metabolic response to the surgical situation. The more acute the surgical condition, the greater the resulting hemodynamic and metabolic destabilization, the greater is this response. Comorbidities and hyperglycemia demand precautions to be taken in order to increase the safety during the entire perioperative period. For that to happen, detailed knowledge of both these conditions is necessary and its perceptive evaluation preoperatively.

3.1 Pathophysiology of Surgical "Stress"

Any major trauma, surgical or nonsurgical sepsis, or factors like massive hemorrhage or massive fluid loss destabilizing the hemodynamic and metabolic parameters induce an endocrine, catabolic, and metabolic response in every patient, with or without diabetes. This is due to an increase in the secretion of the so-called stress hormones, also called the counter-regulatory hormones (CRH).

3.1.1 Endocrine and Metabolic Response to Trauma

The major afferent neural impulses for this response arise from the surgical site, starting from the skin incision and continuing with the tissue trauma, resulting from surgical dissection, retraction, cautery, etc. Another important stimulus is the hypovolemia which may occur due to loss of body fluids and blood from the surgical site.

The net result is an increase in secretion of pituitary adrenocortical hormone (ACTH) (stimulus for which is the afferent neural impulses) and consequently cortisol; increase in secretion of catecholamines (both epinephrine and non-epinephrine); increase in secretion of glucagon; all these changes will result in suppression of insulin secretion and insulin resistance both as shown in Table 3.1. The cellular mechanisms of insulin resistance which as a consequence increases are described later.

An increase in secretion of ADH occurs, for which in addition to neural impulses from surgically afflicted areas, hypovolemia plays a major stimulating role. In hypovolemic situations, volume considerations override the plasma osmolarity consideration, thereby retaining water maximally. It leads to dilutional hyponatremia leading to SIADH, a diagnosis almost never made, and futile fluid overloading with normal saline continues worsening the fluid overload without correcting the hyponatremia. More detailed management is discussed at couple of other places. ADH by itself does not increase insulin resistance.

Fall of perfusion pressure results in increased secretion of renin and angiotensin resulting in increased secretion of aldosterone. It will lead to an attempt to retain sodium. Elevation of renin and angiotensin will cause vasoconstriction thereby attempt to increase the systemic blood pressure. Neural impulses and blood loss also serve to stimulate the hypothalamic centers resulting in increased secretion of growth hormone.

The net metabolic response of the increase in these hormones is hyperglycemia. Cortisol causes net protein breakdown, leading to an increased flow of gluconeogenic precursors, i.e., the amino acids. Catecholamines promote both gluconeogenesis and lipolysis thus leading to hyperglycemia. Catecholamines have yet another undesirable effect, viz., they inhibit the release of insulin through alpha 2 neural inhibition of the beta cells to which anesthesia also is complimentary. Ketosis can

Table 3.1 Preoperative emergency laboratory evaluation

For all patients presenting in emergencies	EKG, X-ray chest, blood urea, serum creatinine, electrolytes, and Hemogram, urine for routine examination, ketones, and protein, urine for culture and antibiotic sensitivity if it is infected. Echocardiography in case of previous myocardial infarction in history or as shown in EKG, Doppler studies where indicated as in diabetic foot gangrene, HbA1c
For selected patients presenting in emergencies	CT scan, in case of head injury, abdominal ultrasound in acute abdomen

The table is composed by the author

occur due to increase in the circulating pool of free fatty acids which are not normally metabolized as explained earlier. Growth hormone also promotes lipolysis. Glucagon has its main effect on the liver promoting both gluconeogenesis and glycogenolysis. In addition, it also promotes lipolysis leading to increased FFAs and ketogenesis. All the above effects lead to an increase in the glucose pool. These hormones are termed counter-regulatory hormones (CRH) and will be subsequently referred to as such. See Box 3.1.

These combined hormonal changes lead to osmotic diuresis and loss of water and electrolytes. See Box 3.2. This loss is over and above the loss of fluids due to tissue destruction during surgery. Obviously, relative or absolute lack of insulin quantity and/or insulin action in a patient with diabetes compounds the above metabolic havoc.

The single hormone which opposes all the above effects is insulin which promotes glucose utilization, thus reducing the circulating glucose pool; in addition, it also promotes protein synthesis, prevents protein breakdown, prevents negative nitrogen balance, and is truly an anabolic hormone. However as explained earlier, the insulin resistance as a result of the high levels of CRH does not allow the insulin to exert its full action to counter these changes. Hence, high levels of external supplementation of insulin are required throughout the three stages of surgery.

The mandatory fasting during the immediate preoperative period further contributes the issue because the fasting period is associated with lowest insulin levels. The

Box 3.1 Endocrine and Metabolic Response to Trauma

↑ ACTH	↑ ADH
↑ Cortisol	↑ Renin
↑ CCAs	↑ Angiotensin
↑ GH	↑ Aldosterone
↑ Glucagon	

Afferent neural impulses for this response arise from the surgical site.

The net effect is decrease in insulin secretion; insulin is the only hormone available to counter all these effects. It is the only purely anabolic hormone.

Box 3.2 Net Metabolic Effects of Surgical "Stress"

Cortisol ↑ = ↑ Protein Catabolism and Substrate Flow as amino acids.
↑ in Epinephrine and Norepinephrine—increased insulin resistance, ineffective Glucose disposal and hyperglycemia, ↑ Substrate Flow.
↑ in Glucagon—↑ in Glycogenolysis and Gluconeogenesis, ↑ Substrate Flow.
↑ in Epinephrine ↑ in Glucagon and Growth.
Hormone = Supply of FFA (Lipolysis).

association of low insulin and therefore higher glucagon in this period result in hyperglycemia in addition to the other effects described above. It enhances hepatic ketogenesis. In diabetes, low or even normal portal insulin levels are ineffective in controlling the hepatic glucose output, a signal pathologic limitation in type 2 diabetes.

Another postulation (which is not fully proven) is that elevated levels of amino acids in plasma, seen as a result of injury, stimulate further secretion of growth hormone to cause changes in heart rate, blood pressure, and vascular resistance.

Thus, against this backdrop, destabilization of the diabetic state can occur anytime—pre-, intra- or postoperatively and quickly. The longer the surgical condition goes unattended or undiagnosed, the grossly uncontrolled hyperglycemia could lead to diabetic ketoacidosis or hyperosmolar hyperglycemic state if not already present and can become worse.

3.1.2 Stress Induced Diabetes and Poorer Surgical Outcomes

These factors exert their full effects even in a person not known to have diabetes. Such a person during illness remains in the diabetic hyperglycemic range. The blood glucose levels will come to normal once the illness is successfully controlled or cured after surgical or medical treatment. This is called stress induced diabetes, (SIH). A paradox is seen in this group of patients with acute illnesses. They seem to be at a higher risk and unsatisfactory outcomes during hospitalization compared with the outcomes of the patients with known diabetes with similar blood glucose levels [8]. The probable pathogenetic changes behind this paradox could be traced to a known observation. Those with impaired glucose tolerance, (IGT) are known to have higher cardiovascular risks. Inducibility of SIH in acute illness could indicate previously undetected IGT. In practice, this is an important point to remember and discuss with patients to underline a possibly worse outcome when the emphasis expressed is that diabetes did not exist prior.

The pathological effect of this tissue trauma, pain, inflammation, or blood loss is to stimulate the sympathetic autonomic system. It results in increase in heart rate, blood pressure, and cardiac output. It increases metabolic rate, protein degradation, and glucose intolerance. In the diabetic context, it is the endocrine and consequent metabolic changes that are of greater importance.

3.2 Emergency Major Surgery

The hallmark of most emergency major surgical conditions is a volume loss be it a stab or blunt injury, roadside accidents leading to fractures, chest injuries, or major abdominal emergencies like peritonitis, perforation, obstruction, etc. The emergency major surgery can be differentiated broadly in three categories:

I. One in which massive volume loss is mainly due to hemorrhage (e.g., stab injuries, some blunt abdominal injuries, etc.).
II. One in which the massive volume loss is mainly fluids (blood loss being only one part of it) as in acute abdomen of any etiology (perforations, peritonitis, intestinal obstructions, severe blunt injuries, pancreatitis, etc.).
III. The one in which an infective process is the emergent problem, where fluid loss may, at times, not be as significant as above; nevertheless, the fulminant infection suffices to create metabolic havoc, as in carbuncles, infected foot, with or without established or impending gangrene, perinephric, appendicular abscesses, etc.

Management of category I is simpler as the metabolic havoc created is within bounds or manageable. Management of categories II and III is much more difficult, not only because there is severe metabolic decompensation but also because very often, the surgical condition in itself is responsible for the precipitation of serious hemodynamic and metabolic instability. Severely infected diabetic foot is one such situation. Such a situation also dictates that unless surgical correction is done as early as possible even when the safety parameters are not achieved and risks are high, it still remains the priority treatment for satisfactory control of the diabetic state and the final recovery of the patient.

It should also be emphasized once again that refusing to take the higher risk is virtually issuing a death summons to the patients. Here exists a vicious cycle wherein the initial hemodynamic and metabolic instability produced by the surgical condition leads to a higher level of disturbance which in turn makes the patient more unsuitable to be taken up for surgery, leading to death through many stages.

Pure head injuries are an altogether different category. There is no massive blood loss, nor any immediate infection, or any spectacular fluid loss. But this is a high hyperadrenergic state with due decompensation of glycemic control. The major issues here are the intracranial accumulation of relatively small volumes, causing detrimental pressure effects leading to massive cerebral dysfunction and raised intracranial tension. The latter produces brain stem compression, neuraxial coning, and possibly ischemia of the neuraxis. It is the later states that decide the urgency of surgical interventions generally irrespective of glucose levels which are to be corrected by and by, intra- and postoperatively.

3.2.1 Presentation of the Patient with Diabetes in Emergency Surgery

1. In the emergency situation, the patient may be a person recently diagnosed to have diabetes. She could be on OHAs or on insulin or one on OHA and insulin combination. Prior to the surgical catastrophe, she may be in uncontrolled hyperglycemia which could worsen.
2. Even in a person known to have diabetes, even if fairly well controlled before the catastrophe, there will still be gross hyperglycemia, with or without hemodynamic

and other metabolic destabilization. Such a patient could well be one known to have diabetes for many years and could also have associated end-organ dysfunction of varying severity and control levels could be suboptimal. These patients are often very likely to present or brought by the relatives without their papers with previous history of a couple of years, earlier diagnoses, investigative reports, and without the medicines that are being taken.

3. Then there are patients who are known to have diabetes but either refuses modern treatment, especially insulin or may be taking alternate therapy. All these are common situations the emergency room doctors meet with.
4. Stress hyperglycemia in one observational study in ischemic strokes was found to be 23%. On discharge, none needed antidiabetic drugs [9]. Some of the adverse outcomes and risks mentioned above in case of stress diabetes are as follows: they were more likely to require more resuscitative efforts, repeat intubation, and a longer duration of the ventilator assistance after the operation. They also had higher mortality levels in perioperative setting than those without and with known DM [10]. This finding, along with those of other investigators, suggests that undiagnosed DM or stress hyperglycemia is an even greater risk factor for perioperative morbidity and mortality than known DM [10].

The primary concern in all these cases is to establish the status of diabetes and end-organ involvement to the fullest possible. With the speed and simplicity of laboratory investigations, the delays should minimize. If delayed, it leads to loss of time and the degree of aggressiveness with which the resuscitation can be undertaken.

In the preceding two chapters, we have discussed the initial management of glucose control and the perioperative diabetic emergencies with all the other metabolic complications with which these patients may present. The next stage of discussion is the preoperative evaluation, the issue of the fitness for surgery, the factors involved in making this decision, the difficulties and the barriers which lead to delay or refusal to take up patients for surgery, and the surgery itself with anesthesia issues. Here we assume that a couple of hours of intensive treatment phase have been undertaken, and the situation for at least the first preoperative evaluation has come.

3.3 Aims of Adequate Preoperative Diabetic Control

- Avoiding hyperglycemia, ketosis, treating sepsis, hemorrhage, fluid loss, etc.
- Control of Hypertension or shock - achieve hemodynamic stability as best as can be to reduce morbidity and mortality.
- Avoiding hypoglycemia.

Traditionally, blood glucoses were maintained in the higher range due to the fear of hypoglycemia. Now, with increasing evidence of the risks of hyperglycemia as well as easily available bedside glucose tests, permissive hyperglycemia is no longer acceptable. There is fair consensus about the upper limit of acceptable blood glucose level of 180 mg/dL. Most problems are noted above blood glucose levels of

180 mg/dL. Obviously, there will be advantages of tighter glucose control than this in some patient groups.

There is however no consensus about the lower limits of blood glucose level. Several examples of various lower blood glucose levels as acceptable are given later in this chapter and elsewhere which vary from 80 to 140 mg/dL, with evidence for and against it. The range which appears suitable for susceptible groups like elderly is a slightly loose glucose control. The most acceptable range to all age groups and patients with many comorbidities seems to be 140–180 mg/dL. In perioperative situations, the blood glucose should be monitored

1. Prior to induction of anesthesia.
2. At hourly intervals when insulin infusions are used intraoperatively.
3. And before and during surgery in all patients.

Perioperative management depends on:

1. Whether patient is on diet control, OHA, or insulin.
2. Major surgery (requiring interruption of oral intake, e.g., bowel surgery for several days) or minor surgery. This is discussed in Chap. 6 in more details.

The obligate glucose requirement to be provided for cells which can only use glucose as substrate are neurons, RBCs, and kidney. It is 2–3 mg/kg/min. This can be provided by giving 5% or 10% dextrose solution. We use 5% solution primarily given at 100–125 mg/h to meet this requirement.

For those patients who are already on insulin, the total dose is divided by 24 to get the hourly requirement. In addition to the Alberti regime and other ways of giving low-dose continuous insulin infusion, one more method can be used. The initial insulin infusion rate should be equal to one half or three fourth of this hourly need. Alternatively, the dose on which the patient has shown reasonable control prior to taking him up can be continued. This method is useful in practical terms. However, doses used during the post-induction period could still be much higher in patients with sepsis, who are obese, who are critically ill and almost always during cardiopulmonary bypass (CPB) or patients on steroids. As emphasized repeatedly in this volume, the glucose and insulin infusions must be used by separate line infusions.

3.4 Preoperative Evaluation

This starts with a thorough preoperative evaluation risk assessment and followed by optimization of these factors. Routine surgery poses no problem in this regard with respect to time available. In emergency surgical patients who need a more thorough preoperative evaluation and risk assessment, time is not in favor of the anesthesiologist. There is a higher likelihood of this patient being unassessed recently, particularly in terms of existence of complications of diabetes. Therefore, a very *serious attempt at evaluation and assessment is* a *must.*

3.4.1 Complications of Diabetes Mellitus

From the point of view of the anesthetist and anesthesia, the important macrovascular complications of long-standing diabetes are coronary heart disease, diabetic nephropathy, and autonomic neuropathy. These are important because of a direct effect on perioperative complications. The mechanisms of injury they share are hypertension, atherosclerosis, increased coagulability, and impaired fibrinolysis.

Diabetic nephropathy, neuropathy, and retinopathy are microvascular complications. The mechanisms of injury they share are the osmotic stress from sorbitol accumulation and formation of advanced glycosylated end products which lead to inflammation. Excess production with reduced capacity to quench these free radicals or reactive oxygen species is due to diabetes. In case of neuropathy, age, hypertension, hyperlipidemia, and the length of the nerves are additional risk factors (see Chap. 9 in this volume for details).

3.4.2 Pathology of Cardiac Complications

The composite findings of this and the other complications described below are summarized from the Joslin's Textbook of Diabetes Mellitus, 14th (special Indian) edition, 2005 by Lippincott, Williams, and Wilkins [11]. Numerous accounts substantiating these findings are available in literature. Since there is vast agreement about the major findings listed below, it is not necessary to go into the specific references.

Diabetes is an independent risk factor for coronary artery disease. It is known worldwide that 80% of all deaths in diabetes are due to cardiac problems. Within it, the atherosclerotic coronary artery disease is the most prevalent. Thus, an increase in incidence of and poorer prognosis of coronary artery disease (CAD) in diabetes are given. Mortality related to cardiovascular disease with diabetes is twice in men and four times more in women with diabetes as compared to persons without diabetes, in carefully matched groups. Prevalence of CAD is as high as 55% in adults with diabetes as compared to 2–4% in general population. Women are protected from CAD as long as they are menstruating. They lose this protection if they develop diabetes in menstruating life [11].

It has an increased frequency of sclerotic coronary artery disease due to accelerated and more malignant atherosclerotic process, at an earlier age and advances more rapidly. Angiographies repeatedly reveal that the lesions in the coronary arteries as well as peripheral arteries, are multiple and in tandem, more diffuse and shaggy, involving multiple vessels in people with diabetes. Hypercoagulable states add to development of CVD events. The restenosis rates after angioplasties are higher in diabetes. Hyperglycemia, impaired insulin action or insulin resistance, insulinopenia, proatherogenic dyslipidemia, vasoactive hormones, cytokines and growth factors, angiotensin II, TNF alpha leading to endothelial dysfunction, vascular inflammation, smooth muscle proliferation, lipid-rich lesions, its rupture, and thrombosis are exaggerated in diabetes [11].

The increased incidence of CAD is compounded by the problem of an atypical presentation in diabetes due to autonomic neuropathy. The patient may not experience the typical pain of myocardial infarction (MI) or angina on exertion as well as severe, serious, or unstable acute coronary syndromes. The possible cause for inability to feel chest pain of MI or angina is the autonomic neuropathy in diabetics. The incidence of "silent" MI in diabetics has been shown to be as high as 25% in the Framingham Study. Atypical symptoms like dyspnea, confusion, fatigue, or nausea and vomiting may be encountered in as high as 32–42% of patients with diabetes. These could however be missed as the symptoms of infarction, causing a considerable delay in the early diagnosis of MI. Individuals with diabetes above the age of 65 years have significantly higher symptomatic as well as asymptomatic coronary artery disease. The sympathetic nervous system failure leaves the heart incapable of responding to stress by increasing heart rate and cardiac output. These elderly individuals therefore stand a definite risk of sudden unexplained death due to sudden dysrhythmias either due to autonomic neuropathy or silent MI [11].

If a person with diabetes also has a peripheral arterial disease, he is likely to have a 70% chance to have CAD as well as cerebral vascular disease, even if it is asymptomatic. Peripheral arterial disease is far more frequent in diabetes.

Hypertension is fourfold higher in people with diabetes. It is due to hyperinsulinism and acceleration of atherosclerosis in persons with diabetes. It leads to left ventricular hypertrophy (LVH). LVH in addition to endothelial dysfunction, obesity, and autonomic neuropathy contributes to systolic and diastolic dysfunction. Thus, patient with diabetes stands a higher risk of development of MI which may be often silent.

3.4.3 Diabetic Cardiomyopathy

This is a definite and separate entity well established by clinical, imaging, and pathologic studies. It is defined as cardiac dysfunction in diabetes. It is diagnosed after exclusion of independent of identified risk factors – coronary atherosclerotic disease, hypertension, and valvular heart disease. It can occur despite well-controlled glycemic levels. Several metabolic abnormalities associated with it lead to changes in the interstitial spaces within the myocardium. Metabolic abnormalities like hyperlipidemia, hyperinsulinemia, and hyperglycemia predispose the heart by changing the structure of cardiomyocytes and interstitial cardiac tissues. The functional abnormalities then develop in the cardiomyocytes [12]. 2D echocardiography and Doppler studies have demonstrated the presence of systolic and diastolic left ventricular (LV) dysfunction in the form of LV hypertrophy, modest increase of left ventricular end-diastolic pressure, and the impairment of the relaxation of left ventricular walls. Congestive heart failure in diabetic men and women is two and five times higher than in the men and women without diabetes.

The final outcome of the cardiac disease in a diabetic patient presenting for surgery can be thus summarized. They stand higher risk for development of MI, the MI may be often "silent," congestive heart failure (CHF), and they stand a definite risk of sudden unexplained death due to sudden dysrhythmias either as a result of autonomic neuropathy or silent myocardial infarction.

3.4.4 Cerebral Vascular Disease

It is also related to the same pathogenic factors described above. In particular the ischemic brain stem strokes lead to death far oftener and are a poorly recognized factor [13]. This is the most devastating (and generally unknown) cause of the fatality that is caused almost exclusively in people with diabetes. The predictor of this is the far more frequently seen in vertebrobasilar insufficiency syndrome. Most commonly, it is seen as transient loss of consciousness under euglycemic, hyperglycemic, and hypoglycemic states. People without diabetes who suffer from fatal strokes, almost always have middle cerebral artery thrombosis affecting two thirds of any one cerebral hemisphere [13].

3.4.5 Gastrointestinal System

Autonomic neuropathy alters the tone of the gastroesophageal sphincter and also causes gastroparesis which may also contribute to aspiration. The altered tone also raises the risk of aspiration due to regurgitation, especially if general anesthesia is given. The ability to coordinate swallowing is decreased. To make a diagnosis of gastroparesis, two criteria are used. The food must remain in the stomach for after 8–12 h fast, and the pyloric sphincter should not be obstructing the propulsion of the food. Routine 8-h fasting thus may not be sufficient prior to anesthesia. History of constipation, frequent explosive nighttime diarrhea without any signs of infective etiology, and fecal incontinence can point to these likely risk factors.

3.4.6 Respiratory System

Early investigations of respiratory system show that diabetes affects the respiratory system, but evidence regarding its impact on functional status of the patient is lacking. The underlying mechanisms hypothesized include impaired lung elasticity, pulmonary microangiopathy, and chronic systemic inflammation of diabetes. Some of the reported lung dysfunctions attributed to diabetes are the decreased lung volume, lung diffusion capacity and reduced hypoxia-induced respiratory drive especially in patients with autonomic neuropathy. People with diabetes may be prone to respiratory depression from opioids and sedative agents due to impaired chemoreceptor activity.

3.4.7 Airway Problems

The "stiff joint" or "limited joint mobility" (LJM) is a syndrome of diabetic cheiroarthropathy. Different joints in the body are stiff or rigid. From the point of view of anesthesia, the temporomandibular, atlanto-occipital, and cervical spine joints are important for extending the neck and to do laryngoscopy prior to intubation. Most commonly involved, these joints support the airway; stiffness in them or difficulties in extending the neck may make the laryngoscopy difficult. In diabetes, any long life protein like collagen protein tends to get nonenzymatically glycated; coupled with abnormal cross-linking of collagen in joints and other tissues, these joints become stiff. About one third of patients with long-term type 1 diabetes have short stature, joint rigidity, and tight, waxy skin. They present with laryngoscopic difficulties and preoperatively can worsen the situation during pre-induction period or induction of general anesthesia. Patients with type 2 diabetes and morbid obesity also undergo difficult laryngoscopy and intubation. Modern flexible laryngoscopes are of value in these situations.

Two tests can preempt the diagnosis of this difficulty prior to anesthesia induction. The "Prayer" sign is the inability to oppose the fingers of the palms as done while praying. The fingers cannot be opposed leaving a gap which can be seen by looking at the ulnar edges of the fingers laterally. Palm print test gives a clearer demonstration of the stiffness of the fourth and fifth interphalangeal joints. To conduct the test, the palm and fingers of the dominant hand of the patient are painted with ink. Then the palm is firmly pressed on a white sheet of paper on a hard surface which gives a print of the palm. The severity is judged by the following observations. Grade 0 is when all phalangeal areas are visible. Grade 1 is the deficient print areas in the interphalangeal areas of fourth and/or fifth digit. Grade 2 is the deficient print area in the interphalangeal areas of second to fifth digit, and in Grade 3, only the tips of digits can be seen.

3.4.8 Diabetic Nephropathy

It progresses from the glomerular hyperfiltration, increased renal plasma flow in the preclinical stage. The kidney size increases. The intraglomerular hydrostatic pressure is increased. It causes glomerular damage, microalbuminuria, and impaired endothelium- dependent vasodilatation. It later progresses to extensive involvement of the glomeruli in the form of nodular lesions described by Klimmelsteil and Wilson decades ago, comprising of deposition of PAS-positive material in the intercapillary and intracapillary regions of the glomeruli. The earliest sign is microalbuminuria. With increasing glomerular damage and involvement, it leads to detection of large quantities of albumin in the urine. Finally, there is an actual decrease in functioning glomerular numbers. It reduces the creatinine clearance and increase in serum creatinine. It progresses to develop end-stage renal disease (ESRD).

Renal dysfunction is accelerated through hypertension, dyslipidemia, high protein diet, infections in the urinary tract, and anemia. Iatrogenic exposure to nephrotoxins and cardiac surgery could lead to worsening of nephropathy. The beginning of renal dysfunction also leads to the development of hypertension. Preoperatively and in particular during radiographic procedures for preoperative evaluation, avoiding dehydration, nephrotoxins, selective and minimum/optimum use of contrast media, and positive rehydration prior to procedure may help to prevent worsening of renal damage. Two classes of drugs, ACE inhibitors and angiotensin receptor blockers, have renal protective action.

Current data is not sufficient to support use of hemofiltration or the low-dose (renal) dopamine infusions. There is no evidence to support osmotic diuresis or calcium channel blockade for renal protection. Use of N-acetylcysteine does not have strong support of evidence but is part of contrast-induced nephropathy prevention protocol in some centers.

Microalbuminuria as marker of renal disease in diabetes or diabetic nephropathy is a common microvascular involvement in persons with type 1 and type 2 diabetic patients. In its earliest manifestation, microalbuminuria is defined as persistent proteinuria of more than 0.5 g/24 h in absence of structural alteration of kidneys and without urinary tract infection. In single urine samples collected after exercise, microalbuminimia can appear. Urine should be tested at least twice in 6 months to confirm it. Like HbA1c, microalbuminimia is a marker for organ dysfunction in a steep linear correlation. Over long periods, both can be considered as a marker for all future abnormalities related to kidney function, hypertension, and cardiac involvement as a consequence. Its importance in early diagnosis lies in the possibility of halting further deterioration of kidneys since it is reversible at this stage.

3.4.9 Issues Related to Diabetic Nephropathy

The issues that complicate management of diabetes in or without a surgical setting in significant renal disease or ESRD are many. Since the urine output is low, volume overload can develop quickly resulting in both cardiac decompensation and peripheral edema. The chances of development of hyperkalemia are high unless monitored in a well-guarded fashion. Nutritionally speaking, protein restriction is required to avoid worsening of renal status. Generally it is restricted to 0.6 g per kilogram body weight. The ability to take adequate and proper nutrition is restricted due to nausea of uremia that causes reduced availability of substrates for neoglucogenesis. Insulin clearance by the kidneys is reduced. The last two factors combined may lead to hypoglycemia. Hence insulin administration needs careful calibration. In fact, a sudden or unexpected hypoglycemia could be the first indication that significant renal disease has developed. In acute conditions, the metabolic acidosis of uremia could worsen a great deal. Any medication excreted by kidneys need appropriate reduction, and withdrawal of metformin is a must along with ACEs and ARBs. In emergency surgery, more often than not, an emergency dialysis option to improve the milieu will not be available. All these factors together increase the risk in any kind of surgical setting considerably.

3.4.10 Diabetic Sensory Motor Neuropathy (DSNP)

Insensate foot is the most common cause for diabetic foot ulcers, infection, abscesses, and necrotizing fasciitis often leading to major amputations. Peripheral artery disease mentioned in the section above adds to the amputation numbers. DSNP in its most common form appears as chronic sensorimotor distal symmetric polyneuropathy. The most common symptoms associated with it are burning and disproportionate sensitivity for low-intensity stimulus called hyperesthesia. Excessive pain for minimal nonpainful stimulation is called allodynia. Tingling and numbness are common. Mononeuropathies involve bigger nerves like sciatic nerve. Mononeuropathies generally are of sudden onset. Diabetic amyotrophy is characterized by severe pain and muscle weakness usually in the thighs, followed by significant atrophy.

Diabetic retinopathy is detectable through dot hemorrhages, hard exudates, microaneurysms, retinal edema, proliferative retinopathy, and retinal detachment.

3.5 The Assessment of Autonomic Neuropathy in Diabetes

Autonomic neuropathy in diabetes is as pervasive as glycosylation. Mechanisms leading to it are hypothesized to be local ischemia due to small arteriolar closure. Accumulation of sorbitol in the tissues and altered activity of neuronal Na^+/K^+-ATPase pump are also the suggested mechanisms. There is autoimmune mechanism which causes immunologically mediated neural damage. 40% of type I and 17% of type 2 diabetic patients suffer from autonomic dysfunction. It affects both the parasympathetic and the sympathetic nerves supplying different organs and its effects on them mentioned above. It starts typically with affliction of the parasympathetic nervous system leading to resting tachycardia due to loss of vagal tone. Sympathetic nervous system dysfunction could also develop before the parasympathetic degeneration. It leads to orthostatic hypotension and bradycardia. It attenuates the ability of increasing the heart rate and blood pressure under the stress. The heart is unable to vary its rhythm in various phases of respiration, an activity under the autonomic control, due to its dysfunction. When both the sympathetic and parasympathetic autonomic nervous systems degenerate, it gives rise to a denervated heart, as in cardiac transplants where it is the denervated heart that is transplanted. Sudden cardiac death in diabetes is also common. All the factors mentioned above are considered to contribute to it. Autonomic neuropathy affects many other organ systems detailed below.

Assessment of autonomic neuropathy, even a quick one, is extremely important since it has the maximum potential to lead to the most serious complications. The signs and symptoms of autonomic disease of different organs could be obvious to discerning physician or could be more subtle. They are as follows:

Cardiovascular signs: Tachycardia even while resting—parasympathetic autonomic failure with sympathetic dominance. Orthostatic hypotension and silent myocardial ischemia and inability to undertake exercise can be due to sympathetic autonomic failure. As emphasized earlier, even in routine surgery, these evaluations are important. In emergency setting, at least a few or any one sign can alert the anesthetist and should be a part of the communication with respect to intra- and postoperative risks.

Autonomic neuropathy of the genitourinary track can be easily diagnosed by urinary retention without obstruction as in neurogenic bladder, or diabetic cystopathy is a sign of parasympathetic autonomic failure and sympathetic over activity with closed internal urethral sphincter. Failure of penile erection or the ejaculated semen going into the bladder called retrograde ejaculation and female sexual dysfunction and loss of vaginal lubrication typically in postmenopausal women are a few signs.

Among the metabolic complication, one must be aware of two of them which are directly related to autonomic dysfunction. Hypoglycemia unawareness is the failure of the sympathetic adrenergic symptoms to appear as hypoglycemia develops. There was a raging controversy at the time of introduction of human insulin which blamed it on these insulins. That is no longer so. Hypoglycemia-associated autonomic failure is the failure of adrenergic symptoms to appear although there is no autonomic neuropathy.

Sudomotor dysfunctions are common and manifest as anhidrosis, i.e., absence of sweating. This is particularly important in the development of diabetic foot ulcers. The common axiom in diabetic foot ulcers is that the moist environment around the diabetic foot by normal sweating prevents ulceration to a great extent. But a dry foot does. Among other discernible signs are the heat intolerance and sweating associated with the mastication called gustatory sweating.

Pupillomotor function impairment decreases the diameter of dark-adapted pupil (which normally should dilate). It is also known as tonic diabetic pupil. In patients with prolonged ventilation, this should be kept in mind while differentiating between opioid injections or pontine hemorrhages. Argyll-Robertson pupil may also be found.

In the tests for diabetic autonomic neuropathy (DAN), the results are valid if end-organ failure, concomitant illness is not present and antidepressants, antihistamines, diuretics, vasodilators, sympathetic blockers, and vagolytics are not used or are withheld before testing.

3.5.1 Parasympathetic Autonomic Neuropathy Assessment

In the initial stages, abnormality of heart rate response during deep breathing alone may be observable. In somewhat later stage when forced expiration against resistance is undertaken for a little time, the Valsalva maneuver, the response may be abnormal. Valsalva maneuver is influenced by both parasympathetic and sympathetic activity and is described in much greater details in the paragraphs which follow. In the most manifest stages, the presence of postural hypotension is seen.

Variations in the heart rate in response to deep breathing and on standing can be lost. This test is more specific. The tests for variability of heart rate however are age-dependent. But these are not dependent on the intrinsic heart rate. These are the standard methods for screening for autonomic dysfunction, described in more detail.

3.5.2 Sympathetic Autonomic Neuropathy Control Assessment

Blood pressure response is intimately connected with an intact sympathetic autonomic nervous system. It is activated by standing and when a supine patient is brought to an erect position in a passive manner, where the individual does not do anything to become vertical. It is called as passive tilting. The sustained handgrip and the Valsalva maneuver partly described above affect with blood pressure a few other parameters. The Valsalva maneuver is first described below in detail.

3.5.3 Standard Valsalva Maneuver

In this test, the patient is lying flat on the back. An EKG monitor and a blood pressure apparatus are connected to him. He then forcibly exhales against a fixed resistance (40 mmHg) for 15 s with an open glottis. This results in an abrupt but short-lived increase in intrathoracic and intra-abdominal pressure. A particular type of blood pressure/pulse rate response follows. It can be described as phases.

In phase I, the blood pressure rises fleetingly, and the heart rate drops. It happens because of the compression of the aorta. The blood is propelled in the peripheral circulation. The changes in blood pressure and heart rate are because of mechanical factors.

In Phase II, the blood pressure at first falls due to decreased venous return during the rise of pressure in the thorax and abdomen. This reduces the cardiac output that results in a reflex tachycardia increase in heart rate and increased peripheral resistance. It recovers itself later in this phase.

In Phase III, when expiration is stopped, there is drop in blood pressure and rise in heart rate.

In Phase IV, the blood pressure goes above the baseline value due to residual vasoconstriction, while the venous return and cardiac output remain normal. There is also reflex bradycardia.

The Valsalva ratio is calculated from the ECG waveform. The longest R-R interval in phase IV after the maneuver is divided by the shortest R-R interval during the maneuver. A Valsalva ratio less than 1.2 is abnormal.

3.5.4 Heart Rate Variability (HRV)

Physiology: The heart rate varies during a respiratory cycle. A beat-to-beat variability is seen. It is called respiratory sinus arrhythmia. It is a physiological response. During expiration, the heart rate decreases due to the vagal input to the sinus node.

HRV is the difference between the maximum and minimum heart rate during the respiratory cycle. Autonomic neuropathy decreases the HRV. Specialized monitors are available to accurately determine the HRV. The patient is asked to breathe quietly but deeply at the rate of six breaths per minute. At this rate, there is maximum variation in heart rate. This is a simple clinical method but is less accurate compared to the HRV monitors.

Normal variability is more than 15 beats/min; abnormal result is less than 10 beats/min.

Aging is associated with decreased RSA due to decreased vagal tone and decreased beta receptor responsiveness, and the criteria may not apply to patients above 60 years of age.

3.5.5 Response to Standing Up (30:15 Ratio)

Physiologically, the heart rate rises quickly when a patient stands up. The rate is highest at the 15th beat after standing, approximately. A relative bradycardia follows. The slowest heart rate is found at the 30th beat after standing approximately. The heart rate should increase normally by 10% on standing. In patients with DAN, the heart rate increases only gradually.

Measuring the 30:15 ratio: first, the longest R-R interval during beats 20–40 is measured. Then the shortest R-R interval between the fifth and the 25th beat after standing is measured. The longest interval is divided by the shortest interval. A 30:15 ratio more than 1.04 is normal, 1.01–1.03 is borderline, and less than 1.01 is abnormal.

3.5.6 Orthostatic Hypotension or Fall of Blood Pressure on Standing Up

Normally, blood pressure is rapidly corrected by baroreflex-mediated peripheral vasoconstriction and tachycardia. The fall in SBP is less than 10 mmHg in normal state. First, the supine blood pressure is taken. The patient is made to stand up, and blood pressure is taken again. By definition, if there is a fall of 30 mmHg or more in the systolic blood pressure and a fall of 10 mmHg for diastolic blood pressure, it is orthostatic hypotension. A drop by 11–29 mmHg is borderline, and a drop of more than 30 mmHg is response to tilting which is a more precise stimulus and may be used instead of standing. The response is similar.

3.5.7 Sustained Handgrip

Strongly exercising muscles in handgrip stimulate a reflex arc which results in increased cardiac output, heart rate, and rise in systolic and diastolic blood pressure. As the peripheral vascular resistance is maintained, the diastolic pressure rises by more than 16 mmHg. A response of less than 10 mmHg is considered abnormal.

The differential diagnosis of diabetic autonomic neuropathy (DAN) should try to establish which of the conditions listed below could be partly or fully responsible for the test results of DAN.

1. Where no causes described below are detected, it is called pure autonomic failure or idiopathic orthostatic hypotension.
2. Multiple system atrophy with autonomic failure as seen in Shy-Drager syndrome.
3. Addison's disease, hypothyroidism, and hypopituitarism uniformly cause an inability to respond through the sympathetic autonomic nerves.
4. Pheochromocytoma and hyperthyroidism cause a purely sympathetic stimulation.
5. Hypovolemia leads to a mixed picture of hypotension and contraction of arterial tree with reflex tachycardia in an attempt to maintain the cardiac output.
6. Medications with anticholinergic will lead to sympathetic and sympathetic blockers will result in parasympathetic and sympathetic autonomic nervous domination respectively.
7. Peripheral autonomic neuropathies (e.g., amyloid neuropathy, idiopathic autonomic neuropathy).

3.6 Management of Diabetic Autonomic Neuropathy (DAN)

Control of blood glucose levels, ACE inhibitors, and β-blockers have been tried for control of the condition. In endocrine hypofunction, replacement therapy is the answer. In postural hypotension, fludrocortisones are often given which may show some improvement. In vasoactive states like pheochromocytoma and thyrotoxicosis, the control of these conditions at least in routine surgery is a must. In emergency surgery, it will add to the risks exponentially.

3.6.1 Autonomic Neuropathy in the Perioperative Course

In addition to the factors affecting the outcome described above, a few more should be noted. It is the increased risks of hemodynamic labaility intraoperatively. Preoperatively in neuraxial blocks under the spinal anesthesia and epidural analgesia also cause hemodynamic labaility. This is also discussed in Chap. 9. There could be major fluctuations in the blood pressure, particularly the sudden fall of it as seen in the spinal shock. It causes sympathetic blockade, and the pulse rate will also fluctuate. Any other form of sympathetic blockade like beta- blockers can also result in hemodynamic fluctuations. This may happen intraoperatively if the position of the patient is to be changed under anesthesia. Postoperatively this can be seen during initiation of positive pressure ventilation and, later, for reasons discussed above. A close monitoring is required. The most important single measure would be to meticulously maintain the intravascular volume. Respiratory arrest is also seen in patients with autonomic neuropathy.

3.7 Preoperative Evaluation

It can be distinctly divided into four parts.

1. In the initial clinical assessment, a clinical diagnosis, with a list of differential diagnosis must be made of the presenting condition outside diabetes which has created the plethora of abnormalities in the milieu. Today this is the most neglected part of an emergency room. The baseline clinical parameters like vital signs should be carefully recorded with a description where applicable. For example, pulse rate could be accompanied by adjectives like thready, week, or the type of breathing, or the sensorium. It will help to develop the clinical sense as one continues to watch the same signs in different and the same patient over days, frequently and over time to assess the improvements that happen. This has a bearing on the issue of fitness for surgery.
2. Second is the evaluation of the diabetic status per se.
3. Third is the evaluation of associated end-organ disease in a person with diabetes or significant hyperglycemia which includes the cardiac status, level of hypertension, the renal status, peripheral vascular disease, autonomic neuropathy, and ocular, skin, and foot disease in an urgent manner.
4. The fourth is to convey the details of the diagnosis and make a provisional prognostication for the relatives and the approximate time required for the next assessment to decide on the further course of action, including those which are being taken up immediately. Neglecting the last and not creating the documentation for it is at the root of all disputes, violent or litigious.

The first table below lists the preoperative evaluation—both clinical and laboratory parameters in brief. The second details the increased risks due to these factors.

Box 3.3 Preoperative Evaluation in Diabetes Clinical and Laboratory 1
Evaluation of diabetic status per se.
Evaluation of associated end-organ disease, viz.: peripheral vascular disease.
Noncardiac autonomic neuropathy.
Renal, GI, respiratory status.
Ocular, skin and foot disease if time permits or is directly relevant.

Box 3.4 Preoperative Evaluation in Diabetes Clinical and Laboratory 2
Cardiac status

- Atherosclerotic CAD.
- Cardiomyopathy.
- Previous infarction.
- Autonomic nervous system dysfunction.
- Hypertension.

Box 3.5 Cardiac Risk Factor Profile in Diabetes Preoperatively 1
Higher incidence and poor prognosis of CAD in diabetics.
Hypertension.
Prevalence 55% compared to 2–4% in nondiabetic population.
Atypical or "silent" MI—incidence is as high as 25%.
Dyspnea nausea and vomiting.
Confusion fatigue.

Box 3.6 Cardiac Risk Factor Profile in Diabetes Preoperatively 2
Increased risk of MI.

Cardiomyopathy—impairment of relaxation left ventricular wall, raised left ventricular end-diastolic pressure leading to increased risk of congestive heart failure.

Blunted cardiovascular responses to "stress" due to autonomic nervous system impairment and risk of "sudden unexplained death" due to dysrhythmias.

Preoperative laboratory evaluation in a patient with diabetes coming for emergency/elective major surgery is to be undertaken concomitantly as the clinical diagnosis is made. Clinical studies like autonomic neuropathy are done as applicable and possible within any surgical situation. In emergency surgery, it will be nearly impossible to carry them out, except fleetingly (see above). The following laboratory evaluations are necessary for complete assessment of all organ systems.

Hemoglobin is a baseline investigation. Anemia may result from renal insufficiency.

CBC: Leukocytosis would point towards infection (see also the discussion on DKA for the same).

3.7.1 Blood Glucose, Glycosylaed Hemoglobin A1c, S. Creatinine and Blood Urea Nitrogen

Blood Glucose, Glycosylaed Hemoglobin A1c, S. Creatinine and Blood Urea Nitrogen: Fasting and postprandial in elective and random glucose in emergency surgery. More extensive charting may be required in those patients who have poor preoperative control especially those who undergo cardiac surgery or those who are on steroids preoperatively as in neurosurgical patients with intracranial space-occupying lesions (SOLs).

Elevated levels of glycosylated Hb (HbA1C) certainly alert the team about poorer control in the past, higher levels, and likely increased number of complications, due to end-organ involvement and risk factors in any surgery. In emergency surgery, it has to left at that. It should not be a deterrent for taking the patient up for surgery. HBA1c is discussed at other places as well for different reasons.

S. creatinine and blood urea have their greatest value in assessing the severity of prerenal azotemia within the established end-stage kidney disease. Creatinine has a dose-related relationship with ACEI and ARB type of drugs and potassium. It is often forgotten that in lean emaciated individuals, the creatinine values may be low, but it does not mean that significant damage to the kidneys has not occurred. Hence, the spot samples of albumin creatinine ratios are important. This has incidentally eliminated the necessity of 24-h urinary excretion of albumin in urine.

3.7.2 S. Electrolytes

Abnormalities are expected in patients with history of vomiting, diarrhea, poor oral intake, tube feeding, intestinal obstruction, etc. aside from renal function and those on diuretics.

3.7.3 Preoperative EKG

It is an absolute must because of high prevalence of previous silent myocardial infarction in patients with diabetes.

3.7.4 2D Echocardiography

Today it is also a must where possible and is recommended even for minor surgical procedures because of the likely involvement of the cardiovascular system in diabetes. It may not be available in remote places where such patients may have to be treated if they cannot be shifted. It should then be considered as situational handicap.

It is a vital tool to reveal presence or absence of regional wall motion abnormalities (RWMAs) and assessment of LV ejection fraction, giving the anesthesiologist vital information regarding cardiac dysfunction. It assesses the status of the inferior vena cava (IVC) with regard to size, fullness, and compressibility which helps guide the anesthesiologist regarding fluid administration intraoperatively.

2D echocardiography is the only noninvasive way of diagnosing diabetic cardiomyopathy. Therefore, 2D echo is a vital and mandatory investigation for a diabetic both for routine and emergency surgery whether major or minor.

3.7.5 X-Ray Chest

Diabetes is an immunocompromised state. Compared to population without diabetes, patients with diabetes likely have tuberculosis four or more times. Tubercular lesions are many times atypical, in unusual locations and may not be cavitatory but proliferative. The routine preoperative detection of HIV AIDS assumes significance in presence of tuberculosis and vice versa. Presence of both in diabetes is a disaster. Patients with abdominal distension may have pneumonia secondary to basal atelectasis or aspiration. In abdominal emergencies, X-ray of the abdomen in standing position is still a valuable investigation for it reveals gas under the diaphragm and obstruction easily.

Most emergencies (except a few neurosurgical emergencies which could pose a real threat to life and may be in case of torrential traumatic bleeds) would allow at least some time for the detailed evaluation.

Today fortunately most of these investigations can be done quickly and at bedside. In places where the patient presents first where all facilities may not be available and there is a need to shift the patients, samples may be drawn, and as many investigations as possible before shifting (which gets delayed on many counts) can be undertaken. This is helpful to reduce time to start management at the referral center, even if the investigations may be repeated. It is equally necessary to send with the patient thus transferred the details of whatever little treatment that may have been done, e.g., insulin administration details or fluid infused. The significance of it has been discussed in the earlier chapters.

After the clinical and laboratory evaluation and the immediate corrective measures are undertaken, a provisional profile of the factors leading to high risk during the surgical intervention emerges. The documentation of this risk profile on the patient papers is a good practice to follow. It should list the abnormalities found and the consequences that may occur, for example, a denervated heart and its association with sudden death. Blood glucose estimation should be carried out immediately prior shifting and starting the anesthetic procedure. Biguanides, alpha glucosidase inhibitors, thiazolidinediones, sulfonylureas, and GLP-1 agonists should be discontinued.

3.8 Attitudes, Obstacles, and Barriers to Early Emergency Surgery in Diabetes

It should be obvious that in the emergency surgery setting, the managing team has but few hours to improve the condition of the patient to a level where surgery can be undertaken. It is in complete contrast with elective surgery where one has as many days as required to bring the patient under safe levels of parameters, minimizing the risk. Thus, it should be obvious as well that the parameter control level in emergency surgery will always be suboptimal.

This raises the most important issue about what could be still acceptable as the maximum/minimum level of parameters within the range of suboptimal levels to the surgeons and anesthetists against the physician's judgment. We will discuss below each parameter and attempt a consensus towards universal acceptance.

The common denominator to all the beliefs, attitudes, or dogmas that these three professionals are likely to be attached to in diabetes is the dominantly unreasonable apprehension about "glucose level." The few other parameters may be viewed as much less threatening. The fear originates in the fact that each considers that his/her risk perception should be addressed adequately. This is an incorrect attitude. The risk is shared by all of them with or without agreements. What is more important is to own the risk together, which is morally and ethically the right attitude but is beset with a few other barriers as well.

The first is to address the relatives together at least during the first encounter and explain all the risks involved in all the three departments and state that it is being shared by all and that they will cooperatively manage the care.

At this juncture, it should be made clear that hereafter one particular person will be the contact point for all the discussions the relatives may want to have. That what will be discussed by the interacting professional will be our common opinion and the relatives should not keep asking the same questions to each one of them should be made clear. The advantage of this arrangement is that the versions which are bound to differ in words, detail, emphasis, and inflections will not take place. The psyche of the relatives today is paranoiac and is exploitative. It results in the relatives trying to establish that all of them are not on the same page and are contradictory to each other. It leads to all kinds of unpleasant arguments and acrimony. This need not be elaborated further.

3.8.1 The Barriers

The first barrier in reaching agreements and joint ownership is the individual ego. Here is a situation not likely to be helped by such ego. The spirit of collaboration, spending time together at least once a day through the period of admission to safety of the postoperative stage is a must. This has been mentioned earlier in the first chapter as well, giving details about what to agree upon and carry on the management.

The second big barrier is the lack of basic minimum knowledge or a deliberately cultivated unwillingness to acquire that in the other two fields outside one's own specialization. Whether one likes it or not, the basic principles must be learnt. It can be effectively done in a few months of working together and spending some time on joint rounds. This will pave way to a much greater understanding where the serious fragmentation of care which is detrimental to the outcome will not only be avoided but a common action plan will evolve.

The third barrier is the lack of or the forgotten understanding of the normal physiology. The body has the capacity to self-correct itself. This understanding must grow in an approach to alter and facilitate fundamental abnormalities for the organs to recover under a benign care. Failure or unwillingness to cultivate these understandings reduces the burden on memory and serves the attitude of not to do so. It also leads to a tendency to simplify and generalize all possible complications or situations anticipated as occurring in each and every patient, a black or white assumption about everything. Medicine may be a science, but it is also an art, and art will always have gray areas. The more each one of the three specialists are able to appreciate these gray areas and learn to discuss them, the simpler will be the task, and the percentage outcome of success could scale new heights. The example of ketonuria discussed above will serve as an excellent example.

3.9 Issues Related to Various Parameter Levels Before Taking Up the Patient for Surgery

The best way is to resolve the differences over the recommended or perceived acceptable levels of parameters for taking a patient for emergency surgery. What is presented below in this regard has been evolved from our own experiences and supported by narrower studies. Some parts of the details are likely to be considered too sophisticated for many of our colleagues working in a much more disadvantageous situation. But, these parts are mentioned with emphasis, meaning thereby that wherever we are, we should create certain facilities and use them to improve patient care. We also believe that cost considerations of whether a patient will be able to pay or not should be put aside. A rational, pointedly optimal, minimal directed care embedded in critical clinical reasoning is the biggest and unfailing method to reduce/optimize costs. The costs may then not be as great as one may believe and will get recovered sooner than later even as it saves costs to the patients. We will also talk about costs, subsequently elsewhere in this volume.

3.9.1 Glucose

The fear of glucose is inordinate and transcends all other fears. It has its root in the fear of infection of the surgical site or the infection getting generalized. Does anyone enquire about the glucose level if a patient goes into respiratory arrest or is coning? Such patients are intubated without any questions. Then why so much objection to high glucose levels which can be anywhere from 200 mg onwards. We have not encountered studies or recommendations about the minimum/maximum cutoff levels of glucose that are acceptable to take a patient up for operation for the acute surgical conditions. Moreover the glucose has not been discussed in the total scenario of the clinical conditions; the trends during emergency treatment and making a projection on the changes which will take place if substantial corrections are done during surgery. The studies by their design are addressed to discrete objectives or end points to be analyzed. The recommendation the authors make to take the critically ill patient up for surgery is less than 250 mg/dL. However this is not an ironclad figure. Much higher glucose levels could also qualify for taking the patient up for surgery in different situations.

It may be quite difficult, but not always impossible, to achieve a blood glucose level of 250 or below in a few hours, as well as to improve the other parameters by administration of fluids, achieving electrolytes, acid base balance, and appropriate antibiotics to bring the infection under some preliminary restriction from either spreading or effectively localizing it. All measures in the short run act synergistically. Almost all surgical procedures can wait for these few hours.

3.9.2 Ketonuria

The correct understanding of ketonuria has already been discussed. Suffice it to say here that there are a few other, simpler criteria which if considered in patients, who have ketones are discussed below. That should take away the apprehension about ketones, and surgical intervention should go ahead.

3.9.3 Disadvantages of Cutoff Levels of Control as Recommended

Instead of looking at the parametric cutoff levels to be achieved absolutely, we recommend that they should be looked at *as a continuum towards normalization* even if they have not reached the recommended, normal or more correctly the physiological level. For example, if the blood glucose from 456 mg is brought down to 260 mg in 3 h, will we hold the 250 mg level as sacrosanct? Or if the pH from 7.19 has risen in 3 h to 7.29 will we hold on to the level of 7.3 and refuse taking up the patient? Both refusals only result in losing more time and an additional costly arterial blood gas analysis. Are we going to ignore the singular fact that taking these patients up for surgery in such situations also will rapidly lead to really normal levels of all the parameters in the few hours after surgery?

That is why we state that the parameters we discuss below should be viewed in the contexts of total milieu of the body. The aim of all the efforts to be undertaken described in such detail in the previous two chapters is to achieve a continuum where the clinical as well as biochemical parameters should start returning towards normal in a steady and continuous manner. Both should be considered together while making a decision to wheel the patient for surgery.

3.10 Monitoring Clinical Goals Towards Fitness for Surgery and Minimum Control Levels That Must Be Achieved Prior to Wheeling the Patient in for Surgery

3.10.1 Heart Rate

Barring those on pacemakers or with a denervated heart, most acutely ill patients will come with tachycardia. The initial heart rate at the time of beginning of hydration and other measures must be recorded and monitored in follow-up. As soon as substantial fluids are administered and insulin started, the heart rate would start decreasing progressively. An hourly record for a few hours will clearly indicate its indubitable progression towards normalization even if it is not completely normal. Appearance of de novo atrial extrasystoles and its disappearance seen on monitor indicate regaining the homeostatic levels.

3.10.2 Respiratory Function

If the respiratory function is described with respect to rate/minute, depth or shallowness, fruity odor, or frank Kussmaul's breathing as the management begins, it will give a clue to what we should be observing. Only some of the abnormalities occur in each patient. Any changes observed that indicate a trend or tendency towards normalization should give an element of added safety to the total picture to feel more confident to take the patient up for surgery. The rate should slow down and the depth should become more normal.

3.10.3 Cognitive Functions

Few patients with diabetes come in coma. Disorientation or drowsiness is more common, and changes for better can easily be detected which add to the safety for surgery. Alertness should improve; disorientation and irritability often seen in hyponatremia should lessen.

3.10.4 Pulse and Blood Pressure

If the modern medical professional cares to put his fingers on the pulse, he may find some age-old descriptions and terms like a thready or week pulse, improving to a strong beat and rising wall tension. These are indicators of a rapidly improving milieu which the cardiac monitors do not tell about. Careful recording of blood pressure frequently is helpful to avoid a patient going into a hypertensive stage if it was a condition already existing. It can then be treated pre- or intraoperatively.

3.10.5 Central Venous Pressure (CVP)

As the hydration proceeds apace, hourly CVP monitoring for just the first few hours indicates if it is rising. Rising trend indicates a return towards a near-normal state of hydration, even if not fully normal. In gross dehydration with or without shock, it is essential learning to see how rapidly CVP column in the manometer drops or gets sucked in the circulation, giving us a direct clue about the speed of rehydration that needs to be undertaken. The CVP of 8–10 cm of water should be aimed at. The two places where the rising CVP does not bode well are failure of the urine output to rise progressively indicating serious renal involvement or end- stage renal disease or a fluid overload resulting in heart failure. The CVP may be higher without reflecting adequate rehydration when the patient is on PEEP, i.e., positive end-expiratory ventilator support. Assessment of fluid status has been described in the preceding chapter in detail.

3.10.6 Urine Output

The hourly urine output is mandatory in managing these cases. After the retained urine is drained by the catheter, hourly urine output of 1 mL/min is reassuring. If it rises rapidly, if the concentrated color of the urine becomes diluted, it is the best guarantee to undertake aggressive fluid replacement, in the first few hours as mentioned earlier.

As discussed earlier in case of urine output not increasing despite proper hydration, no renal involvement, or signs of congestive heart failure, a clinical diagnosis of SIADH is made. It is confirmed by high urinary osmolarity, hyponatremia, and a normal creatinine. Appropriate steps should be taken then to normalize the milieu.

Preoperative considerations of clinical and biochemical parameters and the aim of all resuscitation are to reach the minimum safety of biochemical goals. In emergency critical situations, some of the important measures are described below.

3.10.7 Arterial Blood Gas Analysis (ABG)

Arterial blood gas analysis (ABG) is an important investigation in managing any acute or critical condition. It is a necessity to fine-tune the management of such conditions. Science has always progressed from approximations to precision. In the context of emergency surgery in diabetes, there are a number of ways in which clinical progress can be judged as detailed in this chapter and a few other places. Yet, a large majority of acute or critical cases with diabetes do not revolve only around destabilized metabolic parameters. They could get complicated by other effects of infections, many other concomitant disorders already present in the patient not just the renal or cardiovascular involvement, or coagulopathy or acute respiratory distress syndrome, to name just a couple.

Box 3.7 Clinical Goals
Consistent reduction in heart rate.
Pulse Characteristics.
Respiratory rate improves towards stabilization.
Alertness improve.
Steadily rising CVP.
Increasing urine output.

Box 3.8 Biochemical Goals
"Acceptable" levels of control.
Biochemical goals:
pH should be >= 7.3.
HCO_3^- should be >15 meq/L.
Blood glucose <250 mg%.
Adequate K^+ infusion (up to 20–40 meq K^+/h) with tendency to eupotassemia.

Once the basic management is initiated and the spectrum of abnormalities starts coming under control, finer assessment of the milieu interior is required. The changes are partly due to the natural progression towards recovery and partly as unintended effects of energetic treatment, for example, metabolic alkalosis, which is a serious complication. In such cases, ABG is of great help. The clinicians should have the capacity to interpret it correctly.

Is the facility of ABG a must? The answer is yes, for places which have got good infrastructural facilities and which routinely manage such critical cases. In places where a patient arrives in a seriously destabilized state where primary resuscitation is all that can be done, ABG is not a must, unless such units handle such cases all the time. The reasons are simple and not far to look for. As mentioned above, the criteria to manage criticality are simple and continue to be useful as they were before ABG and after ABG availability. One may however be inclined to add that today among the basic laboratory investigations, electrolyte estimation be considered mandatory and utilized frequently even in peripheral units described above.

Arterial blood gas analysis readily gives many a parameter status, some of which are indicative but not accurate. Arterial blood pH within the normal is a fundamental requirement of life, like normal plasma volume, osmolarity, or respiratory exchange of oxygen and carbon dioxide. A single sample of ABG will give us tremendous information about these components. It gives the pH, concentration of PCO_2, PO_2, and HCO_3, i.e., bicarbonates, electrolytes, hemoglobin, and calcium as well. The last two are indicative but not as accurate as the others. The human body is remarkably adaptive to survive even in the worst state of homeostasis. In the modern era, the greater precision one offers the better are the chances of survival. Individual life is the single most sacred factor today.

In critically ill patients, the first arterial blood gas may be done after a few hours of treatment after identifying all the other metabolic and systemic complications. Doing it at the beginning adds to costs. What it shows in more precise quantitative terms is already known from the grosser evaluation. It is better to judge the progress clinically rather than doing ABG frequently. Its real indications for more frequent estimations are an unstable patient in spite of all the effort or in case of mixed pictures of acidosis where one would like to get to know which components are varying and in which direction or in very long surgeries.

Blood pH remains in the narrow range of 7.35–7.45. Any increase in it is called alkalosis, and decrease is called acidosis. Three body processes maintain the pH. The exchange of CO_2 with oxygen in the lungs removes CO_2. If it is retained, it dissolves in the plasma water giving rise to H_2CO_3 or carbonic acid anions which make the blood pH acidic. This is called respiratory acidosis. Any pathology in the lungs significant enough to lower the gas exchange will result in this condition. To name few commonly met with are the extreme bronchoconstriction in asthma and acute respiratory distress syndrome with large-scale inflammatory changes at the alveolar level, pneumothorax on one side and diseased lung in the other. This is also called hypercapnia revealed in blood gas analysis as PCO_2 of 55–90 mmHg compared to the normal of 45 mmHg. The PO_2 in these cases will plummet to low levels of anywhere near 60 or less against the normal of 95–100 mmHg.

In metabolic acidosis like diabetes or uremia, accumulation of acidic molecules lowers the pH. In pure metabolic acidosis, typically there is an attempt to combat it by increasing the respiratory drive that results in considerable lowering of CO_2, thereby reducing the possibility of the carbonic acid formation. This may compensate but does not fully correct the acidosis. Hypotension due to dehydration and insulin deficiency as in DKA reduces the perfusion pressure of the tissues resulting in hypoxia which leads to incomplete combustion of pyruvates causing and aiding the development of acidosis by forming lactates. The PO_2 remains high.

Once the reperfusion of tissues under adequate pressure as a result of aggressive rehydration is initiated with insulin administration, the lactates get converted back to pyruvates and enter the Kreb's cycle to get fully combusted in aerobic oxidation creating ATPs for energy. The renal tissues then create bicarbonates from carbonic acid which is alkaline in nature to further combat the acidosis. Now the meaning of the criteria for taking up a patient with relatively much higher safety will be easily understood. A pH increased from a previous low of 7.1 or 7.2 to 7.29 (even if it does not reach the criterion of 7.3) indicates that further restoration of milieu will now be facilitated by surgery. Similarly if bicarbonate level, low on admission, increases substantially to a value approaching 15 will indicate that surgery can be undertaken.

In mixed pictures of respiratory and metabolic acidosis, an ABG sample is likely to reveal a lowered pH, hypercapnia and hypoxia, and lowered bicarbonates at the beginning. If a blood gas analysis is done after substantial efforts to combat both conditions, it may not be able to give an indication about the contribution of each acidotic component to the total picture. That is a judgment which the clinician has to arrive at (e.g., which one is on the decrease or increase or resolving, etc.) by using the array of investigational information he will have collected by then.

Metabolic alkalosis is mostly caused by liver disease, excessive diuretic use, or overfeeding of the patients and could be dangerous. Administration of normal saline and withdrawal of all offending causes is the treatment. Respiratory alkalosis could be caused by overenthusiastic ventilation which washes out CO_2 to a great degree. There could be an increase in bicarbonate levels.

Once other parameters start improving rapidly, an arterial blood gas analysis goes a long way to decide the safety. If the pH rises to 7.3 or more, the safety to take the patient up for surgery increases. In such situations, the bicarbonate levels will also generally rise. Any bicarbonate level equal to or above 15 meq can be considered as another safety indicator to undertake surgery. Improvement in the blood pressure, resulting in higher perfusion pressure at the tissue level and adequate PO_2 as seen on the blood gas analysis, will correct lactic acidosis rapidly, and the bicarbonates will rise.

Where ABG analysis is not possible, one may have to rely on ketonuria and hope that reducing ketonuria should indicate a possibility of reduction of level of acidosis. This will have to be supported by a continuously improving clinical betterment of patient. However, this is not fully reliable. In centers where ABG facility is not available and if the improvement on other parameters is not as expected should be referred to a higher center after the initial resuscitation the patients.

ABG becomes mandatory in case of mixed acid-base disturbances (viz., respiratory and metabolic) where it is not be possible to discriminate and decide about the contribution, severity, and significance of each without ABG. In major surgery, such situations do arise.

3.10.8 Potassium

To maintain near-normal potassium level, it is mandatory to add 10 or 20 or 40 mmol of potassium with every infusion with glucose or saline. The ideal level to maintain is 4 meq/L. In an acute decompensated surgical condition even in mild forms of attendant DKA, the total body potassium requirement should be considered to be as high as in any DKA, i.e., −210 to 350 meq. To replace, it will require 20–40 meq/h over 3–6 h for immediate replacement. The immediate goal is not necessarily to achieve eupotassemia but to continuously infuse adequate potassium so that the intracellular potassium content continues to improve.

The subsequent management of such patients presenting with acute emergency surgical issues, i.e., the intra- and postoperative management, are discussed in Chap. 4 of this volume.

References

1. Umpierrez GE, Isaacs SD, Bazargan H, et al. Hyperglycemia: an independent marker of in-hospital mortality in patients with undiagnosed diabetes. J Clin Endocrinol Metab. 2002;87:978–82.
2. Gill G, Benbow S. Managing surgery in the elderly diabetic patient. In: Sinclair AJ, Finucane P, editors. Diabetes in old age. 2nd ed. Chichester: Wiley; 2000. p. 177–85.
3. Capes SE, Hunt D, Malmberg K, et al. Stress hyperglycemia and prognosis of stroke in non-diabetic and diabetic patients: a systematic overview. Stroke. 2001;32:2426–32.
4. Van den Berghe G, Wouters P, Weekers F, Verwaest C, Bruyninckx F, Schetz M, Vlasselaers D, Ferdinande P, Lauwers P, Bouillon R. Intensive insulin therapy in critically ill patients. N Engl J Med. 2001;345:1359–67.
5. Van den Berghe GH. Role of intravenous insulin therapy in critically ill patients. Endocr Pract. 2004;10(Suppl. 2):17–20.
6. Van den Berghe G, Wilmer A, Hermans G, et al. Intensive insulin therapy in the medical ICU. N Engl J Med. 2006;354:449–61.
7. Van den Berghe G, Wilmer A, Milants I, et al. Intensive insulin therapy in mixed medical/surgical intensive care units: benefit versus harm. Diabetes. 2006;55:3151–9.
8. Egi M, Bellomo R, Stachowski E, et al. Blood glucose concentration and outcome of critical illness: the impact of diabetes. Crit Care Med. 2008;36:2249–55.
9. Kelkar SK. Analysis of a series of 77 diabetic and 77 non diabetic ischemic strokes; Poster Presented in Novo Nordisk Update, Kolkata, 1998.
10. Lauruschkat AH, Arnrich B, Albert AA, et al. Prevalence and risks of undiagnosed diabetes mellitus in patients undergoing coronary artery bypass grafting. Circulation. 2005;112:2397–402.
11. Joslin PI. Joslin's textbook of diabetes mellitus. 14th Special Indian ed. Philadelphia, PA: Lippincott, Williams and Wilkins; 2005.
12. Bordun K-AM, Jassal DS. Metabolic alterations in diabetic cardiomyopathy. New York, NY: Springer; 2014.
13. Kelkar SK. Cerebrovascular circulation in patients with or without diabetes and ischemic strokes, a series of 144 cases presented as poster in Novo Nordisk update 1999, Kolkata.

Additional Reading

Preoperative testing and medication management by the OHIO State University Wexner Medical Center.

Intra- and Postoperative Management in Diabetes

4

Contents

S. Kelkar et al., *Towards Optimal Management of Diabetes in Surgery*,
https://doi.org/10.1007/978-981-13-7705-1_4

4.1 Preamble

These two stages have been separated from all the earlier chapters for ease of description and understanding. It will cover the intra- and postoperative management not only in emergency major surgeries but also day care surgeries or procedures which may last for more than 2–4 h in diabetes till the discharge of a patient and subsequent follow-up for a reasonable time. The next three chapters will deal with other operational aspects of routine surgery, followed by the special situations in surgery in diabetes in two parts. We did not want to divert the attention in the control of blood glucose and accompanying parameters which are the most important aspects of making a patient as fit for surgery as can be. Now we will look at other monitoring aspects more from a clinical perspective in the intra- and postoperative management.

Intra- and postoperative management in emergency as well as other surgical situations falls into two categories: the anesthesia management with particular reference to people with diabetes and the attempts at further normalization of all the parameters mentioned above which went in, in deciding the patient to be taken up for surgery. This chapter discusses issues related to general anesthesia in all emergency surgeries, major procedures lasting for more than 4 h, and all elective surgeries that require general anesthesia.

4.2 Few Specific Issues with General Anesthesia

Anesthetic drugs in the era gone by were sympathomimetic hence could disturb the hemodynamics causing higher risks. The newer anesthetics are metabolically and hemodynamically much safer. A patient well under anesthesia is actually in a much less stressful state, without pain leading to reduced catecholamines and insulin resistance, which facilitates glucose level reduction. However under intubated conditions under general anesthesia, the blood glucose can still rise to about 200 mg/dL as discussed earlier. In either case there are other risks that continue. Difficult intubation is discussed earlier. Sudden substantial rise of systolic blood pressure in both hypertensive and nonhypertensive persons may result in postponing surgery for hours or a day. Anesthetic management should take care of these as well as the other risk factors in dealing with any major surgery [1].

4.3 Intraoperative Management: Broad Principles

The patient with diabetes needs insulin to counter hyperglycemia due to surgical "stress." The insulin to be used is rapid-acting human insulin. Frequent glucose monitoring intraoperatively has *no, repeat no, substitute* for the maintenance of glucose within the desired range under anesthesia.

4.3.1 Intraoperative Glycemic Management

There is no consensus target range that currently exists. In general the literature suggests as optimal to keep blood glucose level between 150 and 200 mg/dL (8 and 11 mmol/L) during surgery [2, 3]. Intraoperative hyperglycemia (glucose greater than 200 mg/dL) as well as relative normoglycemia (glucose less than 140 mg/dL) was found to be associated with significant morbidity and mortality. Glucose levels ranging from 140 to 170 mg/dL had the lowest risk of adverse outcomes [4]. During surgery, glycemic levels can be sufficiently monitored by utilizing blood glucose measurement systems designed for inpatient bedside use [3, 4].

Additionally, anesthetists must take the approximate length of time required to complete a procedure into consideration when determining an intraoperative glycemic control strategy. For short, minor procedures, preoperative glucose maintenance protocols may still be employed. For more complex procedures, variable rate IV insulin infusion has been highlighted as a more effective method for achieving glycemic control [5].

4.4 The Principles of Anesthesia Management in Patients Having Diabetes

4.4.1 Timing

Patients with diabetes should be placed first on the operating list. This shortens their preoperative fast and the risk of hypoglycemia and ketosis. A couple of matters should however be considered in this regard.

4.4.2 Fasting

Patients having type 1 diabetes are more prone to diabetic gastroparesis, to the tune of 50%. It causes delay in gastric emptying after the night meal. Undiagnosed gastroparesis either due to absence of or not reporting of the symptoms or ignoring this information is not uncommon. It may increase the risk of regurgitation and aspiration. Some studies have shown beneficial effects of preoperative oral erythromycin on gastric motility. However, other motility stimulants have not been shown to be effective. Metoclopramide is still used routinely and is fairly effective. A 12-h fast may be beneficial in patients with diabetes before surgery in this condition, proven or suspected. These patients should be tested for hypoglycemia preoperatively, discussed later.

4.4.3 IV Fluids

Lactate in Ringer's lactate undergoes gluconeogenesis in the liver and may complicate blood glucose control when given in large volumes. Ringer's lactate is discussed in much more detail in Chap. 2 on perioperative diabetic emergencies. Normal saline infusions if large volumes have to be used to correct dehydration may be safer. There is no ideal solution, and either solution may be used judiciously.

4.4.4 Monitoring

Under anesthesia the blood glucose levels and insulin requirements are somewhat unpredictable. Both hyper- and hypoglycemia may go undetected. The only safeguard is judicious blood glucose measurement intraoperatively. The best way is to use reliable rapid assay meter which gives accurate results.

4.4.5 Standard Monitoring During Anesthesia

ECG, percentage saturation of oxygen (SpO) blood pressure, end-tidal carbon dioxide (ETCO), and temperature monitoring should be instituted. Advanced monitoring is guided by the seriousness of the comorbidities present. It is discussed in detail in the Chap. 2.

Glycosylated hemoglobin (HbA1c) measurement is considered too important to be ignored by the surgeons and anesthetists. Without doubt it is a valuable guide to long-term glycemic control with or without operative situations. However it has *no particular significance* during preoperative evaluation or in the intra- or postoperative period, especially in emergency surgery. Even in routine surgery which needs to be undertaken in weeks more important is the good control of blood glucose level (see more about it in Chap. 6).

4.4.6 Glucose Control

The desirable control levels of blood glucose today are narrow as mentioned above. Any glucose level beyond that will influence adversely the postoperative wound healing and possibility of infection is higher. "Permissive hyperglycemia" which is a term used earlier indicates higher levels of blood glucose mainly due to the concern of hypoglycemia developing intraoperatively. It is not justifiable in current practice. The rapid assay meters widely available today are quite accurate and give results within seconds and easy on technique, and tests can be repeated many times. This is of help in keeping the glucose control in a narrow range intraoperatively without hypoglycemia.

4.4.7 Glucose Supplementation

Longer-acting insulin preparations are more likely to cause hypoglycemia. This can be avoided by glucose administration under judicious monitoring. In major surgeries, it is better to delete the long-acting insulin the night before to avoid inadvertent hypoglycemia. Institution of safeguards against excessive catabolism by the use of regular/analogue short-acting insulin is strongly recommended. Starvation ketosis should be avoided by long fasting. Perioperative situation is catabolic. The energy supplementation should be higher. Administration of glucose with insulin intraoperatively followed by the relief from the surgical condition will then lead to enhanced quantity of glucose utilization postoperatively and meet the energy requirements also. This is emphasized in many chapters in this volume.

4.4.8 Insulin Supplementation

It is essential to prevent lipolysis and proteolysis with resultant ketosis in patients with absolute/relative insulin deficiency with infection perioperatively. It can be done only by adequate insulin administration intraoperatively, under anesthesia. It will reverse these adverse effects which cause suppression of insulin secretion.

4.5 Anesthesia

There are a number of anesthetic drugs, each of which has a variable effect on glycemic control. The effect on blood glucose is minimal in case of most intravenous (IV) induction agents routinely used.

4.5.1 Induction

The major determinants for anesthetic consideration are severity of coronary artery disease, nephropathy, hypertension, and autonomic neuropathy. A careful induction with etomidate or high-dose fentanyl (4–5 μg/kg) with midazolam and/or thiopentone should be performed. There may be an exaggerated hypotension due to autonomic neuropathy which is common. A rapid sequence induction should be performed for patients with GI symptoms. Awake fiber-optic bronchoscopy would be a preferred technique for an anticipated difficult airway.

Succinylcholine should be avoided in patients with extensive peripheral neuropathy due to risk of increased potassium release. Atracurium and mivacurium are preferred in the presence of renal dysfunction. Rocuronium may be used in rapid sequence induction.

Maintenance of anesthesia is with isoflurane or sevoflurane in an air oxygen mixture. The normal insulin production is in response to glucose administration. It is dependent on the quantum of glucose infused and rises as more glucose is given. Volatile anesthetics like isoflurane and halothane inhibit insulin production leading to a hyperglycemic response [6, 7]. This has been observed however in in vitro studies. There is no certainty about this effect in clinical situations.

Nitrous oxide may be used, though it should be avoided in intestinal obstruction due to bowel distention. Patients with perforative peritonitis and sepsis should be ventilated postoperatively to optimize their oxygen delivery. Bowel distention and a tense abdominal closure also make postoperative ventilation desirable. Airway pressures after abdominal closure should be observed to decide about the mode of postoperative ventilation. Less severe cases can be "reversed" and extubated at the end of surgery. The patient should have adequate recovery of airway reflexes prior to extubation.

Etomidate is known to cause less hypotension during induction and generally fewer hangover-like effects upon recovery. Acute adrenocortical insufficiency and crisis may occur after a standard induction dose of etomidate [8]. However, due to diminished cortisol secretion, etomidate triggers a subsequent decrease in the hyperglycemic response to surgery [9]. Review of the etomidate mechanism shows suppressed adrenocortical function mediated by blocking the activity of 11-beta-hydroxylase, ultimately causing decreased steroidogenesis [10].

The sympathetic nervous system output is inhibited by the use of high doses of opiates in postoperative period of recovery. The hypothalamic-pituitary axis also is similarly inhibited. The sympathetic outflow is reduced which in turn decreases the hyperglycemic response to surgery. Anesthetic techniques that use high-dose produce hemodynamic changes for similar reasons [11].

Epidural anesthesia inhibits catecholamine release. The level of the spinal segment to which it acts has no effect on that. As a result noradrenalin and cortisol concentrations do not increase. Epidural anesthesia tends to have a nominal effect on glucose metabolism [12].

Epidural analgesia may be instituted after due consideration to autonomic neuropathy, IHD, and peripheral neuropathy. It should be avoided in sick patients with sepsis. Epidural analgesia may help to attenuate neurohormonal response to stress and may decrease the need for systemic nonsteroidal analgesic/anti-inflammatory drugs and opioids which may have serious side effects in a patient with diabetes.

4.5.2 Anesthetic Drugs and Blood Glucose Control, Induction Agents, and Glycemic Excursions

Ketamine may cause significant hyperglycemia. Cortisol synthesis decreases in etomidate administration as it blocks adrenal steroidogenesis. The decrease in the hyperglycemic response to surgery in patients without diabetes is approximately 18 mg/dL. In patients with diabetes, this effect is not established. Similarly the effect on insulin secretion in administration of propofol is not known. Patients with diabetes show a reduced ability to clear lipids from the circulation. It should be taken into account when prolonged sedation is to be given in the intensive care unit with propofol as it may cause hyperlipidemia.

Benzodiazepine and midazolam are often added in high doses during surgery. Benzodiazepines decrease ACTH secretion and reduce sympathetic stimulation. Both the effects will decrease the hyperglycemic response. Benzodiazepines stimulate release of growth hormone release which may increase the glucose level [13]. If midazolam is given in normal sedative doses, these effects are marginal. However, midazolam and fentanyl may cause hyperglycemia by reducing glucose clearance.

Box 4.1 Choosing Anesthetics in Systemic Diseases Accompanying Diabetes

Assessment of the severity of systemic diseases, like CAD, nephropathy (DN), hypertension, and autonomic and peripheral neuropathy (DAN and DPN) needed to choose agent and manner of anesthesia in diabetes.

Epidural—avoided in sepsis, in presence of DAN and DPN, IHD.

Succinylcholine avoided in extensive peripheral neuropathy.

Nitrous oxide avoided in intestinal obstruction.

Ganglion-blocking agents—caution against hypoglycemia with frequent monitoring.

Beta-blockers delay recovery from hypoglycemia.

High-dose opiate anesthesia produce hemodynamic, hormonal, and metabolic stability.

Box 4.2 Metabolic Effects of Anesthesia

Less important than the surgical procedure.

Ketamine—may elevate glucose.

Etomidate reduces hyperglycemic response.

Halothane, enflurane, isoflurane, and sevoflurane effect on insulin secretion in clinical practice—not known.

Prolonged propofol use for sedation in diabetes with caution due to reduced lipid clearance.

Benzodiazepine in high doses reduce the glycemic response to surgery Midazolam is safer.

Midazolam and fentanyl may cause hyperglycemia.

Ether and especially cyclopropane induce greater metabolic changes as compared to halothane and enflurane.

Spinal and/or epidural anesthesia causes least metabolic disturbances.

The liver is known to have a sympathetic-mediated mechanism for hepatic neoglucogenesis which is hypothalamic in origin. It is in addition to the glucagon response. Ganglion-blocking agents previously used for hypotensive anesthesia may block this glucose output leading to hypoglycemia. The sympathetic outflow reduced similarly by beta-blockers will lead to delayed recovery from a hypoglycemic episode.

4.5.3 Further Normalization of All the Parameters During Anesthesia

In short the preoperative management of both glucose and the other parameters continues to apply the same methods extensively dealt with in the first two chapters. On completion of surgery, the same management methods continue on a modified scale if necessary in the postoperative period till the patient can start taking adequate nutrition orally. Additional relevant remarks are placed below as broad principles of intraoperative management in emergency surgery.

4.6 Intraoperative Management of Glucose Control

This issue revolves around the minimum or maximum permissible levels of glycemia to be maintained during intraoperative period. The method of choice, needless to say, is by continuous intravenous insulin with human crystalline insulin. The same can be achieved by using rapid-acting insulin preparation of aspart or lispro with the same efficiency, but it unnecessarily adds to the costs. The net effect on blood glucose can be best managed by glucose monitoring and adjusting the rate of continuous intravenous insulin. Thus, a preoperative and post-intubation blood glucose level becomes a matter of necessity.

4.6.1 Intraoperative Target Blood Glucose

Over the optimal blood glucose range or level intraoperatively, there is lack of general agreement. The issue has been dealt with teleological ways by taking into consideration the mortality and morbidity statistics under different series or trials. The literature suggests the range of glucose level as 150–200 mg/dL (8–11 mmol/L) during surgery. Intraoperative hyperglycemia (glucose greater than 200 mg/dL) as well as relative normoglycemia (glucose less than 140 mg/dL) was found to be associated with significant morbidity and mortality. Glucose levels ranging from 140 to 170 mg/dL had the lowest risk of adverse outcomes [4]. Many studies have attempted to decide the optimal level of intraoperative blood glucose level. The consensus from all of these studies is a level between 150 to 200 mg/dL. However, the authors would suggest a slightly lower level of 180 mg as a buffer against the blood glucose accidentally shooting beyond 200 mg since there is evidence to suggest that blood glucose above 198 mg/dL results in greater mortality.

One may note in this connection that the critical blood glucose level above which the neutrophil functions get affected has been lowered by the Australian Diabetic

Society (ADS), 2012, to 198 mg/dL, instead of the earlier figure of 250 mg and above accepted by the fraternity [14]. This may also contribute to mortality. During surgery, glycemic levels can be sufficiently monitored by utilizing blood glucose measurement systems designed for inpatient bedside use [2, 3]. In patients with type 1 diabetes, the insulin infusion rate begins at roughly 0.5–1 U/h, whereas infusion rates are typically increased in type 2 diabetics to approximately 2–3 U/h or higher [15].

4.6.2 A Word About Tight Glucose Control

Tight glucose control refers to the maintenance of blood glucose within a narrow range of 80–110 mg/dL [16]. This was advocated more rigorously for postoperative ICU glucose controls consequent to the finding of much improved outcomes with regard to ICU stay, postoperatively, infective complications, and lesser number of ventilator days especially in cardiac surgical setups. However, this has not been substantiated for all subgroups of surgical patients. In addition, there is a real risk of hypoglycemia with consequent neurologically detrimental outcomes. Hence, the general consensus for intraoperative as well as postoperative blood glucose level appears to be to maintain levels around a broad range of 108–180 mg/dL certainly not above 200 mg/dL or below 80 mg/dL.

4.7 Intraoperative Fluid Management

Intraoperative fluid administration depends entirely on fluid losses incurred preoperatively, detailed extensively earlier, and intraoperatively. Active fluid loss and blood loss are replaced according to standard anesthetic guidelines and hence are the same as for any patient undergoing surgery whether diabetic or nondiabetic. The type of fluid used for these losses would usually be the replacement type of fluid (i.e., without glucose) and blood as required. In a person with diabetes, these operative losses are likely to be much higher due to the osmotic diuresis which may have occurred earlier.

4.7.1 Management of Hypovolemia

This is the second crucial factor in the intraoperative period. The continued fluid losses due to hyperglycemia and osmotic diuresis however may have reduced by the time the patient is taken up for surgery. But the fluid loss during the corrective surgery in itself could be massive, and the anesthetist should be trained to estimate the same approximately and replace them with nonglucose-containing fluids and other fluids like packed red cells or blood components or plasma expanders as may be necessary. The replacement is easily guided by the central venous pressure which should be maintained. In the intraoperative setting in bowel surgery, for example, the volume losses could be as high as 10–15 mL/kg/h. The balanced salt solutions with multiple crystalloid additions which almost always contain glucose are hypertonic which is disadvantageous at least in the early stages of rehydration and glucose control for reasons mentioned earlier. However they are useful for specific compartmental losses if they are replaced for glucose saline with fixed rate infusions as has been repeatedly exhorted in these pages. Having glucose in them is helpful in supplying calories under insulin administration.

4.7.2 Evaluation of Fluid Losses and Guide for Replacement

A common clinical experience, about volume management, is a fixation to 2.5 L of IV in 24 h. We do not know from where this fixation has arisen, but we submit that the needs for volume replacement in a hot country like India with additional losses due to the acute conditions and intervention are much higher; with diabetes the losses are even higher in magnitude. It is in our experience rare to see notes describing the status of dehydration, presence of thirst, and oliguria with appropriate increase in the nonglucose IV fluid quanta. Hence the proper action is to judge the adequacy of rehydration by clinical decision-making and other more refined ways than by the above volume fixation[1].

4.7.3 Correction of Acidosis

It should not be a major issue since the patient is likely to have reached the recommended pH of 7.3. As the surgery proceeds and the offending conditions are rectified, further optimization would or is likely to follow as a natural consequence, rapidly. Correction of acidosis could be guided by ABG estimations only if necessary. In all cases of diabetic ketoacidosis in acute or critical medical or surgical situations, correction of acidosis by using bicarbonates is completely contraindicated. If a patient presents with a pH of 6.9 or less and if the immediate aggressive correction of dehydration and insulin infusion does not start improving pH beyond 7, then bicarbonates may be used discretely. What it means is that they be administered in small doses well diluted in a drip over many minutes for it to be taken up by the tissues as the blood circulates. The bicarbonates will by and by push the pH of blood up. By allowing the tissues to take it up the source of acidosis is being contained which is a much more fundamental way of correcting acidosis in a steadier and longer lasting manner. Bicarbonate solutions are highly hypertonic. Even the intravenous solutions of crystalloids which are hypertonic are not preferred in the initial resuscitation so will the bicarbonates not preferred as boluses.[2]

---

[1] Like poor efforts at hydration are the minimalist calorie supplements which do not meet the requirements to prevent catabolism. This has been discussed elsewhere much in detail.

[2] Severely infected diabetic foot or a large carbuncle could bring the patient a full-blown acidotic state where neither blood glucose control nor the acidosis looks amenable for control even after hours of struggle to reach the "safe" criteria described in this volume; the outcome would be refusal for surgery. In cases of such suboptimal control, it is desirable, and an act of commission would be to deliberately undertake to operate on such causes under regional anesthesia. This will save lives since these procedures can be completed in short periods of time. Otherwise patients will surely be lost. Secondly, these and some other situations, there cannot be any control since the cause of surgical condition is so powerfully responsible that unless that is removed even under suboptimal conditions, life and often the limb cannot be saved. See the chapter on regional anesthesia in this volume. There will be cases where they will have to be taken up under general anesthesia.

4.7.4 Management of Electrolyte Disturbance

Mainly it is the potassium, and repeated monitoring may be necessary as extensive surgical dissections with long operative periods are associated with potassium release into the circulation.

Even in the intraoperative period in surgery with diabetes, separate intravenous infusions for rehydrating fluids, IV medications, PRBCs, plasma rich with platelets, fresh frozen plasma, and such others must be maintained. Steady-rate glucose-insulin infusions should be used by a separate IV line. The glycemic, metabolic, and hemodynamic management becomes progressively easier as the surgery proceeds and the precipitating cause is taken care of. Insulin requirements may suddenly crash in the postoperative period anywhere within 6–12 h.

4.8 Elective Major Surgery or Procedures Lasting Over 4 h

Intraoperatively, the general guidelines for management remain the same as for any "major" emergency surgery. We recommend the use of insulin infusions as the method of choice for glucose control intraoperatively. A syringe pump is not always necessary but recommended and may become mandatory in special situations even if the surgery is elective, where severe glucose fluctuations would be encountered as discussed in a later chapter. For more details see Chap. 6 on Management of Routine Surgery in Diabetes.

4.9 Postoperative Period and the Residents

During the intraoperative period, a patient is in a much more controlled situation, and much of the monitoring is being done by the anesthesiologists. When the patient is wheeled into the ICU or wards, maintaining euglycemia becomes the responsibility of the surgical resident, for which he is generally ill-equipped. Such a patient will have a blood glucose reading done in the immediate postoperative period, if extubated, and a corresponding insulin infusion would be running with a fair to good control of blood glucose. When the postsurgical state is also stable and on road to recovery, the surgical medical resident team should be able to perform better to maintain euglycemia while maintaining other parameters well under control. For them (as well as the consultants to facilitate this process), we are giving below a number of perspectives that change after the surgery.

4.10 For the Sake of Basic Agreements in Postoperative Periods

In the chapters on the role of residents in glucose control, perioperative diabetes emergencies, and emergency surgery in diabetes, we have emphasized on the three major caregiver consultants to work in coordination and in tandem so that certain minimum agreements on fluids, electrolytes, acid-base balance, and ancillary therapeutic measures are reached. We have also explained the reasons behind the necessities in concrete medical situations that are bound to arise if such agreements are not reached. This requirement cannot be adequately emphasized.

The action that will help the residents most in practical management is sending clear-cut instructions on some immediate actions to be undertaken in the ICU or wards for the next few hours. Sent along with the patient, it gives the anesthetist and the surgeon some time before revisiting the patient in ICU or the surgical ward. This visit is useful for planning in more detail and more accurately. On both occasions the therapeutic strategy should preferably be discussed by the surgeons and the anesthetists jointly. The most important would be about the type and the rate of rehydration intravenous fluids to be administered over the next few hours among other things before the patient is again attended by the surgeon and the anesthetists. This and the varying rate of insulin infusions is the most complex of the treatment dynamics which varies from hour to hour.

Whether one likes it or not and what the ego state says, the greater such collaboration between these two and later in the day with the attending physician, the easier is the management and better the outcomes. Joint decisions taken for the next 12–24 h will lessen the burdens and useless irritating communications mid-work and late nights. For this to be achieved, some time must be spent with the residents and nurses if not so much with the patient by all of them.

What we mean by that is that the rationale behind the orders issued if explained to the residents and nurses, the management will become so much more intelligent and learning will happen. The plea that these residents are going to be there for an unpredictable short interval will not understand the rationale, cannot be taught or is the stupid lot that has come to us, and is untenable on every count. At every stage teaching must happen, predominantly at the bedside. Since it is not happening anywhere, every setup which treats complicated cases gets the same lot they describe as stupid.

Emergencies, having no time for all this, and tiredness are the stock excuses which are also untenable since these works do not take as much time as may be thought. It is unwillingness or reluctance. Over just a couple of months of this approach, the time needed actually will get limited to a new situation which has not been experienced by the residents and nurses before. The dividends over the effort are enormously high. Sitting on the fences of ego, not relating to each other, results only in borderline situations for patients. The areas of agreement are few. In determining them, the measures taken so far, the intraoperative losses and particular events during the operations, must be the context in which these are considered. These are the optimal levels of hydration to be achieved in the next 12/24 h, for the patient, the other being rate of calories fixed for the patient.

To state the obvious again, no rehydrating fluids should have dextrose. It is a general and well-accepted dictum that in the initial stages of such patients' rehydration is the single most important measure which facilitates the subsequent actions of blood glucose lowering and improves clinical condition. The fluid may have to be administered at the rate of 200–1000 mL/h depending upon the surgical situation and state of hydration before taking up the patient for surgery. Therefore, dextrose at such rates is certainly uncalled for even if backed by high insulin concentration, which to say the least, will never lead to smooth blood glucose control, is most difficult to obtain in the rush especially in acute surgical losses, and hence must be avoided.

The next agreement should be about the total calorie requirement over 12-/24-h period and its uniform spacing as discussed earlier. Unless usable calories are supplied, the hypercatabolic state will continue and worsen. Similar agreements have to be reached if and when a decision on total parenteral nutrition (TPN) is taken. The details of TPN and related issues have been separately discussed under "Commonly Asked Questions" in the last chapter. Agreement on electrolyte management should also be reached.

4.10.1 Postoperative Insulin Management and Transition to Subcutaneous Insulin

The intraoperative IV insulin infusion may now become either excessive or inadequate. Since the offending cause for which surgery is undertaken is removed, there could be a significant drop in the insulin infusion needs. On the other hand, the pain of incision and wakeful state may actually demand greater IV insulin administration. In the immediate postoperative period, one has to continue IV insulin alongside a dextrose infusion until the patient can tolerate food without difficulty. This management in all its nuances has been described in detail earlier.

Initially the patient is given test feeds, and the quantities are increased as may be seen fit. The subcutaneous insulin may then be started once the intake stabilizes. Subcutaneous insulin has a disadvantage—it cannot be retracted or reduced in case of hypoglycemia which IV insulin can be. IV insulin has a disadvantage that it does not result in stable basal insulin levels as the subcutaneous insulin does. It is important to ensure that basal insulin levels remain stable. Aside from the usual scenario of glucose-insulin infusions going at certain rate, this shift to subcutaneous insulin achieves the basal levels of insulin round the clock. The intravenous infusions have to be tapered slowly till can be terminated and glycemic control procedures employed before surgery may be reinstituted.

The shift can be undertaken in two ways. A low level of insulin infusion is continued for 12–24 h after subcutaneous insulin is also begun, once the patient starts eating satisfactorily. This seems particularly relevant in patients with type 1 diabetes as it ensures an adequate baseline insulin concentration in these patients before IV insulin is stopped. Thus it will also significantly reduce the chances of diabetic ketoacidosis. It also helps to get heightened glycemic control in type 2 diabetic patients. It is not an absolute requirement to continue glucose-insulin infusion. Other nonglucose fluids can be instituted to correct other parameters or to hold them stable. The other way is to simply discontinue IV insulin and begin subcutaneous insulin. There is no consensus in literature as to which method to follow. The authors prefer continuation of low-dose insulin infusions for 12 h after subcutaneous insulin is begun.

Insulin may continue after discharge for patients never before on insulin. Education for patients and care givers about taking insulin injection, matters related to it is must. Symptoms of hypoglycemia, precautions to take and self monitoring of blood glucose must be taught. Explanations about how to interpret and respond within a limited range to hypo- and hyperglycemia and when to seek medical attention are important inputs to be given before discharge.

Many insulin regimens are possible in the postoperative period. The effective ones have a component of long-acting or intermediate-acting insulins with rapid- or short-acting insulins in various combinations which are described more fully in Chap. 11. Calculating doses of insulin for upscaling and downscaling of insulin is also described in Chap. 13. As would be obvious, each element of care is not always simultaneous but sequential.

4.11 Observations Residents Have to Carry Out: The Other Clinical Parameters

Some of the aspects of monitoring have been discussed at the stage on acute surgical case getting admitted, from the pathophysiological basis. Now we will discuss these from the clinical standpoint. These aspects cover both the preoperative stage when the patient is being made as fit as can be for surgery and in the postoperative period early and later periods as well. With all the complexities of modern medicine, the fundamental clinical monitoring aspects remain of utmost importance and are constant. In the preoperative period with optimal management, these parameters should show a trend towards normalcy. None need to become completely normal. This will not happen for many days even after the surgery is over.

The parameters are the heart rate, respiratory rate, blood pressure, and the cognitive functions. The more frequently the residents watch all these parameters as the treatment proceeds, the more refined will be their judgment about whether the patient is improving or not and how to accelerate or optimize treatment further. If there is improvement, one has to think about when and in what gradual and manner he has to reduce the various measures that are being taken. If the patient and the parameters are not improving, how and what to modify, in the various treatment modalities, becomes a serious concern. Only a few of these parameters are discussed.

4.11.1 Central Venous Pressure Monitoring

The residents and the nurses should train themselves in techniques of central venous pressure measurement, keenly watching the cardiac monitor for rhythm abnormalities since these modalities are now much more widely available than they were 20 years ago. The column should oscillate freely with each and every breath and descend till it becomes steady, that is, in equilibrium. If this does not happen, then the central venous catheter needs flushing or replacement in other veins. With normal kidney function, a central venous pressure of 8–10 cm of water should be maintained. In patients on ventilators, with positive end-expiratory pressure (PEEP), the central venous pressure may go up as a reflection of mean intrathoracic pressure and will not be the true pressure.

When the central venous pressure is high, the extremities cold and clammy, blood pressure sounds low, and no pulmonary edema or immediately apparent cardiac failure, the most likely cause would be gross acute dehydration with severe vasoconstriction of capacitance vessels. This gets automatically reduced often quickly, once substantial hydration has been corrected in the intravascular compartment as the capacitance vessels dilate.

High CVP may be observed if heart failure sets in, in this period, or if renal insufficiency gives rise to oliguria. Hydration gets corrected initially, but the continued infusion once distributed in the various bodily compartments cannot be retained fully in circulation, and edema formation starts. Interim it will cause circulatory overload leading to congestive failure since the fluid is not getting excreted by the kidneys to maintain the balance. Hence during the rehydration phase, it is necessary to frequently monitor patient clinically to see the signs of circulatory overload and watch for the rate of urine flow and moderate the rehydration efforts.

4.11.2 Placing Central Venous Catheters

In perioperative situations in a patient with diabetes, each resident or consultant is exhorted to avoid femoral central venous catheters as much as can be, for several reasons. Femoral CVP line is more likely to coil up and is somewhat more difficult to pass. But the most worrisome part is the thrombophlebitis, if and once it occurs.

Equally to be avoided at almost all costs is cannulating the saphenous vein and inject intravenous glucose and drugs. The venous thrombophlebitis and subsequent abscesses that are caused could be a highly morbid situation that can be easily avoided. If competent help is available, it is better to get a subclavian or jugular placement of a central venous catheter even if it is going to be delayed by a few hours. Adequate and fast enough hydration can be achieved by a simple intravenous cannula as wide as the veins can accommodate. Within a couple of hours, the venous constriction will resolve to facilitate the flow further.

4.11.3 Laboratory Parameter Monitoring

Right from the beginning, the first sample of blood drawn usually covers the hematological, hepatic, and the renal status with electrolytes. In many places, blood gas analysis for a patient in a serious condition can be done now. The residents must learn to interpret it since it gives a much deeper insight in the patient's condition and is very reliable in monitoring the progress and for prognostication.

The repeat investigations required at 4 and then 8 hourly intervals would be the electrolytes. Postoperatively the intervals will be 12 and then 24 hourly once the substitutions are found to be adequate. Even as the bedside glucose monitoring is on all such samples should also include blood glucose to intermittently match the bedside readings. As the patient starts taking orally or enterally, the whole monitoring game changes, and the activity shifts to wards. We will elaborate on that as in this phase of ICU at a later place.

4.11.4 Monitoring Urinary Parameters

At the outset it must be made clear that urine glucose monitoring may be given up completely. Routine testing of urine (for some uncanny reason, it has disappeared from the clinical practice as a whole) for infection on admission and after catheterization is a must. Any sample of urine to be sent for an investigation should be collected from the catheter and not from the bag. The first urine sample for routine testing and culture and antibiotic sensitivity gives an idea of the urinary sepsis already existing. At times it may be desirable to do culture sensitivity especially if one has a good microbiology support even when the evidence for infection is somewhat slender. Uncontrolled diabetes, perioperative setting, and urinary tract sepsis are loaded situations for septicemia and acute renal failure and poor outcome. Catheterization is not an inroad to infection as is generally supposed. It prevents stasis of the urine in the bladder in sick or elderly or any patient, a ripe precondition for the infection to set in with an accentuated possibility in presence of glucose in urine. It also eases the patient care a great deal and is a must for hourly measurements. Catheter care thus becomes important as dose the removal of it as soon as can be.

The input of electrolytes is lost either in urine, due to fever and sweating or the presence or absence of ADH as described in earlier chapters. While it is possible only to make an estimate of the losses from other causes, urinary losses can be accurately measured. The concentration has to be calculated by noting the urinary volume in liters. In addition, the simple test of specific gravity of the urine tells a good lot about the level of hydration. In some clinical situations, testing a catheter sample of urine for abnormal losses of either water or electrolytes like potassium and sodium can be useful. Few such situations are described below.

Diabetes insipidus is commonly seen in fracture base of the skull, pituitary tumor surgery, hypothalamic hamartomas or tumors, or hemorrhage in the pituitary hypothalamic region, the last often accompanied by severe diabetes mellitus as well [17]. In clean pituitary surgeries, it is transient and less severe and passes over in a week or 10 days as the edema of the hypothalamic region reduces. In more traumatic situations where the tissue damage is of severe degree, it may take a long time to settle, and the management of sodium and water balance is a minute to minute struggle.

Any urinary output above 500 mils/h should raise this suspicion,[3] especially if the urine is diluted. This happens due to complete absence of ADH and is called central diabetes insipidus. A serum sodium value above normal range and urine-specific gravity 1003 or 1004 are enough to make the diagnosis. This should be vigorously counteracted in order to avoid lethal hypernatremia. It is done by using the clinical analogue of antidiuretic hormone desmopressin subcutaneously at a frequency from 6 to 4 h depending upon the volume control of urine output it achieves. One of the ways to avoid dangerous hypernatremia is to pass a nasogastric tube and replace all the urinary volume lost by plain potable water till the urinary output is brought to some reasonable level like 100 mils/h or so or if the sodium gets normalized.

SIADH should always be suspected, far oftener than it is done in clinical practice, when an unexplained hyponatremia even after trying to correct it aggressively with normal saline persists. If it is accompanied by low urine output with highly concentrated urine in spite of volume replacement, the suspicion should be stronger. The creatinine will usually be normal. Hyponatremia is often attempted for correction by infusing 1.8% or 3% saline in variety of regimens like 100 mils in 4 h with a gap of 4 or 6 h of infusion-free periods, and the same infusion rate of hypertonic saline with the same interval is repeated. It can be given continuously. The advantage of hypertonic saline is that it reduces the volume of infusions even if no conscious diagnosis of SIADH is made.

The actual necessity here is to restrict fluids. How we do it is immaterial. Oral excess salt or excess salt through the NG tube will also achieve the same result. If glucose infusions are being used, then 10% dextrose reduces the volume by half as it doubles the calorie intake at half the speed. In SIADH however it will increase hyponatremia since 10% dextrose with normal saline is generally not available. In these situations it is advisable if the clinical condition permits to use high calorie small volume feeds intermittently. Using lipids for that is desirable. As was seen in an earlier chapter, the Leuven protocols relied heavily on lipids to replace 25–30% of all calories. This should be accompanied by much higher levels of insulin administration in acute situations through intravenous route. Postoperatively glucose control can be done by adjusting subcutaneous insulin doses, as dictated by the blood glucose levels and the caloric intake by mouth or NG feeding. There are many subcutaneous insulin regimes, described in Chap. 11.

In other situations when the sodium may be on the higher side with low urine output, obviously the patient is in need of more fluid without saline. The need for

[3] The other situation in which a sudden spurt in the urine output may occur is during the recovery phase of acute renal failure. As the tubules regenerate, there could be really copious urine output sometimes. Such a situation can or at least should immediately discernible in contrast to diabetes insipidus on the basis of the descriptions given above. One characteristic of this recovery is the unregulated and at times heavy losses of electrolytes which have to be regulated under frequent monitoring of the same and by appropriately changing the concentrations of the intravenous fluids.

more fluid in another situation could also be indicated by the high blood urea nitrogen to creatinine ratio, normally 10:1. A fixed specific gravity of urine at 1010 called isosthenuria may indicate chronic kidney disease.

4.11.5 Ketonuria Electrolytes, EKG, X Ray Chest

Once the clinical improvement has set in the postoperative period, it would become much less significant. A spot sample of urine collected for albumin creatinine ratio gives an indication of the levels of irreversible renal impairment and some idea of correctible elements in renal status like prerenal azotemia.

Electrolytes monitoring[4] in the postoperative situation is continued 12/24 h with renal parameters till the patient starts taking orally. Replacing some of the potassium or sodium can be easily undertaken then. In patients not improving, the frequency of these estimations will be dictated by the various parameters, renal function and the overall clinical situation.

Initial electrocardiogram and a plain film of the chest and in many places an abdominal ultrasound are desirable in visceral afflictions. Other investigations like CT or MRI will depend upon the basic surgical conditions.

4.11.6 Interpretation of Data

It is necessary to understand that exact significance, utility, and meaning of the parameter tested and its limitations. A sense of a continuously changing metabolic process, disequilibrating and equilibrating itself as the intervention proceeds, should be developed and held in the background. That will facilitate the interpretation divulged by the monitoring systems and take appropriate steps to correct or sustain situations. This should also lead to eschewing too much monitoring in the name of routine checks.

4.11.7 Factors Influencing Intra- and Postoperative Course

These are factors limiting, moderating, or permitting the aggressive intervention on these three stages of operative course, on a short- and a longer-term basis, i.e., over a period of days or months. They are listed below.

Infection is more common and many factors facilitate it. Caregivers should take extra precautions to see that the infection is not introduced through them and to avoid nosocomial infections with utmost care.

Cardiovascular abnormalities are extremely common making the patient prone to acute myocardial infarction during the course, congestive cardiac failure under fluid

[4] A common dictum in serious surgical or acutely ill medical cases, particularly in Neurosurgery is that if a patient's electrolytes can be maintained in a stable level the likelihood that he will survive will improve.

administration, or existing diabetic cardiomyopathy or autonomically denervated heart leading to rhythmical aberrations and/or sudden death.

Significant renal disease, hypertension, and coronary artery disease go together. Significant renal disease calls for adjustment of drug dosages to avoid drug toxicity and is always a seriously limiting factor in correcting the state of dehydration and electrolyte imbalance and is an impediment for good recovery.

Autonomic neuropathy comes with diabetic cystopathy, urinary retention, orthostatic hypotension, abnormal gut functioning with either diabetic diarrhea or constipation, and respiratory and cardiac arrest.

The surgical resident, to whom the patient will ultimately be transferred after acute phase management is over, must have all the above points in mind while looking after his patient over the course of his stay in the hospital.

4.12 Role of Residents in Transition from Post-ICU to Ward and Blood Glucose Control

The discussion so far has been presented pertaining to the immediate postoperative, intensive care unit phase. This can be 1 day, few days, or even many days, the last being, for example, in traumatic neurological surgical conditions or life-threatening cerebral hemorrhage surgically treated. Now we will present an overview of post-ICU postoperative period in which a slow transition from parenteral support to enteral support to normal oral intake is seen. In people with diabetes, it has some relevance because insulin administration frequency and routes change.

Over the first 5 or 6 postoperative days, the oral intake slowly increases. As a rule it should be resorted to as early as possible. It could be either through the nasogastric tube[5] or directly oral. In situations where these two routes are not indicated, it is advisable to use total parenteral nutrition, the details of which are given in Chap. 13. As quantum of nutrients through the nasogastric or oral route increases, the intravenous fluid rate and the quantity would both proportionately go down. In pancreatic or liver surgeries or major bowel resections, it is advisable to use liberally digestive enzymes through the oral or NG route. This will increase the absorption of the nutrients which will be complex starch, proteins, or lipids and would be used to counter catabolic state and facilitate tissue buildup. Substantial diet and higher doses of insulin are required for healing the tissues after surgery and control glucose. Such does will also prevent further catabolism, increase anabolism by protein synthesis, lipogenesis and restore glucose stores. As a corollary, high-value liberal nutrient supply (see Leuven above and elsewhere) and higher insulin doses are more beneficial than low nutrient supply with an obsession to keep blood glucose in control.[6]

[5] One of the early lessons we learnt from our professor was when he said—I am a great believer in Nasogastric tube.

[6] We have described some aspects of the passage of nutrients through the body and its interactions with the body tissues with insulin and glucagon. More detail will be found in Chap. 11. In the same chapter, we will also describe the various subcutaneous insulin administration regimens pertaining to any patient who has recovered enough to start oral nutrition.

As the oral intake begins, stabilizes, and continues to increase, the intravenous route is not required anymore. In fact, it is of less value since infused insulin does not give tissue storage. The SC insulin with continued absorption gives higher basal levels of insulin which serve all the functions of insulin listed just above. This is called stacking of insulin. The continuous substantial level of basal insulin with insulins designed to serve this function has been a landmark development in diabetes management in most situations.

There are two limitations to the efficacy of high basal level of insulin in glucose homeostasis. One is its inability to control the prandial glucose loads to maintain euglycemia. The second limitation is the frequency and degree of hypoglycemia they can produce especially during the night. It is now known for decades that 3% of all deaths in bed are due to severe hypoglycemia in the night [18]. In fact this is the area intensely investigated by active comparator trials since 2010 as to which basal insulin has the least and least dangerous potential for nocturnal hypoglycemia. More details about this are given in the Chap. 11.

On the other hand, as the surgical condition improves and sepsis is controlled, the insulin requirements may also come down, and as the oral intake increases, the requirement of the glucose infusion rate will also go down. Thus, the insulin requirements themselves being in the flux, here a more flexible and mixed approach, can be suggested as follows:

- Situation A: Intravenous support continues as before, and low-volume calorie intake begins orally or through nasogastric tube. This is the time extra insulin may have to be given as intravenous infusion. Alternately, when oral intake gets tolerated, additional twice in a day intermediate-acting human insulin is begun subcutaneously by giving a low dose of 6 U twice, 12 h apart, and may be increased by 4–6 U daily depending upon fasting and two or more random blood glucose levels and reduce the insulin infusion rate (see below).
- Situation B: Oral intake dominates/intravenous support declines substantially. At some point, the intravenous nonglucose-containing fluids continue to be administered to facilitate other intravenous administration of drugs by keeping a vein open. At this point as the controls become adequate and no evidence of infection is there, patient can be switched over to MSII, i.e., multiple subcutaneous regular crystalline insulin injections, in addition to the intermediate-acting/long-acting insulins being used. In ICU or in ward, multiple injections are only a mild botheration to patients but achieve much better controls. There are many different and effective protocols for subcutaneous insulin injections for which see the note on this issue elsewhere.
- Situation C: No intravenous support for maintenance, full oral supplementation. MSII/basal-bolus or premixed insulin is a reliable option and should be used boldly by increasing insulin doses by 2–4 U each time hyperglycemic reading appears. This has a few caveats which will be explained in the discussion on insulin pharmacokinetics and pharmacodynamics as well as in the various insulin regimens used in most situations requiring insulin, a stage called insulin-requiring diabetes mellitus.

- Situation D: In patients with only NG feeding, the biggest issue is the variability of the glycemic index of the feed. This happens in an attempt to supplement vitamins, fiber, and minerals also by giving vegetable soups, lime or fruit juices, or buttermilk. These are given either as base for the solids or are given as such. Such feeds invariably result in faster absorption of glucose and swings in the glycemic excursions.

The simplest way to avoid this is by fixing all feeds in one base fluid which has no particular ability to cause swings in glycemia. The base can be fixed as water only, which has zero glycemic value, for better dissolution of solids or thin buttermilk that is skimmed to avoid intrinsic fats in thicker buttermilk. Then the feed can be constituted as balanced a mix as possible. It should have more or less common glycemic index to avoid glycemic excursions. It is done by using ready-made mixtures wherein the proximate principles carbohydrates, proteins, and fats are held constant on a per-scoop basis. Depending upon the volume of the feed ordered, these should be dissolved in the maximum possible quantity without losing the liquid enough character to pass through the NG tube. However, the ready-made feeds available are extremely costly. This situation can be helped by preparing these mixtures "in house" by the dieticians by mixing varieties of powders of cereals and lentils and many other ingredients including fats as well and will be found to be much cheaper to the patients compared to the ready-made feeds.

4.13 Postoperative Infection, Glucose, and Insulin Therapy

The possibility of wound infection on the first postoperative day and the then prevailing glucose level have a rising and proportionate relationship. Within the range of blood glucose of 99–144 mg/dL, it was 1.3%. When the blood glucose level rose above 252 mg/dL (14 mmol/L), the rate of wound infection rose to 6.7% [19]. Careful glucose management for patients undergoing major procedures including cardiac and orthopedic surgeries will help improve the general outcomes.

Utmost precaution with intravenous lines, catheters, Ryle's tubes, and ventilator tubes cannot be overemphasized generally and particularly in patients with diabetes. Thus prevention is better. Intravenous catheters should not remain even a minute longer than necessary. Inability to keep blood glucose well below 200 mg/dL is an equally important measure since higher levels result in the immune failure described in detail in Chap. 12. In people with diabetes, urinary catheter is needed in DKA and hyperosmolar nonketotic state (HHNS) or in acute renal failure only. Cystitis, pyelitis on catheter, is one of the most undesirable and avoidable complication. Urinary infection by hematogenous route causing pyelonephritis and septicemia, quickly leading to acute renal failure, is common in diabetes, and surgical residents are cautioned against them.

Infection immediately produces several problems on an accentuated scale in people with diabetes. It produces fever, enhances catabolism, may cause vomiting and nausea, and may suddenly interfere with the prescribed diet being followed.

Infection passes through its several stages of bacteremia and endotoxemia through the polysaccharides after localization, septicemia, DIC, multiorgan failure, and death. The only way to treat the infection and the increased insulin resistance is to treat its cause and give higher and higher doses of insulin till one overcomes it. Thus, it must be clear that at the beginning of infection itself, insulin therapy must be stepped up by at least 20%. Too obvious and needless to state, for infection control, diabetes control with extremely aggressive insulin therapy with multiple monitoring is a must.

On the face of it, all of them especially the last may indicate a decline in the requirement of insulin, but it is not so. If the postoperative patient who is by and large on oral feeding and subcutaneous insulin experiences vomiting and nausea, one has to apply to "sick day rules" as given in the Chap. 13. Reducing insulin is not the answer.

Insulin, as mentioned in Chap. 12, has "anti-catabolic" properties. Therefore in this hypercatabolic insulin-resistant state, its requirements will go up. These requirements also go up because catecholamines, cytokines, and endogenous steroids released therein cause further elevation of insulin resistance. Infection adds to it substantially, pushing the requirements much higher.

4.14 On Achieving Control/Eliminating Infection

While on high insulin doses, at a point of time, the infection/inflammation resolves, better and easier control is achieved, and the blood glucose readings may be near normal. That could also indicate that it is time for reduction in insulin doses. This association of hypoglycemia after infection control is real and frequent enough to keep one alert to the possibilities.

4.15 How Long Insulin Should Be Used Postoperatively After a Major Surgery and When to Discontinue the Same?

This question presupposes that the patient was under good control preoperatively on a said dose of OHA. It is essential to check that premise. In minimal access surgeries, these patients can go back to OHAs if they were earlier well controlled with it. Routine ophthalmic surgeries have become far less time-consuming and are safer. In most minor noninfective surgeries, ward procedures lasting less than 1 or 2 h, all such patients can go back to OHAs within a day or two or mostly on the same day. One may note that the use of insulin in such cases will be transient if at all used. Absence of infection in the intra- and postoperative periods by good glycemic management can accelerate switching the patients back to OHAs. Antimicrobial prophylaxis in the immediate preoperative and intraoperative periods is generally helpful in uninfected cases.

In cases where the oral intake is irregular and is likely to be low postoperatively, repaglinide could actually be a good choice. We find in practice this drug is underutilized in spite of the reality that inability to maintain timing for food or skipping meals is common. Repaglinide need not be taken if meal is skipped. If it is delayed, repaglinide can be taken with the delayed meal. In case of skipping meals, other SUs which have been consumed earlier in the day may exert hypoglycemic effects in a more pronounced way. This risk is absent in repaglinide since its effects do not last for more than 4 h. Glipizide may have a better place in such situations as its hypoglycemic potential is much lower.

4.15.1 A Case for Longer Insulin Use Postoperatively

The issue is more varied in case of major surgeries with tissue trauma, long incisions, sternotomies, etc. Many of these patients are put back on OHA after stitch removal and can be if there is good healing and no infection in the wound. There is no fixed guideline for this. We will however put forward a few considerations and practices that we follow after a major emergency/elective surgery, for the reader to make his own decisions.

Considering the singular effects on cell growth, proliferation, the regulated protein degradation, anti-catabolic effects, and enhanced protein and collagen synthesis under adequate insulin administration, insulin could be continued at least for a month. The most preferable duration would be to allow for full healing of the scar and the operated tissue to get full benefits of actions of insulin.

In any surgery with considerable tissue trauma, handling and long incisions, and long duration of surgery, in sternotomies in CABGs, the minimum most period is till the wounds have healed completely with a firm scar. That will place the timing to about 3–6 weeks or more. Insulin use has other advantages not in just wound healing and is required in minor wound sepsis and so on. Trials like DIGAMI I have shown that longer use of insulin up to 3 months or more reduces cardiac deaths in patients with myocardial infarction extended period of 1 year. The details of various physiological actions of insulin are given separately. In the light of these observations, the duration of postoperative post-discharge continuation may be decided by the consultants. The longer it is given the better.

In diabetic co morbid conditions flexible small dose insulin use is safer. In end stage renal disease, oral antidiabetic drugs may precipitate hypoglycemia or add to acidosis, interfere with precarious food intake. In heart failure thiazolidinediones are contraindicated, acarbose is not well tolerated; in advanced hepatic cirrhosis, in post-operative radiotherapy when tissue breakdown continues, nausea and vomiting may cause low levels of food intake small insulin doses may be preferred.

The haste to remove insulin after a major illness the professionals show is both undesirable and not justifiable. Irrespective of all the effort to stop catabolism and promote anabolism during the illness healing from a major surgery and normalization of the system takes a long time. That is best facilitated by supraphysiological levels of insulin. One would be tempted to say that if the patient is comfortable with insulin postoperatively, there is no particular reason to hurry to stop insulin for all its nonmetabolic effects to which we refer to again and again.

In case of those who were on insulin before, the acute illness developed in most situations will continue to need insulin. In routine surgery it depends upon the cause and nature of illness. If an infective process has been dealt with, there is every likelihood that the patient after due interval for healing will not need insulin. If the condition responsible for undertaking surgery has in any way lowered the nutritional intake over a long period, as may be seen in gallstones or a chronic appendicitis, and if the nutritional intake improves considerably, the chances of such patients requiring insulin postoperatively are less, and the decision is with individual case and the consultants.

The experience informs us that in the post-discharge periods, the requirements of insulin go down progressively in a large majority of cases as these patients go in mild to moderate hypoglycemia frequently. If the total insulin dose comes down to or below 20 U/day, it is advisable to discontinue insulin and appropriate oral drugs given.

4.16 Metformin

If the patients have been on metformin prior to surgery, the recommendation to restart the same is resounding in literature, in the postoperative period [15]. More optimum, i.e., higher doses of the long-acting metformin variety coinciding with major two meals, without combining it with any other oral hypoglycemic agents in a single tablet, would give the optimal results. The resumption of metformin should be decided on the merits of each case and the postoperative parameters. Significant renal and hepatic disease, grossly underweight uncontrolled patients, and intolerance to metformin are the only real contraindications. In extensive bowel resection, reintroduction of metformin as a choice lies with the consultants. In all situations where metformin can be used, it is the drug of first choice as it reduces the insulin doses, improves hepatic sensitivity to insulin action, and interferes with nutrient absorption, among other actions. This is of importance since it helps prevent undue weight gain under ever-increasing insulin doses if glucose remains uncontrolled and may help to reduce weight as well. Metformin acts in combination with gliptines, sulfonylureas, alpha-glucosidase inhibitors, and glitazones also. Alpha-glucosidase inhibitors with metformin may increase gastrointestinal upsets. The issue of using glitazones at all or in low dose has remained more an individual preference than dictated by science from which no specific conclusions can be drawn. Metformin is also discussed in more details in Chap. 6 in this volume.

4.17 On Stitch Removal and at Discharge

If insulin regimen needs to be continued, it would be ideal if we can continue MSII for some time after discharge. However, these regimens mean at least three injections per day, with two different types of insulin used. It could be cumbersome, unreliable, or difficult for the patient or his relatives at home after discharge. The patient's relatives may not be able to learn injection techniques and may continue to rely on paramedics and doctors. It is not uncommon. This however causes difficulties in adhering to the timing, more difficult if multiple injections have to be given and may cause a drug-diet mismatch, the most important cause for dangerous hypoglycemia or hyperglycemia which so much effort has been spent to avoid. In such cases split-mixed, twice a day, regimen can be adopted (see protocols in Chap. 8.). Suffice it to say that once-daily insulin is almost always inadequate for good control in postoperative settings.

Some suggestions are made by the Surgical Care Improvement Project (SCIP). Performance Metrics are developed to cover and prevent as many complications of perioperative complications [20]. It is a simple checklist which can be implemented for this purpose.

1. The use of beta-blocker class of drugs in the perioperative period will reduce the risk of cardiovascular episodes. Traditionally considered to be raising blood glucose levels hence refrained from using the benefits outweigh this risk in high proportions.
2. Prophylactic antibiotic selection for surgical patients prior or within 1 h of incision is important since in clean surgeries with assured operation theater asepsis, it will go a long way to reduce costs and development of secondary or nosocomial infections.
3. Prophylactic antibiotic discontinued within 24 h will serve the same purposes as above.
4. In Cardiac Surgery in diabetes, normal fasting glucose is beneficial in intra and postoperative period. Normalizing the fasting glucose first leads to better overall control. In cardiac surgery hyperglycemia is clearly linked with increase infection and mortality perioperatively (see Chap. 7 in this volume).
5. Patients with appropriate hair removal before surgery. The trend occasionally noticed in neurosurgery is minimal hair removal. Surgeons and anesthetists should consider this.
6. Removal of bladder catheter 2 days after surgery is advisable.
7. Keeping temperature in normal range in the perioperative period.
8. To start the preventive treatment to avoid venous thromboembolism either prior to surgery or within 24 h postoperatively. It would have particular reference to orthopedic surgeries where per force a patient may have to be immobilized for a few days as in polytrauma. However most clean orthopedic surgeries may call for a less generalized approach since very early mobilization has been the rule.

In the next chapter, we will consider the possibilities of hypoglycemia in the postoperative stage and after discharge.

References

1. Kim RP, Edelman SV, Dennis D. Musculoskeletal complications of diabetes mellitus. Clin Diabet. 2001 Jul;19(3):132–5. https://doi.org/10.2337/diaclin.19.3.13.
2. Peters A, Kerner W. Perioperative management of the diabetic patient. Exp Clin Endocrinol Diabetes. 1995;103(4):213–8.

3. Gill GV, Alberti KGMM. The care of the diabetic patient during surgery in international textbook of diabetes mellitus. New York, NY: John Wiley & Sons; 2003.
4. Duncan AE, Abd-Elsayed A, Maheshwari A, Xu M, Soltesz E, Koch CG. Role of intraoperative and postoperative glucose concentrations in predicting outcomes after cardiac surgery. Anesthesiology. 2010;112(4):860–71.
5. Furnary AP, Zerr KJ, Grunkemeier GL, Starr A. Continuous intravenous insulin infusion reduces the incidence of deep sternal wound infection in diabetic patients after cardiac surgical procedures. Ann Thorac Surg. 1999;67(2):352–62.
6. Desborough JP, Jones PM, Persaud SJ, Landon MJ, Howell SL. Isoflurane inhibits insulin secretion from isolated rat pancreatic islets of Langerhans. Br J Anaesth. 1993;71(6):873–6.
7. Lattermann R, Schricker T, Wachter U, Georgieff M, Goertz A. Understanding the mechanisms by which isoflurane modifies the hyperglycemic response to surgery. Anesth Analg. 2001;93(1):121–7.
8. Lundy JB, Slane ML, Frizzi JD. Acute adrenal insufficiency after a single dose of etomidate. J Intensive Care Med. 2007;22(2):111–7.
9. Fragen RJ, Shanks CA, Molteni A, Avram MJ. Effects of etomidate on hormonal responses to surgical stress. Anesthesiology. 1984;61(6):652–6.
10. Forman SA. Clinical and molecular pharmacology of etomidate. Anesthesiology. 2011;114(3):695–707.
11. Hall GM, Lacoumenta S, Hart GR, Burrin JM. Site of action of fentanyl in inhibiting the pituitary-adrenal response to surgery in man. Br J Anaesth. 1990;65(2):251–3.
12. Wolf AR, Eyres RL, Laussen PC, et al. Effect of extradural analgesia on stress responses to abdominal surgery in infants. Br J Anesth. 1993;70(6):654–60.
13. Desborough JP, Hall GM, Hart GR, Burrin JM. Midazolam modifies pancreatic and anterior pituitary hormone secretion during upper abdominal surgery. Br J Anaesth. 1991;67(4):390–6.
14. Australian Diabetes Society. Peri-operative diabetes management guidelines, July 2012, ADS working group of Vincent Wong, Glynis Ross, Jennifer Wong and David Chipps (chair).
15. Marks JB. Perioperative management of diabetes. Am Fam Physician. 2003;67(1):93–100.
16. Van den Berghe G, Wouters P, Weekers F, Verwaest C, Bruyninckx F, Schetz M, Vlasselaers D, Ferdinande P, Lauwers P, Bouillon R. Intensive insulin therapy in critically ill patients. N Engl J Med. 2001;345:1359–67.
17. Kelkar SK. Cranial diabetes a concept and its pathogenesis, Endocrine symposium, JIPMER; 2000.
18. Williams G, Pickup JC, editors. Handbook of diabetes. Hoboken, NJ: Blackwell Scientific Publication; 1992.
19. Zerr K, Furnary A, Grunkemeier G, et al. Glucose control lowers the risk of wound infection in diabetes after open heart operations. Ann Thorac Surg. 1997;63:356–61.
20. Stulberg JJ, Delaney CP, Neuhauser DV, Aron DC, Fu P, Koroukian SM. Adherence to surgical care improvement project measures and the association with postoperative infections. JAMA. 2010;303(24):2479–85.

5 Hypoglycemia in Postoperative Setting

Contents

5.1 Preamble

In the postoperative period, many different situations arise in which for fear of hypoglycemia, the blood glucose is allowed to remain higher. There are situations which could however lead to hypoglycemia which need to be appreciated. Majority of these will arise on account of the quality of care and operationalizing the instructions. More important however is to monitor care closely enough and be aware of what could go astray due to the multiple measures of management undertaken and the potential not only for hypoglycemia but also for hyperglycemic swings.

By definition hypoglycemia is any blood glucose level below 60 mg/dL with symptoms of hypoglycemia and recovery from the same after glucose administration. Adrenergic symptoms are usually the first to appear—sweating, palpitation,

S. Kelkar et al., *Towards Optimal Management of Diabetes in Surgery*,
https://doi.org/10.1007/978-981-13-7705-1_5

tremors, and severe hunger pangs. Neuroglycopenic symptoms arise after this consisting of confusion, headache, disorientation, instability, drowsiness, visual auditory disturbances, and coma. Significant hypoglycemia on glucose insulin drip in the present setting (or any setting) can occur if the majority readings are in the normal range. To put it another way—if the patient is in hyperglycemic ranges the day round, it is rare for him to experience true hypoglycemia, except under one condition. If the rate of lowering of blood glucose, for some reason, is too rapid, there will be hypoglycemic symptoms without the blood glucose reaching the hypoglycemic range.

In the perioperative setting, hypoglycemia can arise from a number of factors. This could happen in situations where infusion of insulin inadvertently runs rapidly or excess dose gets included in the syringe pump by mistake. Hypoglycemia in any critical clinical situation particularly in the postoperative period either in ICU or in the wards (which is the focus of this chapter) is caused by a few specific mechanisms. The frequency of the hypoglycemia may not be high in these situations and may vary in all aspects. It will be instructive to understand the mechanisms under which it may be caused should be understood and detected and corrective measures taken. The different situations in which hypos may occur in acute postoperative care are the following.

5.2 Patients Fully on IV Supplementation of Calories and Insulin

Situation A: These patients can go in hypos if the calorie supplementation for some reason stops but insulin infusion rate is not altered. For example, the surgeon may order Ringer's lactate or normal saline, replacing dextrose infusions but continuing by oversight, same rate for insulin infusion. This situation is avoided by administering any fluids that do not contain glucose by always giving them by a separate line. The other line or the first line should infuse glucose at constant rate which has been balanced against the rate of insulin infusion on units/hour basis as demonstrated amply in the preceding pages.

Situation B: Sometimes two or more dextrose infusions are running at different speeds for corrections of other abnormalities, e.g., magnesium. One or both of these infusions with the additives may become unnecessary once delivered and withdrawn, either without substituting them with plain DNS or without scaling the insulin infusion rate down. Multiple dextrose infusions with different infusion rates, the differential timing with which they may be started, create considerable difference in blood glucose. These situations are best matched by a syringe insulin pump. Depending upon the drip rate of the ongoing or withdrawn additional dextrose solution, insulin infusion may be arbitrarily increased or reduced once discontinued, respectively. Glucose level is checked in both the instances in an hour or two to find whether the insulin infusion rate balances the remaining infusions. It can then be scaled up or down. It is not uncommon to find hypoglycemia in these situations. However the response to both elevation and lowering of glucose levels may not meet action. More than 50% of the patients complaining of hypoglycemic episodes were not advised in the reduction in daily insulin doses by 20% [1].

Situation C: More often than not, the severe stress on the patient comes down swiftly with effective surgical intervention, for example, control of sepsis, drainage of intraperitoneal pus, or when polytrauma settles down. This results in the marked decrease in the insulin-resistant state wherein the insulin requirement of the patients may drop quickly and considerably. Intelligent monitoring will help solve this problem. Contrarily if glucose level in a high-stress situation starts coming under control rapidly with the same insulin infusion, it is an indication that the patient may go into hypoglycemia. A cycle of lower glucose level leading to stepwise reduction of insulin doses starts once stress starts disappearing often rapidly. Other parameters also improve indicating rapid recovery. With experience, detecting it, maintaining normoglycemia and avoiding hypoglycemia becomes easier.[1]

The usual precaution in this is to assure that the normalization or lowering of blood glucose is occurring while the calorie supplementation is going on at the steady rate. There would be few situations, if at all, where continuously improving glucose control would indicate otherwise as in situation D below.

Situation D: Two general situations where insulin sensitivity is high could land the patient in a hypoglycemic state: subacute or unsuspected or undiagnosed hypothyroidism or Addison's disease—hypocortisolism, from any cause. Under the operative stress, these two organs may function even more subnormally (or unable to respond to the stress) and fail to respond to the needs of the body. Both these states are highly insulin sensitive. These two responses may continue to fail even after the surgical stress is removed. Both conditions are likely to be accompanied with hypotension not getting corrected. The authors have faced these situations a few times, but timely and instinctive suspicion and historical exploration have saved these patients from all sorts of diagnostic interventions.[2]

Situation E: At times serious liver disease makes its appearance during the treatment phases. This is likely to happen if the ultrasonography fails to describe the

---

[1] To illustrate—We had a male patient 65 years of age, with diabetes who was diagnosed to have a massive streptococcal bacterial pneumonia, was put on insulin and intravenous antibiotics (the symptoms resolved quickly even when the radiographic changes remained), and was sent home on split-mix insulin twice a day. On the seventh day after discharge, he was admitted with severe hypoglycemia. The radiological recovery was complete and diet as well as insulin regime was maintained well. This is how infection and its resolution play a role in controlling glucose or in producing hypoglycemia.

[2] To illustrate—A middle-aged woman whose preoperative investigations did not show any abnormality was operated for a large abscess on the back under GA who remained drowsy for an unduly long period. Upon checking her thyroxine levels done a few months ago, it was normal but was revealed that she had for some reason discontinued the tablets after that.

In another and rather remarkable case, a stable fit-to-operate young man underwent closed mitral valvotomy and was otherwise stable but grossly hypotensive after surgery. On exploring it was revealed that prior to the operation, he was treated for fairly extensive pulmonary tuberculosis and was fully cured prior to operation. A random sample of blood for cortisol was drawn, and cortisol was started without waiting for the results with dramatic improvement in the blood pressure. The reasoning given was an occult tubercular adrenalitis which had left it suboptimal in response. The cortisol level was found to be lowest normal, which under the serious operative stress was considered hypoadrenal response.

structure or portal vein diameter is incorrectly reported. In liver failure there is reduction in the mass which reduces the glucose-storing capacity. There could be an increase in the insulin resistance reducing glucose deposition. Both the situations will result in increasing the quantum of glucose passed into the blood and hyperglycemia. In decompensated failure hypoglycemia will be due to the reduced capacity of the liver for gluconeogenesis. Since the insulin clearance will be decreased due to either resistance or reduced cell mass, higher levels of insulin can cause hypoglycemia [2, 3].

Situation F: Kidneys degrade the circulating insulin and are part of the gluconeogenic processes. In advanced disease the mass of functioning tissue is reduced. In uremia the food intake is also less. These two mechanisms result in hypoglycemia. In chronic kidney disease, undiagnosed but significant nephropathy or kidney injury (AKI) hypoglycemia is likely [4].

5.3 Patients on Part IV and Partly on NG Feeds

Situation G: In diabetes with an acute or routine illness, an often-forgotten assessment is that of gastroparesis. A complaint of fullness in the stomach after eating relatively less, refusing the next feed, or some evidence of regurgitation are enough to suspect it. It is caused by the parasympathetic loss or the vagal tone, responsible for the propulsion of the stomach contents. To complicate the matter, the pyloric sphincter under the influence of sympathetic nervous system and the weakened stomach contractions together may result in ineffective emptying of the stomach contents. Sympathetic autonomic nervous system generally degenerates later compared to parasympathetic; hence its effects can be felt in such a situation.

While sophisticated tests cannot be undertaken in acute or non-acute surgical situations, often a plain X-ray of the abdomen can sufficiently demonstrate gastroparesis. It is here that the common postoperative surgical practice of carefully aspirating the stomach contents and not a cursorily performed one becomes important. It gives an idea of the slower rate of propulsion but also the quantum of the remaining feed. This calls for spacing the feeds further, making the feeds smaller with higher calorie density and lower the insulin administration. It also avoids the most unfortunate happenstance of vomiting and aspiration. The insulin regimen in such patients may be subcutaneous or a mix of IV and subcutaneous insulin.

5.4 Three Different Mechanisms Causing Hypoglycemia on NG Feeding

Situation H: The NG feeding becomes unreliable. This happens commonly if a 2-h NG feed is advised. The insulin units are ordered accordingly under the assumption that the patient is going to be fed every 2 h and that the patient will be in a position to accept it. In patients with obtunded consciousness, other sicknesses, those receiving chemotherapy, in bowel surgery or metabolic encephalopathy, the gastric content may not empty in 2 h. A large volume then will be aspirated as a standard precaution before the next feed. No feed is then (rightly so) given for a variable period. It is not easy to maintain a 2 or 3 or 4 hourly check on gastric aspirate before each feed and then to give the next feed, in ICUs and even more so in wards. Such patients can miss their next feed, or it may get postponed by a couple of hours. But the insulin given especially subcutaneously (which makes sense in such situations) cannot be withdrawn or reduced and continues to act. As a result there will be hypoglycemia.

This situation is avoided by a slower feeding rate of 4 h in which larger quantities up to 250 or 300 mL of total feed can be given. Four hours would be an adequate time for the stomach contents to empty. The chances of regurgitation may be less with less frequent feeding. Use of short- or rapid-acting insulin in multiple small doses, withdrawing the intermediate- or long-acting insulin in lieu of it, or use of a short-acting oral drug like repaglinide could solve this issue. Use of properistaltic drugs like metoclopramide and alginates given to improve the gastroesophageal sphincter tone would be helpful. These drugs occasionally produce extra pyramidal reactions which are quite frightening but can easily be treated with slow and diluted IV diazepam within minutes. Erythromycin would be safer as it will not produce cholestatic jaundice and extra pyramidal signs in the short run.

Situation I: It is a common practice to stop feeding in the night by 10 p.m. and start feeding again in the morning by 6 p.m. Even with a 4 h spacing, hypos do keep occurring because a long gap of 8 h results from this practice. Even with the use of regular insulin, the last dose of which, given late in the night, may still produce early- or late-morning hypos. The solution to this situation lies in feeding the patient which may be once at 2 or 3 a.m. with the same or even reduced quantity of the daytime feed. NG feeding is an artificial situation where conscious recognition and action for correction of hypo are not expected to be initiated by the patient.

Situation J: Depending upon the volume of the feed ordered, all the ingredients should be dissolved in the maximum possible quantity without losing the liquid character to pass through the NG tube easily. The ready-made feeds available are prepared with these ideas of uniformity and balance of proximate principles, vitamins, minerals, etc. However they are extremely costly. This situation can be helped by preparing these mixtures in the house, by mixing varieties of powders of cereals and lentils. Agencies in many places have and do prepare such standard mixtures including fats as well and are much cheaper to the patients. This will maintain the uniform calorie supplementation rates as well and avoid hypoglycemia on a given regiment of insulin or in stable (medical) or some surgical cases even with OHAs.

Situation K: Several other examples of preventing hyperglycemia during the preoperative period of routine surgery have been given in Chap. 6 which could also serve as prevention of hypoglycemia. Postoperatively also procedures like a CT scan or percutaneous enterogastrostomy or PEG for short may be undertaken. In such situations the oral or nasogastric feeding will have to be withheld. Care should be taken to avoid administering any hypoglycemic drugs prior to such procedures to prevent hypos unless the glucose is high.

5.4.1 Patients on Normal Diet Postoperatively Requiring Hypoglycemic Agents

These patients undergoing major surgeries with long incisions or considerable bowel handling and so on could be on insulin. But many in today's era of minimally invasive surgery could go back on oral hypoglycemic drugs as soon as they start taking orally. These patients may go into hypos due to drug-diet mismatch, mainly because patients do not always eat the prescribed diets. To avoid this drug-diet mismatch, the oral drugs with minimal hypoglycemic potential may be given on discharge. These drugs may also be given after the patient has eaten and has retained food. All drugs in a particular class do not have the same hypoglycemic potential. The details about the pharmacokinetics and pharmacodynamics with other drug-to-drug interactions have been discussed in Chap. 6. Here their relative hypoglycemic potential is discussed.

1. Glibenclamide tops the list on all four parameters—frequency, severity, long duration, and recurrence of hypos [5]. Glimepiride and glipizide have much less potential to cause hypos. Gliclazide in conditions like hepatic/renal diseases where insulin degradation is delayed or may be inadequate may have a higher propensity for hypos.
2. The non-sulfonylurea drug repaglinide has least potential to produce hypos. Since it is excreted by the liver, it is safe to take even with early nephropathy and irregular dietary habits or even for elderly whose intake is less than usual.
3. Metformin as monotherapy as a rule does not cause hypoglycemia. It would be individual judgment when to restart it after major bowel surgery. Alpha-glucosidase inhibitors, gliptines, and thiazolidinediones are classes of drugs who also do not cause hypos in monotherapy.
4. It may be useful to remember that oral sulfonylureas of older varieties are still in use, and occasionally the second- and third-generation sulfonylureas produce hypoglycemia which is difficult to correct and may take as many as 2–3 days. In any major or acute surgical setting, all the oral hypoglycemic drugs should be discontinued as soon as the preparation for surgery starts, and the patient has to be brought to as optimal a condition preoperatively.

5.4.2 Preoperative Hypoglycemia with the Minimum 6–8 h of Preoperative Fasting

Preoperative hypoglycemia however is rather infrequent a phenomenon. The patient is tense and stressed and therefore unlikely to easily go into hypoglycemia unless preoperatively the patient has been starving for too long and is emaciated (i.e., with low intrinsic energy stores to counter hypoglycemia) and has received hypoglycemic drugs. Normally such hypoglycemia is not possible. In fact, in most patients with diabetes, because of increased hepatic glucose output, the longer a patient fasts, the more insulinopenic, hyperglycemic, and gluconeogenic he will become. In the following situations, hypoglycemia could still arise:

1. Preoperative ingestion of long-acting OHAs, unbeknown to the treating team followed by preoperative starvation.
2. Preoperative ingestion of long-acting OHAs or intermediate-acting insulin in the usual doses but not eating food as is common during the night preoperatively, due to anxiety leading to morning hypoglycemia.
3. Incorrect administration of various types of insulin—especially long-acting ones—followed by preoperative starvation or the mismatch between insulin concentration and syringe used. Various reasons for insulin mismatch are discussed in detail later.
4. Some physicians or specialist diabetes physicians routinely start glucose-insulin infusion as a standard protocol irrespective of the value of FBS. it may be often started by the surgical/medical resident doctors or may come as a routine instruction. If the blood glucose is already on the lower side, it may precipitate hypoglycemia.
5. The patient has either forgotten to tell about the scheduled oral or injectable dose taken or the doctors have not checked on the night before or a patient who has not brought his medicines while getting admitted by night/evening when many of the OHAs or injections have been already taken. These are different preconditions leading to hypoglycemia.
6. Bedtime or pre-dinner intermediate-acting insulin is a common practice among diabetologists but is viewed with some reservation as the cause of hypoglycemia among primary care providers. A patient settled on that regime needs to have no fear of hypoglycemia on the day of surgery unless he unnecessarily reduces his food intake drastically on previous night.
7. In acute situations such a development is unlikely. The plasma concentration reached by using longer-acting basal insulins does not cause hypoglycemia if the diet is properly controlled. In this respect glargine and the newer long-acting insulin analogues like detemir are compared in Chap. 11 in this volume.

   In these cases it is advisable to use constant low rate low concentration glucose solutions at a determined rate to maintain the blood glucose around 140–170 mg. High-concentration glucose infusions push blood glucose levels high resulting in excess pancreatic insulin secretion, cause hypoglycemia, perpetuating the hypo hyper cycle. In Somogyi phenomenon hypoglycemia is followed by reactive hyperglycemia destabilizing the control.
8. In case of tapering of steroids given in high doses, there is generally a lag of 24–36 h when the blood glucose gets lowered. If the insulin doses are not reduced proportionately and in an anticipatory manner, hypoglycemia is likely

5.4.3 Hypoglycemia Due to Diet and Drug Mismatch

At this stage the patients are often not in a position to eat full diet for a variety of reasons. In case of inadequate intake compared to the prescribed one, one has to have a mechanism to adjust insulin doses. Such situations can be minimized in two ways. One is to monitor the blood glucose before the three major meals, that is, to say a fasting or a pre-breakfast, pre-lunch, and pre-dinner glucose. The values obtained give an idea of how much more the blood glucose is likely to rise vis a vis the quantum of food the patient is able to consume. This helps to increase or decrease the insulin dose prospectively. For example, if a patient is on basal-bolus therapy and his pre-lunch glucose is 130 mg/dL and the dose of the regular insulin prescribed before lunch is 16 U, there is reason to raise this by another 5–6 U in anticipation of lowering his postprandial one. If it is 80 mg/dL, there is little reason to raise or lower it.

Another solution is to give the insulin after ascertaining that the patient has taken his meals adequately enough or not and if he will retain it. Short-acting insulins are more suitable here. If the intake in this recovery phase is inadequate, it is a common sense practice to reduce the insulin dose by either 20% as recommended in literature or 4 or 2 U from all doses daily till the hypoglycemic episodes disappear while not allowing the glucose to go far outside the limit. On the contrary, if the pre-lunch glucose is 300 mg/dL, the real solution is to raise *the morning pre-breakfast dose substantially* or change a premixed preparation to regular- or rapid-acting insulin to a much higher level.

Two well-recognized operational aspects of insulin injections causing severe hypoglycemia are discussed below.

5.4.4 The Mismatch Between Insulin Syringes and the Concentration of the Insulin in Vials

Insulin syringes come in two capacities of 40 and 100 U. In the 40 U syringe, the figures are in red. These syringes should be used to draw insulin from 40 U/mL vials of insulin. Thus when the syringe is fully loaded, it will deliver 40 U of insulin. The same holds for the 100 U syringe of which the lettering is in bold black. These syringes should be used to draw insulin from 100 U/mL vials of insulin. When the syringe is filled fully from a 100 U/mL vial, it will have 100 U.

(a) If by mistake insulin from a 40 U/mL vial is drawn in 100 U syringes, it will contain only 40% of the intended dose resulting in unacceptable hyperglycemia, the sudden rise remaining unexplained. This however is the less dangerous situation.

(b) The type of insulin syringe, extremely commonly used and is universally available in India, is the 40 U insulin syringe because in India, 40 U/mL insulin vials are universally used. Supposing that by chance insulin is drawn from a 100 U/mL vial by the 40 U syringe, it will have a dose 2.5 times more. If this is administered, there is every chance that significant hypoglycemia will develop.

(c) There are five high-risk medicines prescribed in wards. The errors in prescription for the top five could give rise to severe iatrogenic adverse reactions. Insulin is among the top five such medications where errors could also be frequent. In case of insulin, the complexity increases for the following reasons. Currently more than 60 preparations of insulin and variety of devices are available in most adequately developed countries. These are single-ingredient and two-ingredient human or analogue preparations. There are half a dozen companies marketing insulin in India alone. The number of brands for each type multiplies. 30–35% of all hospital deaths in first 48 h, are due to incorrect number of units drawn, using short hand for brand confusing staff, mismatch of insulin ordered/injected, mismatch between the insulin strength/corresponding syringe, and mistakes in preparing the insulin infusions[6]. Delay in the prompt correction of infusion rates with glucose monitored could also be a cause. Use of prefilled syringes of insulin for infusion may reduce the risk but will not eliminate it [Author].

(d) Thus it behooves on the administrative authorities to see that the insulin concentrations in vials that are ordered for daily use should be accompanied by the purchase of only corresponding insulin syringe strength *throughout the hospital.* It can be 40 or 100 U. Availability of multiple types of same classes of insulin should be seriously curtailed to just one brand. As the experience in India goes, the usage of 100 U/mL insulin strength has remained confined to the cartridges prefilled with that concentration and corresponding insulin-injecting pens. For routine use in wards, 40 U vials have remained the norm.

 The authors also recommend that once particular brands of insulin from a company are chosen, *brands from another company should not be ordered* in a hospital setting over short interval of time or keep on changing for reasons rooted or not rooted in quality. Rapid alterations or changes in brands cause confusion at all levels. From the doctor ordering the brand he is used to and the dispensing pharmacist giving a different wrong brand, the same brand coming to the wards and the ICUs, with nurses from novices to more experienced ones and getting administered is an entire chain prone to finally give the wrong composition to the patient.

(e) Some of the longer-acting insulin preparations are clear. It would not be desirable if it is given intravenously. Most others are milky. Yet it is not uncommon to come across a nurse preparing to fill the syringe pump with intermediate-acting insulin or at least has no idea that it is not to be given intravenously. The nomenclatures of which is crystalline insulin R or what does NPH will stand for will be confusing to all. The bigger easily readable brand names and miniscule letters of the chemical composition are confusing enough. If multiple brands are also freely circulating, the situation becomes complicated and precarious.

5.4.5 Reversing Hypoglycemia

Insulin-induced hypoglycemia is quickly reversible. Such significant hypoglycemia as is conventionally advised is treated by a 50 or 100 mL bolus of 25 or 50% glucose and another 50–100 mL of it added to the running drip. This reverses hypoglycemia fairly satisfactorily and quickly but is not advisable. These are high concentrations. We would prefer to avoid even 10% or higher glucose concentration to be given intravenously even as a small bolus since their thrombophlebitis potential is high. The high blood glucose levels achieved in turn may stimulate the pancreas under the effects of OHAs, which will cause a relapse in hypoglycemia creating a viscous cycle for 2–3 days and creating a total disorganization of the main area of treatment. A simple 5% DNS drip initially rapidly and then on a maintenance rate will avoid the situations described above.[3] One mg glucagon injections are rare if ever required to reverse hypoglycemia. Glucagon will work only and only if there is sufficient glycogen store in the liver.

The quantities mentioned above are a rough guideline and will essentially be dictated by the blood glucose level, insulin concentration, speed of infusion, patient characteristics, surgical process, level of consciousness, stability of correction, and so on. Therefore as is obvious, innumerable shades are possible while managing.

In spite of several reasons described above till now, hypoglycemia may still occur only infrequently since the blood glucose control is nowhere near optimal and glucose generally is on a much higher side. Even then if the managing team is tuned to it, it is much less dangerous than thought, as explained elsewhere. We have considerable experience of handling hypoglycemia even in patients neurologically already obtunded and of hypoglycemia in many other serious situations. The ability to spot it quickly and treat it quickly in a measured way and not excessively over and over if required is what is needed. It may be emphasized again and again that too frequent glucose monitoring without intervention is unreasonable and is no guaranty that it will detect hypos early or at all. Hypoglycemia is easy to spot even with when the monitoring is at its minimum (see below).

This situation can be further avoided by using intermediate- acting insulins in lowered doses, twice a day. These are absorbed more slowly and once the peak is achieved over 4–6 h they continue to decline in their levels. This is more likely to match the 4 h feeding and absorption cycle. However NPH produces the maximum number of episodes of hypoglycemia. Glargine and insulin detemir are peak less and safer. Glargine and detemir are never given IV. Alternatively crystalline insulin or short-acting analogues can be used four times in 24 h (see more detailed discussion in Chap. 11 in this volume).

During postoperative recovery the most versatile regimen to get tight control and avoid hypoglycemia is the basal-bolus therapy which can then be converted in two premixed insulins on discharge discussed elsewhere. The dose of insulin on which they are stable in the wards may even be reduced by a few units if there is apprehension about the intake at home. The rapid-acting insulin analogues are distinctly superior in both these aspects.

[3]An acutely hypoglycemic brain produces bizarre EEG wave patterns. For the EEG waves to normalize, it takes no more than 22–25 s even with a 5% dextrose drip much before full recovery of cognition in minutes to follow. In investigating a case of excessive morning drowsiness suspected of malingering, we strapped the patient to an EEG machine and did his blood glucose which was 20 mg/dL. After the first waveforms were recorded, we started a glucose 5% dextrose drip at 100 mils/h. The EEG normalized in 25 s and recovery of consciousness within minutes. This patient was later diagnosed as having insulinoma.

5.4.6 Reiterating a Few Points About the Practices and Hazards of Intravenous Insulin Route

Human insulins in this regard are more predictable, mathematically, in intravenous route. It means that an approximate function could be established between the numerical value of blood glucose under x U of insulin would reduce to a lesser range or greater range if the infusion rate is raised or lowered to $x \pm y$ U. It is this programmable predictability that can be used to keep postoperative patients euglycemic.

Monitoring without action and action without monitoring are two unacceptable acts in any situation. It is common to see 24 blood glucose testings done in a day without the orders being changed even once. Monitoring does not have as its motto to check if the patient is in hypoglycemic range. It is to continuously adjust the insulin doses to keep all readings in a euglycemic range as per the goals set. It is wasteful, involving high costs, and is unnecessary and painful to the patient. Optimization of monitoring and insulin dose is the key. Methods to acquire and practice it are described in this volume.

Typically, in situations of hypoglycemia, all the next doses are reduced, and the preceding dose is left as it is. At its best or worst, this will lead to either normoglycemia or hyperglycemia in the readings of the post-hypoglycemic event. It is the preceding dose that causes hypoglycemia and not the next dose coinciding with the next meal.

5.5 Minimum Most Monitoring

Once the balance of insulin administration and calorie supplementation is achieved, strict glycemic control can be achieved with just three glucose readings in 24 h—viz., 6 a.m., 2 p.m., and 10 p.m. The morning reading gives us a clear picture of whether the night doses of insulin have covered the period properly or whether any decrement or increment is necessary in the night dose. The 2 p.m. blood glucose readings tell us the effectivity of the morning insulin doses, and the 10 p.m. blood glucose reading tells if the morning and the afternoon doses of insulin have controlled the glucose adequately or it needs to be increased or decreased. This way in 24 h, the night dose of insulin is changed in the morning of the next day. The 2 and 10 p.m. doses are changed, by the second morning and evening fixing all the insulin doses, till a significant change in the status of the illness, for better or worse, occurs.

The three conditions needed to be fulfilled for reliable control in minimum most monitoring are strictly timed testing for blood glucose, constant rate of supply of calories, and strictly timed insulin/OHA administrations. This works best when the patient is on nasogastric feeding, but it works with any form of calorie supplement and any route of insulin administration in any patient of any severity of illness once the frequent blood glucose monitoring has achieved a round-the-clock balance as long as the feeding schedules are constant. Excellent controls can be obtained.

References

1. Mathioudakis N, Everett E, Golden SH. Prevention and management of insulin-associated hypoglycemia in hospitalized patients. Endocr Pract. 2016;22:959–69.
2. Pfortmueller CA, Wiemann C, Funk GC, et al. Hypoglycemia is associated with increased mortality in patients with acute decompensated liver cirrhosis. J Crit Care. 2014;29(2):316.e7–12.
3. Changani KK, Jalan R, Cox IJ, et al. Evidence for altered hepatic gluconeogenesis in patients with cirrhosis using in vivo 31-phosphorus magnetic resonance spectroscopy. Gut 2001;49:557–64.
4. Arem R. Hypoglycemia associated with renal failure. Endocrinol Metab Clin N Am. 1989;18:103–21.
5. Kelkar SK. Analysis of 18 consecutive cases of severe hypoglycemia in coma admitted to CIIMS. CIIMS bulletin 1997.
6. National Patient Safety Agency. The fourth report of the Patient Safety Observatory. Safety in doses: medication safety incidents in the NHS, Jan 2007. www.nrls.npsa.nhs.uk/resources/patient-safety-topics/medication-safety/?entryid45=59822&q=0%. Accessed 8 Nov 2015.

Management of Routine Surgery in Diabetes

6

Contents

S. Kelkar et al., *Towards Optimal Management of Diabetes in Surgery*,
https://doi.org/10.1007/978-981-13-7705-1_6

6.1 Preamble

Routine or elective minor and major surgery in diabetes must be taken equally seriously as the emergency surgery, in each and every aspect related to it. In emergency surgery, each stakeholder is prepared for a certain element of adverse or untoward happening. There is no guarantee that something similar may not happen in the elective cases, be it minor or major surgery, a distinction between the two made below. If any such untoward incident not discussed preoperatively happens, it reflects extremely adversely over all those involved in care and the hospital set up. It can result in unseemly incidents which undermine the morale of all concerned. In particular, explanation, documentation and communication of the risk factors and percentage possibility for complications in an elective surgery would be the paramount, among other factors of care.

In emergency surgery an array of facilities to tackle most complications, and trained personnel like intensivist, or ICU in charge, residents and nurses exposed and tuned to intensive management of serious situations are easily available. The anesthetists and surgeons would be more likely to play a part in the pre-, intra-, and postoperative states, although it may not be a guarantee on account of their busy schedules and long hours of surgeries especially of the emergency nature.

In routine surgery this paraphernalia is more peripheral. It necessitates that some one person has to be overall in charge of a case, a contact point for all concerned. This is often either ignored or is never properly realized, resulting in fragmentation of the care as well as communication which can even turn or interpreted as contradictory as explained in Chap. 3.

6.2 The Social, Cultural, and Ethical Side

In the medical or hospital culture today, the tendency is to compartmentalize care and the responsibility of the consequences. The surgeons will say that surgery was without any complications or they have been taken care of; hence any complication that may develop is not their responsibility. The anesthetists will say that they have given back a patient stable and conscious; hence their responsibility is over.

Surgeons or the anesthetists do not seem to realize or deliberately want to deny the concrete fact that if the patient had a potential risk of a complication, it has got precipitated due to the surgical stress the patient has undergone and is still reeling under it, however smooth it may have been. It is not easy to bring this home to these powerful individuals, and the medical personnel who are not in a position to make others equally responsible are left to face the ire of the relatives. It is made to look as if the creation of the complication, however trivial or serious, is a doing of the medical management.

The gestalt of the human suffering as a whole and the responsibility to care for it as a whole, thus, has got divided in its parts, the value of which will always be less than the whole. This attitude among other consideration is also reflective of the social reality of narcissistic behavior brought about by the technology. It is immune to pain and indifferent to the suffering of those who is the cause for their service. This is compounded by the cryptic, jargonistic, condescending, or paternalistic explanations which have become the fashion of the day. The sense that the communication should lead to assuaging the fear, empowering patient and the others, to face the reality is not manifest.

There is a flip side to it also. It is to deliberately overstate the likelihood of all or any untoward happening that may result in the three perioperative periods and to scare everyone out of their wits. A legitimate question may be asked here. Should a technical scientific monograph of this nature indulge in clarifying these issues as well? This question if raised as an objection is not legitimate today. It is now long established that the entire medical milieu is deeply contexted in the social realities which should be taken care of by ethical and empowering communication, a matter rarely practiced properly. We have not raised these issues in the setting of the emergency surgical situations but here since the gravity of the situation in routine surgeries is far too serious.

A number of smaller issues that arise in this setting must also be discussed. It relates to eleventh hour cancellations, to unexpected hypoglycemia, and to routine instructions being issued without precision and clarity, leading to confusions, irritability, disappointments, loss of time, energy and money for the individual patients and his family, and so on. It is compounded by the fact that surgical theaters often find it difficult to observe the times for many reasons – legitimate and illegitimate. The concern for those suffering is lost in the self-satisfying egoistic explanations dished out to the patients offhand. The fact is that in most situations, there are no fixed protocols to establish clean instructions and mechanism to tackle the time deviations arising out of different situations. Most frequently unprofessional time management also compounds the miseries of those undergoing elective surgery.

6.3 The Technical Side of Elective Surgery

1. The medical/paramedical staff unless particularly trained have limited experience of treating diabetes. In the perioperative management of diabetes, the limitations will be more obvious. Advice given is often in an ad hoc fashion or piecemeal.

The primary limitation is lack of basic understanding of issues related to diabetes and its management. Put it differently—there is logic in all the branches of medicine, not just numerous unconnected million datum. It includes diabetes. The understanding of that logic or an effort to transfer it to all caregivers is not there. The professional is more and more unwilling to learn the logic, reluctant to coordinate and cooperate or are plain disorganized to effect better care.

2. Increasing the use of day care procedures or as early a discharge from hospital as possible has become the norm. To shorten the stay matters most; diabetes control is done on an outpatient basis. That in itself should be an invitation for greater and more coordination between surgeons and physicians.
3. Yet, situations where a patient is admitted under other exigencies and all investigations, therapeutics, controls, fitness scheduling are extracted in a hurry.
4. As a result of this, in most places the physicians are called in as an emergency rescuer to manage the blood glucose control in record time, expecting efficiency since the surgeon anesthetist team is in a hurry to get it over with.
5. Yet at other times if it is not convenient, no one listens to the physicians who try to explain the feasibility of taking a patient up for surgery, raising all kinds of objections under the cover that it is their final responsibility.
6. And as seen above, the moment complications develop, the physician is then to take care of it.
7. The shortening of stay or early discharge however is mainly for economic reasons. The hospitals want to increase the turnaround time, do more and more work in a hurry, and get as much more out of the waiting lists as possible. Insurance have added to these hasty attitudes.
8. It has resulted in discarding the ideas or rest, tranquility, stress reduction, familiarity with hospital atmosphere, rapport, and post-discharge periods.
9. Early and hasty discharges result in inadequate instructions to the patient and their caregivers for the management of diabetes. They are ill prepared for it. A detailed dialogue, answering their concerns and questions, may not happen. The way discharge is handled, the likelihood of readmission for either control or complications is frequent. Adequate medical support after discharge may not be available to the fullest degree.
10. In this hurry of reducing the turnover time, a long-standing malady of the indoor management has suffered even further. In this hurry of reducing the turnover time, an important care function - a properly written discharge summary of day care or admission has suffered even more. In India, the supportive staff of wards and ICUs under the consultants, majority consists of limited period round-the-clock graduates of alternate medicine which never really allows them to come to the grips of any patient issues in these two settings. Neither do they have an elementary knowledge of the logic of modern medicine. They know the pharmacology but hardly anything more of modern medicine.
11. It is these doctors who write the discharge summaries, and consultants go over it in hurry. Qualitatively they are poor. The situation is bound to worsen if the same has to be carried out for day care patients, as other major patient issues getting priority.

12. This analysis is not to say day care should be abandoned. It is to say that a mechanism has to be found to improve care. How it could be done is discussed in great detail in my volume of Reorganization of Public Health Care Delivery.

6.4 Need for a Framework to Operate

To avoid the unexpected and untoward outcomes in routine surgery particularly in diabetes, it would be fruitful to be aware of all the major and minor issues in this area. To do that certain clear guidelines about how to operate in these situations would go a long way. We have extensively made use of the guidelines developed by the Australian Diabetes Society [1]. These are both evidence based and experience based, not prescriptive but indicative; hence we found them to be the most useful for this volume.

In the management of the routine or elective surgeries, decisions are made relying on common sense, at times even arbitrarily. This is reflected in the guidelines which state that considerable body of advice given is not backed by adequate evidence. To expect that such clear-cut evidence-based advice could be available is not likely in the long run. At its best any guideline is merely a unanimous opinion of few experts [1].

More importantly these guidelines state the protocols developed by different countries would be suitable more for that country for the way their hospitals run. One cannot and is not expected to replace a guideline with another from somewhere else. Advice in other guidelines will need changes when applied at some other places. The overarching idea is to improve perioperative diabetes control and reduce complications in this period [1].

However, there is enough evidence now gathered, much of which has been presented in Chap. 3 and the first two chapters preceding it; it can be said that more definitive advice can be given which is much more than consensus, arbitrary, or just common sense. (Authors) A few caveats can easily be laid down in the light of such evidence.

These are primarily intended to assist many situations which are commonly prevalent in many South Eastern, Middle Eastern, and African Countries. (Author) Briefly these guidelines are also meant for:

1. Practitioners who do not have special training in diabetes but look after the patients with diabetes are in large numbers in these geographical areas. The guidelines could provide basic assistance to them.
2. These professionals who in majority of places have no backup for perioperative diabetes management in the form of a well-trained diabetes physician.

The authors also have adopted few of these guidelines to as simple stratified action plan as could serve many different areas in the developing world. Few points may be noted herein under:

1. Unless stated otherwise the following discussion applies to all routine, elective major surgeries or day care procedures or minor surgeries which may take longer than 2 h, in adults *and* in the nonpregnant state. In the elderly patients discussed under special surgical situation, these rules are more relaxed.
2. In all the three phases of routine operative setting better the control of hyperglycemia to as near normal as possible, the better it is. It prevents/reduces the risk of complications both in intra- and postoperative phases for people with diabetes. Given the evidence sited earlier and given below, a few more aspects in the context of routine surgery in diabetes will become clearer.
3. At places however the evidence is not obtainable. It will need management by common sense or consensus.
4. Preoperative clinical assessment and laboratory investigation as already detailed in Chap. 3 are the same for routine major surgery, except that here it can be undertaken more leisurely and adequate time is available to make corrections and document risk evaluation and communication with all concerned.
5. The quality of communication would also decide the frame of mind of the patients and their relatives with which further undertakings are expected to proceed more smoothly.

6.5 Admission for Routine Surgery

At the time of admission, the patient should bring all their diabetes and other medicines being taken for various reasons—hypertension, hyperlipidemia, coronary artery disease, anxiolytics, and so on—not just prescriptions. With 73,000 plus brands in the market, prescriptions alone do not tell the exact composition and ingredient concentration. This will facilitate the control preoperatively and resumption of the patient's usual and corrected therapy in as short a time as possible postoperatively. The treating physician then can use his experience to set or modify doses to gain good control of blood glucose and other parameters across 24 h.

The golden rule in diabetes control is the three Fs. Fix the Fasting First. Without this diabetes control is simply not possible. There are many subcutaneous insulin administration regimens detailed in Chap. 11. Experience in using them is necessary to fix the fasting and then the other hyperglycemic spikes associated with food intake. In routine or elective major surgery defined below, using insulin in one of these regimes is considered desirable, since it helps in controlling the high, normal, or even low glucose levels in all phases of surgery. It stands to reason that as good a control as possible should be attempted prior to admission and fine-tuned in the few days after admission so that homeostasis could also be achieved and a steady state is obtained. The handling of the oral medication during this period will be detailed per context at different places.

6.6 Twenty-Four-Hour Glucose Profile and Continuous Glucose Monitoring System

It is not infrequent to be ordered to control blood glucose in a short span for an admitted patient scheduled for surgery. In such situations both these techniques are extremely useful to control the blood glucose rapidly. Continuous glucose monitoring system (CGMS) is a costly and technologically intricate blood glucose control technique which the patient may take days to learn. It is usually applied to those patients whose insulin doses have to be carefully monitored and administered. Such patients usually have brittle diabetes with wide fluctuations in both directions with many other severe systemic disorders. The greatest utility of CGMS is in monitoring gestational diabetes, where tight control is the norm, since occasional hyperglycemia can also affect the fetus in a variety of ways. CGMS overall is applicable to a few patients who can afford it.

The 24-h blood glucose profiling is extremely low cost and technologically simple and therefore has universal applicability. It is a simplified modification of CGMS. The 24-h glucose profiling estimates blood glucose in states of fasting, post-breakfast, pre-lunch, post-lunch, if necessary at 5 or 6 p.m., pre- and post-dinner, and blood glucose at 3 a.m. This technique can be applied to any person with diabetes on any kind of dose regimen from simple OHAs to complex insulin regimens with or without OHAs. At one go these six or seven readings tell the glucose levels in periods that matter. The significance of each of the timings of monitoring is explained below.

The fasting is important since that is the first to be fixed.

Post-breakfast glucose is not done normally but if it is high, it is one of the most difficult glucose levels to control. Among the various reasons, the common one is a late breakfast. The other reason is the practice of taking medication including regular or premixed insulin before lunch and not at breakfast. The other issue is a relatively short interval between breakfast and lunch, common in India. In such cases the blood glucose rises due to this crowding, while the medicines are not able to exert their full potential a result of their pharmacokinetics. At times this interval becomes too long in patients who are not able to control their dietary timings. At times these are simply unavoidable situations and are legitimate. At other times it is simply carelessness. These are classic examples of drug diet mismatch.

The pre-lunch blood glucose is particularly important for those who complain of pre-lunch hypoglycemia. It also gives an idea of how the morning fasting doses should be modified to get a normal/acceptable post-lunch blood glucose level.

The post-lunch blood glucose is the standard way of monitoring. To remove any doubt about the timing, it should be done 2 h after beginning a meal. The rule holds for all prandial glucose estimations. In India oftentimes the lunch is the most major meal, and the pre-lunch hypoglycemia and the post-lunch hyperglycemia therefore are common and difficult to control and challenge the drug regime to be administered.

It was not then and still is not a practice to test pre-dinner and post-dinner blood glucose. About two decades back, no laboratories would be open at those times.

Today in spite of widespread availability and patient awareness about rapid assay glucose meters, it is still not done since it is not prescribed by the clinicians. With the rapid assay glucose meters, it is still a botheration to many. That is the reason why one would just not know how high these two blood glucose could go and the reasons why the fasting would never come under control.

The 3 a.m. blood glucose is likely to rise consequent to a high post-dinner level producing high fasting readings. This happens also because at this time, there is a surge of pituitary growth hormone which being an insulin antagonist will cause a further rise of blood glucose. Insulin secretion also tends to be lower during late evening and night.

Alternatively the blood glucose may fall on account of the medication at the nighttime. If that happens, then the Somogyi phenomenon comes in force with a surge of other counter regulatory hormones to push the fasting levels again high.

The 5 p.m. blood glucose has several significances. In India, the working conditions, travel back home, dietary habits, and in particular the OHA consumption peculiarly combine to create hypoglycemia at those hours. In the consulting rooms if probed, this becomes obvious indicating drug diet mismatch and calls of adjustments [2]. At times the pre-dinner blood glucose is found to be high but no care to adjust, particularly the pre-lunch administration as well as the morning administration of medication is taken. This is a direct consequence of the lack of insulin pharmacokinetics and pharmacodynamics of insulin as well as OHAs.

In such situations a short-term addition of regular insulin is given at 5 p.m. subcutaneously to control pre-dinner and hopefully post-dinner as well. If this additional insulin is being given, it becomes useful to know the level of blood glucose at the time of administration. If it is found to be high, modification of the medicines with altered pharmacokinetic properties may have to be done.

Before we go for a theoretical/hypothetical problem-solving, we need to understand a couple of things. Any blood glucose level is *not* controlled by the *immediately administered* dose of medication but by a dose prior to that. For example, high pre-lunch blood glucose can never be brought down by increasing pre-lunch regular insulin or OHAs taken pre-lunch. It is controlled by the morning pre-breakfast doses. A high post-lunch will therefore generally mean that the pre-breakfast dose is not able to control the pre-lunch and therefore not the post-lunch either.

The second principle is that before applying the 24-h blood glucose profiling, the dietary spacing must be properly done and implemented. In its absence, adjustment of doses and its timing with even the 24 h profiling is likely to fail. Then a complex regime will have to be invented where most of the medicines, particularly insulin would be short acting, would go for multiple insulin dosing with a basal long-acting insulin like glargine making the regimen costly and still leaving gaps in which the hypo/hyperglycemic seesaw continues to swing up and down.

In the example below, let us assume that the patient is taking his breakfast lunch and dinner at 8 a.m., 1 p.m., and 9 p.m., with some irregular snacking which is variable in timing and quantity.

Let us put him on the most ideal basal-bolus regimen of three regular insulin injections at a dosing schedule of 16, 12, and 10 U at 8 a.m., 1 p.m., and 9 p.m.

subcutaneously with basal long-acting insulin at bedtime of 20 U. The 24-h glucose profiling has given us the following readings:

Fasting: 190 mg	Post-breakfast: 270 mg
Pre-lunch: 125 mg	Post-lunch: 200 mg
5 p.m.: 85 mg	Pre-dinner: 140 mg
Post-dinner: 212 mg	3 a.m.: 190 mg

- Step 1—Fix the Fasting: Since the pre-dinner glucose is high, it will have to be brought under control by increasing the pre-lunch insulin dose from 12 to 16 U or more of insulin as well as increasing the long-acting basal insulin.
- Step 2—Since the post-dinner is also high and so is the fasting, it therefore stands to reason that the pre-dinner dose also should be aggressively increased to 20 U. This will not affect the 3 p.m. level since by that time, this rapid/short-acting insulin levels would have reduced, but the blood glucose post-dinner will be under control. The continued presence of basal insulin given in the night at bedtime will continue to exert its effect maximally, and the fasting will drop to a reasonably acceptable level. Alternatively a small dose of rapid/short-acting insulin at 5 p.m. would also solve the problem.
- Step 3—The moment the fasting comes down, and the dose administered at breakfast which is fairly substantial, 16 U of regular insulin, both pre-lunch and post-breakfast, will drop down to a reasonable level.
- Step 4—Since all blood glucose levels are on the higher side except 5 p.m., given the higher level of insulin resistance in the preoperative setting, a simultaneous increase in the basal dose of insulin from 20 to 25 or even 30 U subcutaneously will increase plasma level of basal insulin over long hours. This increase in the basal level of insulin will cause greater disposal of blood glucose to lower the average blood glucose level.

By the time a 24-h glucose profile is completed, we have been able to modify almost all the doses of insulin. Continued monitoring will guide us to fine-tune the dosing schedule. As more experience of glucose profiling accumulates, it is possible to modify an existing schedule without waiting for all the readings to appear. For example, a high fasting could dictate increased dose of basal as well as pre-dinner insulin in the morning itself; a high post-breakfast which is sure to result in high post-lunch can dictate an increase in pre-lunch insulin by two to four to six units. It is like an online real-time control. We will not discuss this further. Suffice it to say that the numerous variations of doses, types of insulins used and the native state of insulin resistance can be managed easily and control established within a short time with this technique.

RABBIT 2 surgery study treatment group was given glargine as the basal and glulisine as the bolus insulin before meals. It demonstrated that this combination improved glycemic control and reduced hospital complications compared with sliding scale insulin (SSI) in general surgery patients. It also concludes that a basal-bolus insulin regimen is preferred over SSI with type 2 diabetes [3]. This however will be costlier than less costly insulin formulations.

6.7 Glycosylated Hemoglobin Level and Fitness for Surgery

Glycosylated HbA_{1c} has emerged as an important prognostic factor in the long-term diabetes care. High levels of HbA1c have been shown to increase the severity and frequency of complications in numerous trials and benefits with reduction [4, 5].

In elective surgery interpretation of glycosylated hemoglobin levels is more academic or at best useful to indicate higher levels of tissue damage. HbA1C screening does allow identification of patients undiagnosed for diabetes till then. It assists in stratification of perioperative risk. However, waiting for it to come down with intensive diabetes control does not contribute to the outcome of the surgery, except delaying it when patient has been brought under control for the same.

Many professionals, including surgeons and anesthetists, place a great deal of concern about high levels of HbA1c which is a misplaced one in surgical setting. On one hand there is a no data to show that delaying elective surgery to correct HbA_{1c} is beneficial. Empirical reasoning also supports this. On the other hand, glycosylation is a chronic process which leads to many abnormalities at the cellular, tissue, or organ levels. Rigidly controlling it may or will prevent further damage as has been shown in DCCT [5]. But that does not guarantee reversal of the tissue damage resulting in structural modification that has already happened. It must also be mentioned that lowering HbA_{1C} in nonsurgical cases in an aggressive manner has not shown decreases in the mortality [6]. In short, once the required levels of glucose and blood pressure control are achieved, the elective as well as emergency surgery should proceed without waiting for the HbA1c to come down. This is discussed elsewhere also.

The variability of measurement of HbA_{1c} across the laboratories was a concern in the early 1990s. It would be reasonable to assume that in India even in 2018, the same or similar variance may still remain, emphasizing that in perioperative setting of any kind, its utility is quite limited. Clinicians should be reminded that the accuracy of HbA_{1C} across laboratories and different assay methods is not a given. Some thought should be given to situations which can vary the HbA_{1c} value like hemoglobinopathies, chronic bleeding, iron deficiency, anemia due to renal failure and recent transfusions, or ongoing hemolysis as well as frequent hypoglycemic episodes [7].

6.8 The Issue of Fitness for Surgery

The universally prevalent practice is to get fitness from the managing physicians who are completely ignorant about what happens and measures taken in the theater under anesthesia. The role of the physicians is to assist the anesthetist in the preoperative period and take over from him/her the postoperative management either in ICU or in the wards. He has already used his skills to prepare a patient by achieving as best levels as can be for all the parameters of risk and instituted therapeutic regimes to treat them with a view to prevent any complications. He continues to be of help to discuss issues for which anesthetists might want more clarification.

In such situations the anesthetist could consult the physician for the same. In case of some intractable difficulty during operation, the physicians could render further service from outside.

To our belief physicians giving fitness does not stand to reason. The authors believe that the question of fitness majorly concerns fitness for anesthesia. It includes the technical difficulties, detailed in the chapter on intraoperative management of anesthesia earlier. It is also about the management of existing complications which may exacerbate under anesthesia. While all the medications are chronically administered to protect or control such eventualities, no one can predict in an individual case what can happen under anesthesia. The best judge, as the authors believe and have so practiced, is the anesthetist to give fitness or express his concerns whether the anesthesia would be under high, moderate, or low risk.

The one area where anesthetists should become highly proficient is Therapeutic Techniques in all the fineries usable in continuous intravenous insulin. Physicians who routinely manage nonsurgical acute illnesses would always know a trick or two. Hence the issue of whose responsibility it is giving fitness is a matter of continuously participating in managing a patient, fitness being just a relative label.[1]

Each surgical facility should train their residents also to be able to take basic decisions about glucose management in all the three phases of surgery. The prevalence of diabetes, gestational diabetes, diabetic foot infections or cardiac diseases is high and rising. At least 25% of people with diabetes undergo surgeries in their life time. Training for better perioperative management for such huge numbers becomes a necessary part of medical education. The lengthy chapter at the beginning will give them the insight of how to manage diabetes to a substantial extent on their own.

6.9 Scheduling Surgery for a Person with Diabetes

6.9.1 The Day Prior to the Surgery

Once all the doses of the medications necessary including insulin are fixed and good control of all parameters is achieved, the same should be continued till the day/night prior to surgery for all those whose surgeries have been scheduled in the morning. In the absence of significant renal disease, attention should particularly be given to hydration. In India and probably in many other countries, the water drinking habits of patients are indifferent; hence this precaution is all the more necessary. It has numerous physiological advantages, and a well-hydrated patient can avoid unforeseen consequences better under the surgical procedures. In case of anxiety-prone patient, there is no harm to give a small dose of anxiolytic for a few days prior to surgery. It helps a great deal. Giving it just a day prior may not give as much benefit as starting it a few days earlier will give for pharmacokinetic and pharmacodynamic reasons.

[1] An aphorism used by one of the authors is no patient is unfit for anesthesia unless dead. He is only at a higher risk.

If a person with diabetes is to be operated, it is better to put him first on the list both for the major surgery or a day care procedure. It will reduce the glucose level variations to the minimum. The control is then easier. The reason is the minimization of the duration of the fasting. It will prevent the excessive hepatic glucose output, catabolism, and insulin resistance. It mimics the daily routine. Adjusting the duration for fasting in a backward manner is also easier if it is the first case. The surgeon and anesthetist decide how many hours prior to surgery the patient should be fasting. It is generally about 6 h for solid food intake. This however may be required to be much longer if a patient has diabetic gastroparesis. It can easily extend to 8–12 h, particularly if general anesthesia is to be given for fear of vomiting and aspiration. As is discussed below, these patients can be managed more easily with monitoring, on the day of surgery. Depending upon the morning blood glucose, insulin or glucose with insulin infusion can be started till the patient is taken up for surgery.

6.9.2 Day of Major Elective Surgery: The Morning List

Omit usual morning insulin and OHAs. If all the doses for the concomitant illnesses are taken in the night before, like antihypertensives, no drug administration for any other medicine is needed. A fasting glucose done in the morning of surgery will decide the preoperative action for instituting the type of infusion and fix the dose of insulin with it. The various possibilities relating to this situation are discussed below.

6.9.3 The Fasting Blood Glucose

The fasting blood glucose preoperatively should be in the range of less than 140 mg or 110–126 mg/dL. This is a goal that can be achieved by admitting the patient a few days earlier to surgery or on an outpatient basis. This level of blood glucose however may be accompanied by transient episodes of mild hypoglycemia in days prior to surgery which is more easily detectable in the ward setting prior to surgery, and dose adjustment could be done adequately.

If the morning fasting is within the acceptable range and if the patient is taken up early, no action is needed. If such a patient is going to be taken up in the morning after 10 a.m., then an insulin-glucose infusion a couple of hours prior to induction would help prevent starvation ketosis and fasting hypo- or hyperglycemia as discussed below.

6.9.4 Variations on the Morning of Surgery: Fasting Hyperglycemia

On the day of surgery 6 a.m., fasting blood glucose could be unexpectedly higher than acceptable in a patient who has been under excellent control. The anxiety-induced stress or the fasting having got prolonged or missing the night doses or reduced doses of the same or would be the causes. In diabetes it happens since hepatic glucose output increases in the fasting state. Instead of handling this situation by many easy ways, this often becomes the reason to cancel or postpone surgery causing great difficulties to all concerned. There is nothing alarming in the situation to cancel surgeries. In a given situation if the surgery is scheduled first and is to start around 9 a.m., an infusion of 2 or 3 U of insulin per 100 mL in normal saline per hour from 6 a.m. will bring it down by the time the patient is shifted for surgery.

6.9.5 Fasting Hypoglycemia

Low fasting blood glucose below 80 or 70 mg/dL on the day of the operation also should not cause panic, and *hasty overdone efforts to correct this* should not be undertaken. Such efforts will undoubtedly bring about hyperglycemia which in its turn cannot be lowered within a couple of hours leading to the cancellation of surgery. One may be concerned with hypoglycemia but that does not give a license to *aggressive* counter effort to correct it. The simple measure is to start a slow 5% dextrose normal saline drip at 50–100 mL/h, check the glucose and add a few units of insulin to the remaining glucose, and make a preoperative check before shifting. By definition the diagnosis of hypoglycemia *must be accompanied by the symptoms of the same* with blood glucose lower than 60 mg/dL. Secondly, such hypoglycemia is extremely common when the patient is under insulin therapy. On the night before the surgery, the patient out of anxiety may not eat adequately.

Whether the surgery is major or minor, defined later below, these instructions will be applicable to both in the morning schedule.

6.9.6 Surgery Scheduled in the Afternoon

Afternoon procedures pose the following difficulties for all patients with diabetes. The longer the duration of fasting, the greater will be the episodes of low or higher blood glucose readings. In case of an infected foot surgery or any other open infection surgery, it is a common practice in India to schedule it later in the afternoon to enable fumigation of the theater after that. Such patients should be instructed to stop taking anything by mouth from 10 a.m. after the usual breakfast.

If the fasting glucose is within limits, the usual insulin taken by the patient can be administered subcutaneously, often in a dose reduced by 20%. Alternatively, depending upon the fasting level and the subsequent fasting state, a small dose of crystalline insulin with 50% of the usual dose of intermediate-acting insulin can also be given. There is neither a hard and fast rule nor a fixed protocol as to what should be given and how much. Since the patient is in controlled conditions and to avoid confusions, in India one could give the same insulin with a reduction as thought appropriate, continuing to monitor glucose every 2 h and deal with the situation.

These steps will prevent both undue hyperglycemia and hypoglycemia during the time he is fasting. A 2–3 hourly blood glucose monitoring will suffice to indicate the movement of glucose level in either direction. It can be taken care of by starting an appropriate infusion described above in the morning schedule of the surgery.

It is becoming a common practice even in India for the patient to arrive in the morning for an afternoon surgery or for a day care procedure. Yet the time maintenance and following up on all the instructions could be undependable. This must be kept in mind.

If the patient is on regular insulin in a basal-bolus regimen where the basal has been taken in the night, or if he is on premixed insulin regime twice a day, in the preoperative control period, he may remain stable on fasting glucose level on the day of surgery. Two hourly glucose monitoring will indicate when to start appropriate insulin-glucose saline infusion. The rate can be decided by the blood glucose level. In surgical theaters in India, time management is difficult generally due to heavy load of surgical patients. This particular infusion will keep the glucose in balance during the waiting period. Pre-intubation blood glucose is routine if the intubation in such patients gets delayed.

The trend to replace the oral antidiabetic drugs being replaced by insulin several days prior to and after the surgery is decreasing because of decrease in the time of postoperative fasting. This has come about due to increased sophistication of techniques in surgery and anesthesia. Hence discontinuation of oral antidiabetic drugs on the morning of surgery generally serves the purpose.

The major or minor surgery needs to be defined. These instructions will be applicable to both in the afternoon schedule.

6.9.7 Postponing an Elective Surgery

In attempts to reduce the hospital stay and expenses, the preoperative control is attempted by the physicians on an outpatient basis, over a week or even more. It works in most cases and the patient is admitted the day before. At times the glucose control may be found erratic or the blood glucose levels highly unsatisfactory. In such situations it is wise to postpone the surgery and keep the patient in the wards for a few days to gain control, and then such a case can be rescheduled.

In case of patients who are on verge of DKA or extremely high blood glucose and should the surgical condition demands immediate operation, the protocols laid down in Chap. 3 should be followed. If the surgical condition can wait for a couple of days, such a patient should be admitted and controlled before taking him up for surgery.

In the literature suggestions have been found to postpone the surgeries if the blood glucose is in the vicinity of 500 mg/dL. This is too lenient a level which is quite unacceptable. Levels lower than this also should be included for cancellation. The patient should then be admitted and controlled and surgery undertaken as soon as possible.

Postponement in patients already admitted who are otherwise controlled may show variation in the morning blood glucose should *not* be postponed as described earlier above.

6.10 A Word About Major and Minor Elective Surgery

The working idea of which is a major and which is a minor surgery is geared toward indicating the complexities of the management in the setting of diabetes as the main confounding factor. So-called minor surgeries are defined here as those after which the patient resumes oral intake within a few hours. Minor surgeries do not pose a major problem as far as glycemic management is concerned and may be managed with OHAs or small doses of subcutaneous insulin for a day or 2.

The simplest definition that can be offered for major surgery is one in which the patient is expected to remain "nothing by mouth" for 24 h or more after the surgery, be it elective or emergency. The "major" surgeries like major abdominal, cardiothoracic, vascular, neurosurgeries, transplants, etc. require close monitoring and glycemic management protocols for an extended period pre- and postoperatively. The complexity it indicates is that of intravenous management of fluids, calories, insulin infusion, and control of blood glucose among other parts of care for 24–96 h or more before full food intake, and earlier regimens which kept the patient controlled are satisfactorily instituted. Ideally this type of care should get extended even in elective surgery. Patients undergoing major surgery in addition could have other serious comorbid conditions, requiring additional management in this period. It calls for closer care, skills, and competence derived from experience and admission for a few days after the surgery.

However, both categories of patients require thorough preoperative evaluation and workup as discussed in detail in Chap. 3 in this volume.

Australian Diabetes Society Guidelines 2012 add to the above that if a day procedure takes more than 4 h of surgical time, then in that context it should be treated as major surgical case [1].

6.10.1 Day Care Procedure

On the other hand, all day care procedures, any surgery which is followed by Nil by Mouth for only a few hours, from diabetes point of view are considered minor. The reasons are obvious. A patient has been under control and has his medication for diabetes, and for other comorbid conditions optimized as best as can be, he starts taking food orally within a few hours and is then back to his routine. This makes the diabetes and other conditions' management little intensive for but a few hours. Such patients are either discharged on the same day or may remain only few days with simple routine ward care and administration of medicine. Thus a hip replacement could be considered minor and a carbuncle with septicemia will become a major case.

6.10.2 Patients on Diet Alone

In India such patients should be as carefully investigated as those on insulin. Such claims of being under control on diet alone are likely to be patient belief than the reality of being totally out of control. Investigations like HbA1c will bust the myth of control. More detailed investigations are not likely to reveal the tissue damage and level of complications, preoperatively. The record of quasi normal blood glucose readings against a high HbA1c performed in standard laboratory will clearly indicate that substantially uncontrolled diabetes and the likely systemic complications and tissue damage are present. The heart and the kidneys would be the predominant features, but one or many others could also be present and may complicate the intra- and perioperative phase by untoward happening.

In such claims the concerned persons must be told about the gravity of the situation.

A genuine case of good control will come to fore with HbA1c well below 6.5% [1]. In such cases the management during preoperative phase will consist of all the methods described above, be it minor surgery or major. Possibly the glucose estimation may have to be conducted more often. The caveat is that if hyperglycemia does surface, it should be treated with regular or short-acting insulins in small dose or during the stage of Nil by Mouth by an IV infusion of insulin with or without glucose as the case may be. Oral antidiabetic agents have no place in this management. Later on after postoperative recovery, such a patient may be shifted to appropriate drug regimen.

6.10.3 Patients on Oral Hypoglycemic Agent (OHA) Medication (Without Insulin) in Elective Major Surgery

1. Management if the level of diabetes control on one or more OHAs is satisfactory.

   All classes of oral antidiabetic and all drugs within each class of oral antidiabetic drugs can be safely continued till the night prior to surgery. Injectable medicines like GLP-1 agonists such as exenatide or liraglutide can be continued up to the night prior to surgery.

   All these are to be stopped on the morning of surgery. It applies to patients placed on the morning or afternoon list. The fasting glucose check on the morning of surgery should dictate the management of glucose as discussed extensively above.
2. Management if the level of diabetes control on one or more OHAs is not satisfactory.

   Such patients will have to be admitted and should be put on any system of monitoring and insulin regime the treating physician is comfortable with to achieve good control of fasting and postprandial glucose levels. On the day of the surgery, all the OHAs and GLP 1 agonists will be stopped as above. The fasting blood glucose will decide the infusion type in the morning list. The night dose of insulin prior to the day of surgery can be safely used.

For surgery scheduled for the afternoon, breakfast should be given at 8 a.m. The monitoring and management should proceed as described in the Sect. 6.9.6 Surgery Scheduled in the Afternoon. These rules will hold for minor surgeries as well.

6.11 Ancillary Ward Procedures and Glucose Control

6.11.1 Bowel Preparation

Bowel preparation is undertaken preprocedurally or a day prior to surgery. Hence it stands to reason to admit these patients for the same. Colonoscopy and bowel surgery both need a clean roughage-free bowel. It is helped by drinking clear fluids for a minimum of 1 day before the surgery or the procedure. Bowel preparation could be lengthy and exhausting. The clear fluids, liberally administered (and made tasteful), must contain glucose to avoid hypoglycemia as well as to maintain good hydration, since regular food is discontinued. With frequent small glucose ingestions therein with the sulfonylurea, oral hypoglycemic drugs will precipitate severe hypoglycemia; hence the latter should be discontinued. The blood glucose measurements should be carried out at least four times and fasting around the usual lunch time, in the evening around 5 p.m., and later in the night. The best way to manage the glycemic excursion probably is the use of regular insulin in small doses, to be modified according to the readings, at 6 a.m., 12 noon, 6 p.m., and 12 midnight at these times.

The regular insulin works for 6 h. By the regime mentioned above, there will be no period which is without adequate levels of insulin in plasma. Short-acting insulin administration is not recommended as it will leave the patient with intermittent periods of low plasma insulin levels leading to hyperglycemic excursions, leading to the common occurrence of chasing blood glucose which is not desirable. It is unpredictable whether the beta cells will secrete insulin in these low insulin-level periods; hence regular insulin for four times is the best way to manage.

Patients on clear liquids will have reduced intake of carbohydrates. As a result, the insulin needs to be given in smaller doses. It may be considered desirable to temporarily stop the ongoing regimen since it is likely to contain intermediate- and long-acting insulin which would be more potent than regular insulin in precipitating hypoglycemia during bowel preparation. Thus instead of going for a flat reduction of 20% or 50% of all doses, four times insulin regime is easier to modify and is self-limiting in time, and the preceding doses with subsequent glucose levels can easily decide the next doses.

6.11.2 Alternate Insulin Regimens for Presurgical Procedures [1]

1. In basal-bolus regimens, a total of four injections are required. This can be continued till the night prior to surgery. On the day of surgery, a single shot of intermediate-acting insulin can be enough. This dose is calculated by adding

three bolus insulin doses the patient is on. Fifty percent of this dose is then given as intermediate-acting insulin in the morning of surgery. Importantly the nighttime intermediate-acting insulin dose is not required to be changed and can remain the same.

2. As an alternate method, the bolus doses with single ingredient of rapid-acting insulin, irrespective of the number of doses, can be reduced to half. The component of the intermediate- or long-acting insulin is given in a dose two thirds of the original.
3. Many patients are on short-acting insulin with intermediate-acting insulin in the morning as well as in the evening. The short-acting insulin dose is excluded, and only the intermediate-acting insulin is given in the same dose as before.
4. Patients on premixed fixed insulin dose combination can decrease all the doses by half without changing the earlier time schedule.
5. A combination of either a nighttime or a morning glargine with short- or rapid-acting insulin with each major meal is a common regime. In such cases the simple way is to continue glargine at the same dose and the same time and stop all short-acting insulins.
6. Twice a day premixed insulin preparations are common and convenient hence may have higher compliance. In Indian conditions however these regimens at home may turn out to be a little more unstable since more frequent BGL monitoring is essential. Similarly those already having unstable glycemic control will find it more difficult to understand reduction to 50% of doses and glucose levels and how they should respond to adjusting the dose. Giving advice on phone may be difficult to give and for the patient to understand. Hence the best way is to admit the patient with a laxative if permitted in the night prior and asked to come to the hospital early.
7. The patients who are on high insulin doses or those with poor glycemic control should be admitted. This should be done as or before the bowel preparation with the ingestion of clear liquids begins. The effective way to control them is to shift to an IV insulin-glucose route, frequent monitoring which should be dictated by the blood glucose and followed by change in the doses.

6.11.3 Radiological Procedures [1]

Similar to those undergoing minor surgery, patients with diabetes who undergo radiological procedures also need to fast prior. If the time of the procedure is in the afternoon or later, 4-h fasting is adequate for most procedures. Morning procedures can be covered by overnight fast. All antidiabetic drugs should be withheld on the day of procedure. IV infusion of insulin doses can be started and modified as discussed earlier if glucose level goes higher. Once the procedure is over and normal diet is resumed, the corresponding oral drugs can be started if the surgery is not imminent or on the very next day. In such cases insulin infusions with glucose saline or subcutaneous insulin from any of the above regimens described under bowel preparation may be continued as per the comfort of the clinician, capacity of the care level in wards, and above all by his discretion.

Sestamibi scans are undertaken to assess coronary artery disease status. It is done at rest and then as a stress study. Together it becomes a lengthy procedure. Hence to avoid the prolonged fasting, the two studies should be done on separate days. For any procedure performed later in the day or afternoon, the glucose control will be done as per the discussion on minor surgery in the afternoon. In particular in patients whose diabetes control is fluctuating, the stress sestamibi study should be performed *within a hospital* having a nuclear medicine unit. The reason for it is to keep the glucose control as optimal as possible using insulin-glucose drips which is easy to organize in hospital setting.

Positron emission tomography (PET) scans use the radio-isotope fluorine-18-fluorodeoxyglucose (FDG.) Acute hyperglycemia and insulin therapy in patients with diabetes during the procedure can interfere with the uptake of FDG in those areas which are being investigated [8–10]. Obviously any patient with diabetes should have a stable control that is an important aspect of the PET procedure.

In radiological procedures, there is a strong common electromagnetic interference. The insulin pumps and continuous glucose monitoring devices have sensors, transmitters, and remote control devices. These are designed to remain unaffected by the electromagnetic fields. Precaution should still be taken so that such equipment is not exposed to this strong field. These equipments however must be removed when a patient is undergoing X-rays, MRIs, and CT scans. It can be done immediately before the patient enters a room which has this kind of equipment/machines.

6.11.4 Logistics of Handling Such Procedures Efficiently

In India the ward staffs and doctors also are not told sufficiently early the exact time of any procedure. They face considerable commonly encountered difficulties like shifting the patient at short notice; if the procedure time gets delayed as often happens, monitoring glucose again; making changes in diabetes and other medicines in a planned manner, feeding/keeping the patient nil by mouth ahead of time of the procedure, insulin dose adjustments, or withholding or reducing/stopping insulin injections to avoid hypoglycemia. Timely communication both ways would be of great help to avoid glucose swings.

To avoid hypoglycemia especially in delayed radiological procedures, it is advisable to start glucose saline infusion at low rates with blood glucose monitoring hourly and insulin added to the infusion if necessary. For calculation of such additions, see the note on Sect. 1.8.

6.12 Metformin in Minor Surgeries and Ward Procedures (ADS, 2012, Abridged and Adapted)

If there is one drug that every treating physician should attempt to continue in glucose management, in above situations as well as major surgery, it is metformin. It need not be stopped for minor surgery. The Indian experience with both metformin and earlier biguanides is long, deep, and satisfactory. Robert Tattersall many years ago regretted that biguanides were removed from therapy. Metformin has the best potential for increasing insulin sensitivity among its other actions which consequently reduces the insulin doses required for control. The main issues related to metformin in surgery and ward procedures including those investigations using radio contrast are briefly summarized below. The central consideration and the common factor in all the issues around surgery or procedures to which, the discontinuity or resumption of metformin is tied up, are the existing renal failure which may worsen. If that is not to happen, resumption of metformin is a given.

1. Continued ingestion of metformin over long periods will help keep the glucose control well within the bounds. If it is discontinued many days prior to surgery or long procedures, it will lead to hyperglycemia. Hence it should be continued as long as possible before surgery. That is to say—till the night before surgery or on the day of major surgery. Postoperatively it should be restarted with oral intake getting established.
2. Stopping metformin the night before a major surgery is a common practice. How long it should be withheld after surgery or whether withholding it before major surgery is not supported by adequate studies.
3. Under the stress of surgery with accompanying hemodynamic metabolic changes, it is often likely that the creatinine level goes higher. In that case or if there were hypotensive episodes during surgery either due to blood loss, sepsis, lability of signs of myocardial ischemia, or anesthetic agents, metformin must be withheld to avoid postoperative lactic acidosis. Once all these parameters settle down and creatinine rises back to its preoperative levels, metformin then can be resumed when oral intake also gets reestablished. If serum creatinine level does not deteriorate postoperatively, it can be resumed with adequate oral intake. Otherwise it will contribute to the development of lactic acidosis [11–13]. Metformin should in particular be withheld before surgery in the presence of sepsis or ischemic heart disease.
4. The anxiety over the development of lactic acidosis if metformin is used is not at all well founded. No doubt the mortality associated with lactic acidosis is unacceptably high. Nearly half such patients will die. But only 0.03 patients per 1000 patient years develop lactic acidosis associated with administration of metformin [14].

Similar anxiety is present when radiocontrast materials are used. If the kidney function is normal, the possibility of developing lactic acidosis is low.

6.12.1 Metformin and Intravenous Radio Contrast

5. Metformin does not worsen renal function. This issue of development of lactic acidosis arises nearly exclusively if the kidney function has already deteriorated to a significant level and metformin is continued. Injecting a radio contrast for investigation will worsen it [15].

6. This assumes significance in its continuation or otherwise during radiological procedures requiring injection of contrast media, particularly in diabetes. Deterioration in the renal status is not uncommon after radiocontrast, especially if the patient is not specifically hydrated before.
7. As said above, metformin is related to higher risk of lactic acidosis in patients already having a markedly deteriorated kidney function. Serum creatinine should be checked pre-procedurally as well as post-procedurally, when intravenous radio contrast is going to be injected. The decision to restart or withhold metformin should be taken after that. Contrarily contrast media injection may precipitate renal failure with subsequent lactic acidosis in patients taking metformin [16–18]. Most radiologists prefer and advice stopping metformin 24–48 h before the procedure time and 48 h after the procedure. These are precautionary practices. Adequate backing by controlled studies is not available for these practices.

Intraoperative management in minor or major elective surgery or procedures follows the same lines as any other described above.

Anesthesia requirements in various routine surgical procedures in diabetic patients can be divided as follows:

1. Diabetic foot surgery.
2. General surgical operations like hernia, hydrocoele, appendicectomy, operations on the lower limbs, etc.
3. Gynecological and obstetrical operations including cesarean section.
4. Head and neck, thoracoabdominal operations.
5. Operations exceeding 4–5 h.
6. Operations in positions other than supine position.

Operations in groups 1, 2, and 3 can be done under regional anesthesia, while operations in groups 4, 5, and 6 will preferably need general anesthesia. Of course, some of the smaller operations can be done under regional anesthesia.

Postoperatively in elective minor surgery or investigative procedures, the therapeutic modality which kept the patient under good glycemic control should be restarted once full oral intake is resumed. Restarting metformin is discussed above. In elective surgeries the blood glucose range could be lower, that is, between 100 and 140 mg/dL postoperatively. In emergency surgery glucose level should be maintained from 140 to 180 mg/dL. In older patients with comorbidities it should be higher than mentioned above especially after emergency surgery.

6.13 Oral Hypoglycemic Drugs

Since these patients are much more likely to go back on their oral hypoglycemic drugs far more frequently, this section will briefly describe the mechanisms of action of these agents.

Sulfonylurea group of drugs, the secretagogues, increases insulin secretion in response to hyperglycemia. Repaglinide and nateglinide, the non-SUs, bind to a sub-unit of SUR 1 receptor and also have the same action but differ markedly from other SUs. Insulin sensitizers like metformin and thiazolidinediones reduce peripheral resistance to insulin which results in more effective actions of available native insulin. Alpha-glucosidase inhibitors interfere with conversion of oligosaccharides in glucose delaying the glucose absorption. Newer class of gliptines prolongs the actions of GLP 1 and causes greater secretion of insulin and increase beta cell mass to some extent. Injectable GLP 1 analogues in addition to these gliptines actions also cause satiety and weight loss as a result.

6.13.1 Mechanism of Action of All Sulfonylureas

All sulfonylureas bind to the its receptor sulfonylurea receptor 1 (SUR 1,) at slightly different sites but all of which results in K-ATP channel closure, and rise in the intracellular potassium and opening of calcium channels with calcium influx in the beta cell. Intracellular calcium is mobilized, the cell depolarizes, and it results in insulin secretion. It is the properties of individual SUs that decide the usage.

Presently the most used SUs are glimepiride, gliclazide, and glibenclamide. Older drugs like Glipizide, its extended release formulation and chlorpropamide have nearly gone out of use. The latter has many undesirable side effects. Glibenclamide has the highest proportion of severe hypoglycemia which after the first 2–3 years of its usage declines as the drug is less and less effective ([19] p. 687–698).

6.13.2 Glimepiride

Glimepiride binds to the SUR threefold faster and dissociates from the receptor nine times faster than glibenclamide and hence produces quicker insulin release of shorter duration. It does not restore the first-phase insulin release (no sulfonylureas do) but increases the second-phase insulin secretion and whole body glucose uptake, increases insulin sensitivity, gives better fasting glucose levels, and has lesser documented hypoglycemia compared to glibenclamide ([19] p. 695). It could be due to 2 to 3 hours the drug takes to reach peak levels. The dose range is 1–8 mg/day, average dose being 1–4 mg, once. However in clinical practice, it is used as 2 mg twice a day 12 h apart.

6.13.3 Gliclazide

Gliclazide is extensively metabolized in the liver to inactive metabolites. It has a short-duration action and is generally given twice in a varying dose range from 40, 60, to 80 mg. Modified-release gliclazide has a hydrophilic matrix that results in progressive delivery of short-acting gliclazide and needs nearly half the dose ([19] p. 695).

6.13.4 Repaglinide and Nateglinide

Repaglinide has its own binding site in the SUR 1 but still closes K-ATP channels. Like SUs it does not directly stimulates insulin exocytosis. It is rapidly absorbed in 45 min, and its plasma levels return to baseline in 3–4 h. The insulin-releasing action starts in 30 min, the effect subsiding in 3–4 h. This is a useful property exploited by clinicians to use it in people who find it difficult to maintain meal timings. If a meal is skipped, repaglinide need not be taken. Despite its short action, it also controls the fasting glucose. The magnitude of hypoglycemic episodes is much lower than glibenclamide. The other member nateglinide also has similar properties but a much large dose of 120 mg/day compared to 0.5–4 mg of repaglinide.

6.13.5 Insulin Sensitizers

The metabolic syndrome of obesity, hyperinsulinemia, insulin resistance, PCOD, increased cardiovascular risk, and dyslipidemia has at its root high level of insulin resistance. The importance of reducing insulin resistance or increasing its sensitivity can therefore be easily understood in both the complications arising and longer indigenous insulin secretion which has its own importance. The principal drugs in this category are the metformin and thiazolidinediones.

6.13.6 Metformin

Individuals with impaired glucose tolerance (IGT) are the most vulnerable group to develop diabetes over the next 5–10 years. This is a group suitable for diabetes prevention programs. Metformin with its anorectic effects causes a mean weight loss of 2–3, which is not seen in any other oral drugs. It prevents or postpones the onset of diabetes in IGT group. The percentage postponement is about 30%. It reduces the abdominal fat tissue. By reducing the hepatic insulin resistance, it reduces the hepatic glucose output substantially. Excess of hepatic glucose output is a putative abnormality in type 2 diabetes. It also decreases the plasminogen activator inhibitor 1 (PAI 1.) It accelerates intravascular fibrinolysis and prevents to an extent progression of the same. Diabetes among other situations is also a hypercoagulable state ([19] p. 695).

The usual dose of metformin is 500–1000 mg twice daily. It does not accumulate in the body and as monotherapy has very little hypoglycemic potential. The newer extended-release preparations appear to be more suitable and with less side effects as the drug plasma levels peak after 4 h and are less by 20% compared to the short-acting varieties. The maximum effects of metformin are found with doses from 1750 to 2000 mg/day.

To avoid the gastrointestinal effects of anorexia, nausea, and abdominal or occasional diarrhea which are transient, it should be used with (preferably the major) meals, starting with smaller doses which are later increased to the limits of tolerance. In these days of combined pills era, it is often given with breakfast which is a minor meal. This does not result in glucose control postprandially. (The innumerable combination drugs invading the market has created multiple anomalies on vast scale in practice of medicine. These are extensively discussed in the first author's monograph on India's Private Health-Care Delivery: Policies for Universal Health Care). Fortunately majority of irrational combinations are now banned by the GoI including those of oral hypoglycemic drugs. The authors unequivocally oppose combination therapies and also believe that prescriptions should be generic in essence with or without the brand names.

Lactic acidosis can occur only if it is used in renal insufficiency. Otherwise it is practically unknown, 3/100,000 patient years ([19] p. 698). Thirty percent of patients on long-term metformin will develop vitamin B 12 deficiencies which should be treated probably with injectable vitamin B 12. The evidence of adverse cardiovascular events is debatable, mostly on account of study designs [19].

6.13.7 Thiazolidinediones

Only two drugs in this class are available, rosiglitazone as 4–8 mg/day and pioglitazone 15–45 mg/day. They act by binding with PPAR gamma receptors which then binds to many nuclear sites, coding many proteins and stimulating the formation of those enzymes involved in glucose metabolism. Insulin sensitivity increases both in muscles and in adipose tissues. The most striking of their effects which were seen in India after their introduction was their potential for increasing the insulin sensitivity to a degree where it was considered to be a certain solution to postponing insulin administration and or withdrawal of the same. The converse of withdrawing these two drugs would lead to a dramatic increase in the blood glucose levels. These drugs also improve dyslipidemia, consistently increase HDL cholesterol, reduce triglycerides, decrease PAI 1 levels (see above in metformin), reduce rates of urinary albumin excretion, and also probably preserve the beta cell mass and apoptosis of beta cells.

The initial enthusiasm started dying when large weight gains of 10–15 kg became apparent in more than would be expected and the use declined among the specialists of diabetes. The weight gain was due to two actions of thiazolidinediones. One was water retention. The other was excessive fat deposition especially over the shoulder areas. It was later found to have potential to produce congestive cardiac failure. Neither the edema nor was weight gain amenable to any treatment. These effects appear to be more frequent in Indians, which probably led to a government action forbidding high-dose glitazone use. Pioglitazone at 7.5 mg/day continues to be prescribed.[2]

[2] In the last 10 years of the practice of first author, there was a hardly a patient with type 2 diabetes who had gained more than 10 kg of weight who was not on pioglitazone with frank edema. Many could relate the weight gain to the beginning of glitazones.

6.13.8 Alpha-Glucosidase Inhibitors

Alpha-glucosidase inhibitors (acarbose 25–50 mg with each meal or voglibose with each meal, (see below)) act by competitively binding this enzyme at 10^4 times more than glucose and prevent the hydrolysis of oligosaccharides (partially digested complex carbohydrates by the salivary ptyalin) to form glucose, reducing the glucose absorption helping to reduce prandial glycemic excursions. It also inhibits the pancreatic amylase which also digests the starch. Miglitol does not inhibit pancreatic amylase but, unlike the other two, interferes a little with glucose absorption also.

Most of its actions take place in the upper ileal region. Lesser quantum of oligosaccharides thus reaches the lower ileal region. This region has less oligosaccharidases leaving the undigested ones that are passed to the colon where many other substances are created out of them like short-chain fatty acids, methane, and hydrogen.

The treatment must start with low doses and gradually increased, beginning with evening meal, increasing over 2 weeks to the other two meals one after another. These doses may be doubled after several weeks, one meal at a time. If gastrointestinal side effects appear, the doses should be reduced and started with earlier smaller doses.

These drugs are effective in the treatment of severe hypoglycemia after major bowel surgery and in reactive hypoglycemia. Given to type 1 diabetic patients with the evening meal, it is effective in preventing severe nocturnal hypoglycemia.

The therapeutic modality used nowadays is simultaneous use of drugs with different mechanisms of action in submaximal doses. There is no significant difference of actions in any drug between submaximal and maximal doses. Instead of stepwise approach as was prevalent earlier, using different drugs correcting different defects will give better results. However as mentioned earlier, giving a combination of more or at least two drugs is not the way. Type 2 diabetes is caused by multiple mechanisms, and each should be taken care of for the best glycemic control.

6.14 Drugs Used for Comorbidities

6.14.1 Hypertension

Angiotensin-converting enzyme inhibitors are the drugs of choice for controlling hypertension. While tight control per guidelines would be beneficial to younger patients, the blood pressure control as well as the glucose control should be much more relaxed in elderly patients. Mortality increases with targets brought nearer to tight control as has been shown by several trials mentioned elsewhere.

Enalapril and ramipril are the most commonly used ones generally 5 mg twice a day. Enalapril is much cheaper and is included in the National List of essential Medicines. Fifteen percent of patients get dry irritating cough which does not get under control unless enalapril is discontinued. Ramipril does not have this side effect but has costs added. This class of drugs increases serum creatinine levels in higher doses by about 30% which must be taken in consideration while changing/increasing the doses. These drugs should be discontinued before pregnancy is contemplated since they produce fetal anomalies. If the creatinine level rises above 3 mg/dL in other situations, these drugs should be discontinued.

These drugs also cause hyperkalemia and hence should not be used with potassium-sparing diuretics. It may be a sound clinical practice to check potassium every time blood is tested either for creatinine or for some other investigation. The hyperkalemia is clinically not dangerous in most situations, but that does not mean it should not be checked frequently and not treated vigorously. Discontinuation of the potassium-sparing diuretics and use of loop diuretics like frusemide will correct it well. In case of irrepressible hyperkalemia, 20 mg of salbutamol sulfate is grounded and used as inhalation by intensive care physicians. It is quite effective.

There are a number of molecules in the class of angiotensin receptor blockers (ARBs) which are more ubiquitous in action and have the same mechanism of action as the ACEs and have the same contraindications. Some of them are associated with weight loss. They do not have the side effect of producing irritating cough as in enalapril. They can be combined with ACEs but are more costly for long-term use.

6.14.2 Other Antihypertensives

Prazosin in doses of 2.5–5 mg is a useful substitute in case ACE inhibitors and ARBs have to be discontinued. The slow-release preparations do not produce postural hypotension and are distinctly superior. Clonidine has wide range of safety. Amlodipine in doses of 2.5–10 mg is a useful adjunct to ACEs and ARBs. In some patients it is a cause for de novo development of peripheral edema.

6.14.3 Beta Blockers

Nonselective beta blockers are *not to be used* in diabetes or diabetic hypertension. They increase the peripheral insulin resistance and can mask the early adrenergic symptoms of hypoglycemia leading the patients directly to a neuroglycopenic stage. They are particularly prone to produce vasoconstriction and severe bronchospasm in higher doses.

Diabetes and coronary artery disease have a high causal and associative relation. The extensive in tandem shaggy coronary arterial lesions in addition to the tachycardia jeopardizes the diastolic filling of coronary arteries. Selective beta 1 blockers should be and are routinely used to control tachycardia in such patients. Nothing is more dangerous to CAD than continued tachycardia or sudden development of the same as it reduces the diastolic filling time of the coronary arteries leading to ischemia of the myocardium. The principle is to increase these drugs gradually titrating with pulse rate. They are also useful in lower doses in case of heart failure. The disturbances in glycemic excursion if any should be handled by increasing insulin or other antidiabetic medication, since the main action is far more important than the glycemic excursions.

Lipid-lowering agents are considered important. They have enjoyed years of popularity and extensive high dose use for years. In diabetes the aim is to lower LDL cholesterol to 130 mg or below 100 if concomitant coronary artery disease is present and lower than 70 mg if a person with diabetes has already had a myocardial infarction. There is some rethinking going about whether to lower lipids to this extent, but no consensus has appeared yet.

6.14.4 New Agents

Diabetes and heart failure with diabetic cardiomyopathy are now recognized to have a frequent association. A new class of drugs, SGLT2, with a number of related molecules from the same class has emerged that increases glycosuria, induces some weight loss, and produces as a result a mild form of ketonemia. These ketone bodies are then utilized by the heart muscle for its fuel requirement. What was unexpected was the early separation of the Kaplan-Meier graphs in the improvement in cardiac muscle function from within a couple of weeks in the trials which continued to improve over weeks to follow, compared to the other arm. These are considered as useful drugs since a couple of years now.

Hydroxychloroquine is in use for autoimmune disorders like rheumatoid arthritis for decades. Many well-designed trials have now shown its effectiveness in blood glucose control as well lately. The most singular effect observed is the stabilization of insulin dose in fluctuating diabetic patients [20].

Uncontrolled diabetes is considered in addition to hypercoagulable or immunocompromised, and such other associated state is also considered an inflammatory state. Hydroxychloroquine, an immunomodulator and anti-inflammatory drug used in rheumatoid arthritis for decades, has been tried in type 2 diabetes for its anti-inflammatory properties. In a study with small number of patients, the control arm was only insulin, and the intervention arm was insulin with hydroxychloroquine (HCQS.) The treatment arm showed that the insulin requirement was decreased in the intervention arm compared to the control arm [21].

The impact of oral antidiabetic agents on changes in lipid levels, either increasing or decreasing, is an important consideration. The lipid-lowering effect should go beyond the lowering that may be caused by glycemic control alone. Hyperlipidemia and atherosclerosis go together. In a head-to-head trial between pioglitazone and HCQS, reduction in the total cholesterol and LDL, cholesterol was found to be significantly lower in the HCQS rather than pioglitazone group [22]. In addition to its effects on the reduction in LDL-C, lowered insulin requirement and better glycemic control, as a result of its anti-inflammatory properties, HCQS is reported to have an antithrombotic property also. Thus HCQS could provide an added advantage in reducing cardiovascular risk [22].

The possible explanation for the glucose-lowering effect of hydroxychloroquine can be given by a series of reactions occurring in the intracellular realm. The insulin-insulin receptor combination is internalized in the cytosol. The parent drug, chloroquine, stabilizes intracellular lysosomes. That leads to the process of lysosomal insulin-insulin receptor combination degradation slowing down. The parent drug chloroquine slows insulin clearance. The cystosolic insulin-metabolizing enzymes are inhibited by hydroxychloroquine. All these reactions lead to a lowering of glucose with HCQS [23].

A considerable literature is now available about significant vitamin D deficiency in high number of Indians and its benefits in diabetes also when corrected, generally with calcium supplementation. This is not surprising at all since every cellular function that involves exocytosis as in the case of insulin secretion or as in muscle contraction has a concomitant need for exogenous calcium to move in the cells and mobilization of cytosolic calcium for this process to occur. Correction of these difficulties is expected logically to be helpful. This has at least brought to attention the need for such supplementations particularly in more susceptible groups like postmenopausal women.

Diabetes patients need drugs acting on several organ systems. There are some important drugs with drug interactions that every clinician should know. They will be found in Chap. 13.

References

1. Australian Diabetes Society. Peri-operative diabetes management guidelines, July 2012, ADS working group of Vincent Wong, Glynis Ross, Jennifer Wong and David Chipps (chair).
2. Kelkar SK. Observations on office staff in a remote thermal electric power plant MP India; 1997.
3. Guillermo U, Umpierrez E, Smiley D, Jacobs S, Peng L, Temponi A, Mulligan P, Umpierrez D, Newton C, Olson D, Rizzo M. Randomized study of basal-bolus insulin therapy in the inpatient management of patients with type 2 diabetes undergoing general surgery (RABBIT 2 surgery). Diabetes Care. 2011;34:256–61.
4. UK Prospective Diabetes Study (UKPDS) Group. Intensive blood-glucose control with sulphonylureas or insulin compared with conventional treatment and risk of complications in patients with type 2 diabetes (UKPDS 33). Lancet. 1998;352:837–53.
5. The Diabetes Control and Complications Trial Research Group. The effect of intensive treatment of diabetes on the development and progression of long-term complications in insulin-dependent diabetes mellitus. N Engl J Med. 1993;329:977–86.
6. Dluhy RG, McMahon GT. Intensive glycemic control in the ACCORD and ADVANCE trials. N Engl J Med. 2008;358:2630–3.
7. Little RR, Rohlfing CL. The long and winding road to optimal HbA1c measurement. Clin Chim Acta. 2013;418:63–71.
8. Lindholm P, Minn H, Leskinen-Kallio S, Bergman J, Ruotsalainen U, Joensuu H. Influence of the blood glucose concentration on FDG uptake in cancer – a PET study. J Nucl Med. 1993;34(1):6–11.
9. Ishizu K, Nishizawa S, Yonekura Y, Sadato N, Magata Y, Tamaki N, Tsuchida T, Okazawa H, Miyatake S, Ishikawa M. Effects of hyperglycemia on FDG uptake in human brain and glioma. J Nucl Med. 1994;35(7):1104–9.
10. Zhuang HM, Cortes-Blanco A, Pourdehnad M, Adam LE, Yamamoto AJ, Martinez-Lazaro R, Lee JH, Loman JC, Rossman MD, Alavi A. Do high glucose levels have differential effect on FDG uptake in inflammatory and malignant disorders? Nucl Med Commun. 2001;22(10):1123–8.

11. Mears SC, Lipsett PA, Brager MD, Riley LH III. Metformin-associated lactic acidosis after elective cervical spine fusion: a case report. Spine. 2002;27(22):E482–4.
12. Mercker SK, Maier C, Neumann G, Wulf H. Lactic acidosis as a serious perioperative complication of antidiabetic biguanide medication with metformin. Anesthesiology. 1997;87(4):1003–5.
13. Chan NN, Feher MD. Metformin and perioperative risk. Br J Anaesth. 1999;83(3):540–1.
14. Bailey CJ, Turner RC. Metformin. N Engl J Med. 1996;334(9):574–9.
15. Thomsen HS, Morcos SK. Contrast media and metformin: guidelines to diminish the risk of lactic acidosis in non-insulin-dependent diabetics after administration of contrast media. ESUR Contrast Media Safety Committee. Eur Radiol. 1999;9(4):738–40.
16. Jamet P, Lebas de Lacour JC, Christoforov B, Stern M. Fatal case of metformin-induced lactic acidosis after urography in a diabetic patient. Sem Hop. 1980;56(9–10):473–4.
17. Klow NE, Draganov B, Os I. Metformin and contrast media—increased risk of lactic acidosis? Tidsskr Nor Laegeforen. 2001;121(15):1829.
18. McCartney MM, Gilbert FJ, Murchison LE, Pearson D, McHardy K, Murray AD. Metformin and contrast media—a dangerous combination? Clin Radiol. 1999;54(1):29–33.
19. Joslin EP. Joslin's textbook of diabetes mellitus. 14th ed. Lippincott, Williams and Wilkins, USA 2005, Indian Edition.
20. Pareek A, et al. Efficacy and safety of hydroxychloroquine in the treatment of type 2 diabetes mellitus: a double blind, randomized comparison with pioglitazone. Curr Med Res Opin. 2014;30(7):1257–66.
21. Quatraro A, Consoli G, Magno M, et al. Hydroxychloroquine in decompensated, treatment-refractory noninsulin-dependent diabetes mellitus: a new job for an old drug? Ann Intern Med. 1990;112:678–81.
22. Krentz A, Bailey C. Oral anti-diabetic agents: current role in type 2 diabetes mellitus. Drugs. 2006;65:385–411.
23. Fessler B, Alarcon G, McGwin G, et al. Systemic lupus erythematosus in three ethnic groups: XVI. Association of hydroxychloroquine use with reduced risk of damage accrual. Arthritis Rheum. 2005;52:1473–80.

Special Surgical Situations and Diabetes Management: Part 1

7

Contents

S. Kelkar et al., *Towards Optimal Management of Diabetes in Surgery*,
https://doi.org/10.1007/978-981-13-7705-1_7

7.1 Major, Elective Surgery in Special Situations: General Principles

It is desirable to admit patients who are not controlled optimally with or without being treated by insulin. Admissions 2–3 days prior to stabilize glucose control and optimize insulin doses will help postoperatively a great deal. The attempt should be to reach a fasting blood glucose level between 80 and 120 mg/dL and a bed time level of 100–140 m/dL. It is desirable to switch the patients on long-acting insulin to intermediate-acting insulin as it provides greater flexibility to alter doses for quicker control. Intermediate insulin is started after the patient is admitted couple of days prior to surgery, or on outpatient basis to achieve good control and then admitted for surgery. In cardiac surgery in particular wide swings of glycemia occur. Hence frequent perioperative blood glucose monitoring followed by action by changing insulin infusion rates or subcutaneous doses or glucose supplementation as the case may be is crucial for better postoperative outcomes.

Preoperatively there is a choice of fluid regimens. One could use glucose-insulin-potassium (GIK) fixed dose infusions. Or glucose and insulin infusion can be started as separate line infusions. Authors prefer the latter since it is easier to change one or the other or both in its quantum or rate with multi-flexibility and quicker control of glucose.

Intraoperatively blood glucose should be monitored hourly in all major surgeries. An immediate postoperative glucose level determination helps in shifting the patient to ICU care with specific instructions to be followed regarding the insulin infusion rate for the next few hours. It also creates baseline guidance for modifications if necessary. There should be at least a 1-h overlap between starting/stopping intravenous insulin and removing/reinstituting subcutaneous insulin, respectively. More will be discussed about it later. We will first discuss below the older method of GIK infusion.

7.2 Standard GIK Solution

Standard GIK solution is 10% solution of dextrose as 500 mL unit to which is added 15 U of short-acting insulin and 10 mmol of potassium chloride. It is to be infused at 100 mils/h over 5 h. Five percent dextrose solutions are/can be used instead of dextrose solution of 10%. Alternatively, short-acting insulin is added at 0.32 U/g of dextrose in the infusion which translates to 16 U with 5% dextrose and 32 U with 10% dextrose if used. Potassium is avoided in patients with renal dysfunction and those with hyperkalemia.

7.2.1 Advantages of GIK Solutions

1. They are inherently safe because glucose and insulin are infused together. In separate line infusions, if glucose infusion is stopped inadvertently, hypoglycemia may occur. If insulin is stopped, then it will result in hyperglycemia. This will not happen with a standard GIK infusion.
2. GIK does not need sophisticated equipment like syringe/infusion pumps.

7.2.2 Disadvantages of GIK Solutions

1. Insulin depends on receptor sensitivity for its action in vivo. Therefore, adjustments have to be made to insulin dose to be added to "neutralize" the dextrose which does involve making many fresh solutions. Many of these solutions may be wasted after partial use.[1]
2. Finer control of glucose level thus is more difficult. Separate infusions are easier and superior to titrate to blood glucose levels.

7.2.3 Brief Note on Intraoperative Glucose Monitoring

The standard practice is to measure blood glucose in the morning while the patient is fasting. These readings could vary, and how to deal with different values during the preoperative period is discussed in detail in Chap. 6. Whatever the fasting value and action taken, hourly glucose monitoring is a must intraoperatively. The dynamics under anesthesia intraoperatively changes so much that hourly glucose monitoring will help change the infusion of insulin or glucose to maintain euglycemia. Any blood glucose level on the day of surgery above 200 mg/dL should be considered suboptimal or poor control. An intravenous infusion of insulin without dextrose for finite period of a couple of hours should be considered to bring it to optimum levels before induction. In special cases, as in cardiopulmonary bypass, these schedules will be completely different as described below, but in other major cases, changes will be much less wider.

[1] The authors faced this problem in the early 1990s. Till then the syringe pumps had not been a routinely available implement. To reduce the wastage as well as to achieve finer control, we devised the mid drip technique described in detail earlier. See also in Commonly Asked Questions for Alberti regime and its evolution.

7.3 Cardiac Surgery and Patients with Diabetes

The most serious macrovascular complications in diabetes are seen in the cardiac, cerebral, and lower limb vasculature. In this chapter, the cardiovascular and cerebral circulatory issues with a few other special situations listed at the beginning of this chapter will be discussed in the context of their surgical aspects, with necessary understanding of the pathophysiology and structural abnormalities and its nonsurgical management.

7.3.1 Coronary Artery Disease in Patients with and Without Diabetes

Patients with diabetes have a significantly higher incidence of coronary artery disease (CAD) compared to those without diabetes. The survival in the latter group is much greater. CAD in diabetes generally requires multiple coronary arteries grafts. CABG has to be resorted to more often than angioplasty [1, 2]. CAD is vastly different in patients with diabetes compared to those without diabetes. In the nondiabetic group, the vascular involvement is much less severe, less number of people with more than one vessel is affected, those affected tend to have smaller number of lesions, and, most importantly, they are often discreet and single. Diabetes-specific cardiomyopathy will not be a risk factor although diastolic dysfunction could be present from other causes. That makes it easier to treat them by percutaneous angioplasty more often than a person with diabetes can be or surgically.

On the other hand, people with diabetes having coronary artery disease as well have more extensive involvement of coronary vessels. As a rule more than one vessel is affected. The atherosclerotic lesions in all these vessels tend to be multiple, in tandem, more diffuse, and shaggy, causing considerable reduction in the intraluminal flow of the vessels in high numbers. Thus, these lesions are more difficult to treat, and the results could be suboptimal compared to people without diabetes undergoing coronary artery disease management.

The intraoperative management of coronary artery disease in diabetes will be discussed under two headings. One is the endocrine response to cardiopulmonary bypass and, second, the carbohydrate metabolism under the same. The preoperative evaluation and its various significances have been already discussed.

7.3.2 Cardiopulmonary Bypass (CPB)

In many types of cardiac surgery, the beating heart is brought to cardiac asystole using cardiopulmonary bypass (CPB) or the heart-lung machine. CPB is used to perfuse the body with oxygenated blood without the use of heart and lungs. It is done under hypothermia. The heart and lung are excluded from the circulation and therefore also removed from participation in hormone secretion and degradation. The type of blood flow used during bypass is non-pulsatile in nature, and this is one of the most potent forces which disrupt the functional hormonal response. The blood flow to organs and the distribution of blood flow within the organs have much reduced perfusion pressure. Moderate to profound hypothermia depresses the metabolic rate of cells. It leads to decrease in the rate of enzymatic processes and other metabolic processes as well.

The level of trauma in bypass surgeries is extremely high. In addition inotropes with catecholamine like action are often used. The CPB pumps are primed by fluid containing glucose. The induced hypothermia, with the above three factors, increases insulin resistance to high levels. Thus, it requires high dosage of insulin perioperatively in patients undergoing open-heart surgeries [3, 4] (See Box 7.1 and Fig. 7.1 below). As a consequence of these aspects of management, when the hypothermia is reversed gradually, the rate of cellular metabolism increases, and large quantities of glucose in the presence of high levels of insulin infused during hypothermic stages could lead to severe hypoglycemia which could be dangerous. Hence frequent glucose monitoring is a must, and a safe range of glucose should be achieved and maintained.

Box 7.1 Insulin Units per Hour Required During CABG

1. Preoperative—1.5 U/h.
2. After skin incision—3.0 U/h.
3. During CPB 5.0—U/h.
4. Immediate post-op.—8.3 U/h.

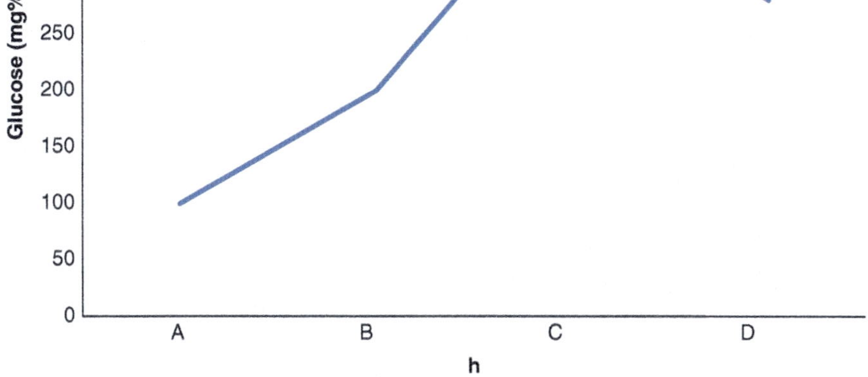

Fig. 7.1 Carbohydrate metabolism during CPB. A, onset of anesthesia; B, onset of CPB; C, well-established CPB; D, off CPB

7.4 Endocrine Responses to Cardiopulmonary Bypass

These responses have been discussed earlier briefly; here we will discuss them in much greater details. Activation of the hypothalamic-pituitary axis and the sympathetic nervous system outflow determines the effects of endocrine response. The afferent nerve input carries pain sensation from area of trauma or injury. It carries both the somatic and autonomic impulses which activate the hypothalamic-pituitary axis. Endocrine system works on a negative feedback. For example, adrenocorticotrophic hormone (ACTH) stimulates cortisol secretion which normally inhibits ACTH secretion. Under CPB, high levels of cortisol fail to inhibit ACTH secretion [5]. Overall, the catabolic hormones like catecholamines are released with other pituitary hormones. The anabolic hormones such as insulin and testosterone are suppressed.

Catecholamines are released from presynaptic sympathetic nerve terminals. It is a response of hypothalamic stimulation caused by trauma [5]. Norepinephrine shows a marked increase, leading to elevating the peripheral vascular resistance. There are also volume changes of blood flow to various organs during cardiopulmonary bypass. Norepinephrine causes tachycardia and hypertension [5]. Norepinephrine levels increase fourfold, and epinephrine levels increase tenfold over the pre-bypass levels and remain elevated for many hours in post-bypass period. Stimulus for increased catecholamine secretion is thought to be the hemodilution and hypotension occurring on initiation of CPB and hypothermia. Epinephrine stimulates glucagon production. The glycogenolysis is also increased directly by it. These two actions make the availability of glucose in the early stages of CPB. Epinephrine also directly increases gluconeogenesis by and through the release of lipids and glycerol. The high levels of epinephrine however as a result of their action result in higher insulin resistance. This inhibits the glucose utilization of other organs as the CPB proceeds.

Cortisol increases insulin resistance. It interferes with binding of insulin to its receptor. The intracellular transfer of glucose is thus reduced. Cortisol also causes proteolysis and lipolysis—the last factor contributes to ketone formation. Finally, growth hormone increases insulin resistance and impairment of glucose use. It also stimulates hepatic gluconeogenesis [6]. Renin is released from the kidneys causing the conversion of angiotensin I to angiotensin II. The latter stimulates the secretion of aldosterone from the adrenal cortex. That increases sodium reabsorption and loss of potassium in exchange. Potassium is secreted in the renal tubules, and then it is lost in the distal convoluted tubules of kidney [5].

7.4.1 Pituitary Response

Hypothalamus controls pituitary function. The hypothalamus secretes the releasing factors. These cause corresponding hormone secretion from the pituitary. It also releases some inhibitory factors also. These inhibit a few of the pituitary hormones. Both the inhibitory and releasing factors are secreted into the hypothalamic-hypophyseal portal system. The secretion of the anterior pituitary hormones like corticotrophin-releasing factor (CRF) releases the ACTH. Growth hormone-releasing factor, somatotrophin, releases growth hormone (GH). The secretion of prolactin is under tonic inhibitory control via prolactin release inhibitory factor. The increased prolactin secretion occurs in perioperative state by release of this inhibitory control. The secretion of thyroid-stimulating hormone (TSH), luteinizing hormone (LH), and follicle-stimulating hormone (FSH) does not change significantly [5].

7.4.2 Salt and Water Metabolism

The hypothalamus has direct neural control of vasopressin release from the posterior pituitary. Vasopressin (ADH) release is large. It is 20 times of basal values. ADH remains at this high level for a long time. Coronary artery bypass graft patients have higher levels of ADH compared to patients undergoing valve replacement. Such high levels result in large amounts of water retention which could cause dilutional hyponatremia and concentrated urine. The excess production of ACTH and renin angiotensin system (see above) retains sodium in exchange of potassium which is lost in urine. This opposes the hyponatremic effects of massive ADH release. The ADH effects may last continue for 3–5 days after surgery. In addition CRF stimulates the production of the pro-opiomelanocortin, POMC, a precursor of ACTH and b-endorphin [5].

ACTH in CPB is *not* switched off by high levels of cortisol also. It is far in excess of that required to produce a maximum adrenocortical response. It therefore continues to stimulate cortisol production within minutes of starting of surgery. Cortisol rises to 1500 nmol/L within 4–6 h once the surgery starts, as against the normal baseline value of 400 nmol/L. The mineralocorticoid effects of cortisol result in sodium and water retention and potassium loss [7, 8].

Increased cortisol and catecholamines increase insulin resistance. High levels of catecholamines reduce insulin secretion. Catecholamines simultaneously increase the secretion of growth hormone and glucagon [8, 9]. High levels of cortisol also cause skeletal muscle protein breakdown. It provides amino acids which are the precursors of gluconeogenesis. It also stimulates lipolysis. Glucose utilization is impaired. These effects are called "anti-insulin effect" causing further increase in the glucose levels. Cortisol effect also decreases the production of inflammatory mediators such as leukotrienes, cytokines, and prostaglandins.

7.5 Carbohydrate, Lipid, Protein Metabolism, and Hormonal Response During CPB

Carbohydrate metabolism during CPB and cardiac surgery is markedly deranged. Blood glucose levels often rise beyond 270 mg/dL (15 mmol/L) even in patients without diabetes [10, 11]. With diabetes, it frequently rises beyond

360 mg/dL (20 mmol/L) [12]. The magnitude depends upon the degree of hypothermia and method of bypass. In a patient without diabetes, the expected insulin response to this kind of hyperglycemia is 500 μU/mL. In a patient with diabetes, once the CPB is established, the serum glucose rises to over 400 mg/dL. The corresponding insulin response in these patients is barely 200 μU/mL. This indicates blunted insulin response to hyperglycemia. These two responses persist during the period of CPB and early post CPB period and slowly come to normal over 12 h or so. Hepatic, pancreatic, and renal functions are also modified [5].

7.5.1 Glucose Levels and Cardiac Surgery

There is no doubt that the toxicity of higher glucose levels in cardiac surgery is as crucial for control as the glucose levels in gestational diabetes mellitus. There is a direct relationship of adverse effects to each mmol rise of glucose in cardiac disease in diabetes. This is even more so under surgical intervention. For example, the risk of adverse events increases by 17% even with a minor elevation of just about 1 mmol of glucose (18 mg/dL), above 110 mg/dL in cardiac surgery [13]. In-hospital death and congestive heart failure in patients admitted with acute myocardial infarction increase if the blood glucose is above 110 mg/dL [14]. Mortality risk after myocardial infarction increased 3.9-fold for a glucose level of 110–144 mg/dL (6.1–8 mmol/L). In a separate prospective study of 336 patients, the same outcomes were observed [15].

With a deficient insulin response, lipid metabolism accelerates under glucagon during cardiopulmonary bypass because decrease in glucose utilization for energy creates the need for alternate sources of energy. This results in fourfold increase in the levels of free fatty acids. Increase in free fatty acid levels also occurs due to increased levels of epinephrine, norepinephrine, and growth hormone. Catecholamines also contribute to the increase in blood glucose. Coronary bypass operations without CPB while the heart is beating normally will bring down the extreme stress CPB induces in the body. However, this is not yet the norm for CABG operations.

High levels of counter-regulatory hormones—catecholamine, cortisol, glucagon, and growth hormone—and unfractionated heparin administration during cardiac surgery promote lipolysis, facilitated by insulin deficiency and ketone body production. Triglycerides are metabolized to fatty acids. The new "cleaner" heparins contribute less to the lipolysis. Oxidation of FFAs to acyl CoA and its conversion to ketone bodies, beta-hydroxybutyrate, acetoacetate, and acetone take place in the liver. These are a useful, water-soluble fuel source for both the heart and brain. Glycerol is a three-carbon structure and is substrate to gluconeogenesis.

7.5.2 Protein Metabolism

In any major surgery involving extensive tissue trauma, protein metabolism is characterized by high degree of catabolism. For example, after major abdominal surgery, up to 0.5 kg/day of lean body mass may be lost. It causes considerable muscle wasting. Skeletal muscle protein is mainly affected. The amount of protein degradation is also influenced by the nutritional status of the patient. Visceral protein may also be broken down to release essential amino acids. Increased levels of cortisol and cytokine are mainly responsible for protein breakdown. Liver also releases acute phase proteins. At the same time, albumin production is reduced. Over a long stressful period, its decline has tremendous significance for optimal intravascular plasma status, extravascular fluid, and high mortality. Amino acids are also used for gluconeogenesis to maintain circulating blood glucose at a level more than 3 mmol/L. The amount of nitrogen can be measured by estimating urinary losses of urea. Nutritional support, enteral and parenteral, and additional substrate availability have not been of much help to prevent protein loss after surgery. It cannot stop the inhibition of protein anabolism, nor can it prevent catabolism [5].

7.5.3 Other Hormonal Responses: Cytokines

Cytokines are low molecular weight, heterogeneous glycoproteins. These are comprised of interleukins (IL) 1–17, interferons, and tumor necrosis factor. These are synthesized by activated macrophages, fibroblasts, and endothelial and glial cells in response to tissue injury, either from surgery or trauma. Cytokines act systemically as endocrine elements. Most of the paracrine effects are exerted locally. Cytokines act on target cell surface receptors in mediating immunity and inflammation, in significant manner. The level of IL-6 response within 12–24 h after surgery is an indication of how much tissue damage has occurred. In addition to cytokines, fibrinogen, C reactive protein, complement proteins, alpha 2-macroglobulin, amyloid A, and ceruloplasmin are the other acute phase reactants secreted. Cytokine effects include fever, granulocytosis, hemostasis, and limiting tissue damage. It promotes healing as well [5].

The immune and the neuroendocrine system affect each other. In vitro systems have shown that cytokines increase cortisol secretion. Raised cortisol levels inhibit cytokine production, limiting the severity of inflammation [5].

7.5.4 B-Endorphin and Prolactin

The role of increased secretion of B-endorphin and prolactin during surgery is unknown, but they may alter immune function.

7.6 Modifications in the Stress Response: Opioids, Etomidate, and Benzodiazepines

Stress responses arise during surgery. Anesthesia may reduce/increase some of the responses. Opioids like fentanyl in high doses, more than 50 mg/kg, are routinely used in cardiac surgery. These suppress the hypothalamic sympathetic outflow. But the stimulatory effects of cardiopulmonary bypass are so strong that these inhibitory effects of opioids are overcome. High opioid doses otherwise prolong anesthetic recovery and need longer ventilator support postoperatively.

Anesthetic drug etomidate causes reversible inhibition of the enzyme 11-b-hydroxylase and the cholesterol side chain cleavage enzyme. These actions decrease the adrenal cortical production of corticosteroids. An induction dose of 0.3 mg/kg of etomidate blocks the synthesis of aldosterone and cortisol for up to 8 h. Benzodiazepines (midazolam 0.2–0.4 mg/kg and infusion of 0.9–0.125 mg/kg/h) may also have an inhibitory effect at the hypothalamic-pituitary level affecting steroid synthesis. However its significance has not been established. Clonidine, a centrally acting alpha sympathetic outflow antagonist may also decrease sympathoadrenal and cardiovascular responses to surgery.

7.7 Mortality in Cardiac (Open-Heart) Surgery

Over years it is well understood that the persons with diabetes undergoing cardiac surgery, mostly need multi vessel bypass. They are also under higher chances of dying. The older literature seems to support this. Over years however the picture certainly has not remained as grim.

An old study compared 340 patients with diabetes and 2522 patients without diabetes on whom CABG was performed. The operative mortality was three times more in patients with diabetes—1.8% vs. 0.6% [16]. A higher-risk group, the kind which is more likely to be found today, consisted of 291 patients of which 95% of them had type 2 diabetes. Retinopathy, nephropathy, or neuropathy was already present in 40% of 291. All of them underwent CABG. The median period of hospitalization was 7 days. There were 54 adverse outcomes like nonfatal strokes, acute myocardial infarctions, and sepsis, or they died. Adverse events were increased by 17% for each 1 mmol/L increase in blood glucose levels above 6 mmol/L [12]. The mortality increased four times if the glycated hemoglobin value was more than 8.6% [17].

7.7.1 Type 1 Diabetes and Coronary Disease

Type 1 diabetes is the more severe form of diabetes. All micro and macro vascular complications are likely to be more serious and may arise at a much younger age. Atypical presentation of coronary artery disease like dyspnea in young age may mislead from making the diagnosis. High threshold for suspicion is needed.

EKG alone is inadequate to detect silent coronary artery disease. Sedentary, asymptomatic patients with diabetes, having hypertension, hyperlipidemia, tobacco use, or family history of cardiac disease, should undergo cardiac imaging/stress testing if they have to undergo a major surgery. It is a recommended precaution to exclude occult coronary artery disease before general anesthesia. In the presence of significant coronary artery disease, it would not be unusual to undergo CABG or angioplasty as a safeguard before going under general anesthesia. This will avoid intraoperative mishaps.[2] Type 1 patient with diabetes for more than 15 years, with other risk factors for CAD and/or unsatisfactory control of diabetes, should be given beta-blockers preoperatively. It is one of the best cardioprotective measure [18].

As discussed earlier a type 1 patient with significant renal involvement cannot tolerate fluid load. The plasma insulin clearance is reduced. Hence fluid and insulin administration should be carried out under caution and strict monitoring for cardiac overload and pulmonary edema and hypoglycemia.

7.7.2 Desirable Blood Glucose Control and Mortality During Cardiac Surgery

Good glycemic control seems to be the best guaranty of reducing mortality of CABG in diabetes. If achieved, the mortality of cardiac surgery in patients with or without diabetes is nearly same [19]. In CABG, mortality is proportional to the level of glucose. The lowest of it is found with mean glycemia less than 149 mg/dL (8.3 mmol/L) [20, 21].

7.7.3 Blood Glucose Control and Other Complications During Cardiac Surgery

Insulin requirements are generally much higher in cardiac procedures; recent studies suggest improved patient outcomes with tight glycemic control during and after cardiac surgery [22]. Tighter control can be achieved by using a fixed dose insulin infusion at 5 mU/kg/min. The concomitant IV glucose administration is varied so that in all stages of operation, the glucose level remains between 72 and 108 mg/dL (4–6 mmol/L). Such combinations with monitoring can be carried out without hypoglycemia developing even in cardiac surgery [23].

GIK administration will almost always cause moderate hyperglycemia with blood glucose concentration ranging between 133 and 171 mg/dL (7.4–9.5 mmol/L).

---

[2] Rarely one may come across a situation wherein cerebral circulation is severely compromised in the form of unilateral complete block of one carotid artery with or without narrowing of the other. In such situations, carotid endarterectomy will take precedence over CABG since in such a situation under non-pulsatile flow of CPB, massive cerebral infarction is highly likely. As a general rule, carotid Doppler may be a useful preoperative procedure in CABG or high-risk major surgery.

GIK however reduces the risk for atrial fibrillation as well as infection in diabetic CABG [24]. Similar proportionate increase in hospital-acquired infections was seen with higher blood glucose level greater than 198 mg/dL (11 mmol/L) [25].

7.7.4 Immediate Postoperative Management in Cardiac Surgery

The postoperative management of glycemia does not differ in any way as discussed so extensively at several places. However, as discussed above, during the reversal of hypothermia, serious hypoglycemia can/will arise. Hypothermia and CPB cause extreme insulin resistance resulting in hyperglycemia. Large number of insulin units is required on an hourly basis for several hours to maintain euglycemia. Postoperatively, when the hypothermia is reversed, the cellular energy level rises rapidly, and glucose enters cells in massive flux, with potassium. At this point, the circulatory levels of insulin becoming high may result in severe hypoglycemia. Frequent monitoring during reversal, moderating intravenous insulin administration against the glucose levels, and awareness and experience of this condition are required to manage the situation without any risk for the patients.

7.8 Postoperative Infection Prevention

It is more than established as will be discussed below that tight glycemic control is an essential. Here are a few comments made in literature about the variety of procedures in cardiovascular system on the prophylactic management of infections in cardiothoracic surgery.

7.8.1 Surgery Involving Median Sternotomies

There is no doubt that sternal or the closed skin incision is more likely to get infected in people with diabetes, and as long as it is minor, it could be made to settle down. Staphylococci are the causative infective agents. Prophylactic antibiotics will reduce postoperative infections after bypass grafting and valve replacement. In case of long duration of surgeries, additional prophylactic antibiotic dose may have to be given to maintain the antibiotic tissue levels at mean inhibitory concentration to decrease the risk of staphylococcal surgical site infection (SSI). Prophylactic antibiotics if continued till all catheters, wires, and drains are removed will lead to higher rates of resistant organisms, if an infection occurs [26].

7.8.2 Placement of Intracardiac Devices and Cardiac Catheterization: Prophylactic Antibiotic Use

The pacemakers, defibrillators, ventricular assist devices, ventriculoatrial shunts, and arterial patches are the most common of the cardiac devices which are placed within it.

Seven randomized studies of prophylactic antibiotic use for permanent pacemaker implantation indicate that the SSI, inflammation, and skin erosion are considerably reduced. Current consensus favors the use of antimicrobial prophylaxis before device placement. Antibiotic prophylaxis before cardiac catheterization is not currently recommended because of the very low rate of SSIs associated with this procedure. An additional dose is often given when patients are removed from bypass machine [24].

7.8.3 Thoracic (Noncardiac) Surgery

Whether to use or not to use prophylactic antibiotics in pulmonary resection has not been decided in any definitive way. Evidence is in favor of prophylactic antibiotics. It shows lesser number of patients getting infected. A single dose within 60 min before operation is advised. For prolonged operations, additional doses may be necessary. Vancomycin or a fluoroquinolones should be given 60–120 min before incision [24].

7.8.4 Esophageal Surgery

Obstruction, decreased peristalsis, or stasis within facilitates growth of oral aerobes and anaerobes in esophagus normally sterile. In turn, the risk of mediastinal infection is increased, and prophylaxis is generally recommended. One prospective, randomized study in endoscopic sclerotherapy of esophageal varices showed no benefit of prophylactic antibiotics in reducing the risk of bacteremia or SSIs [26].

7.9 Metformin in CABG[3]

Metformin has retained its position as the first choice for people with diabetes for over two decades now despite the advent of newer and finer drugs. We have discussed the various issues related to metformin in Chap. 6 in this volume. Here are a few specific details about metformin in CABG. Continuing metformin through the period of cardiac surgery seems to be advantageous. The outcomes have been found to be better among them compared to those who stopped taking it [27]. It is as expected. The third arm in UKPDS (2000) Metformin, added later in this long trial, showed a distinct advantage against macrovascular complications. It increases insulin sensitivity with more physiological levels of insulin and no hyperinsulinemia. Hyperinsulinemia is a factor in the development of cardiovascular disease [28]. Insulin requirements are generally much higher in cardiac procedures; recent studies suggest improved patient outcomes with tight glycemic control during and after cardiac surgery. Metformin as one of the best sensitizers could be of considerable help [20].

[3] It has not been fully established if the metformin benefits in cardiac surgery are also found in general surgical patients. It is preferred to continue metformin throughout the perioperative period in all patients. Normal kidney function should be ascertained.

7.10 Emergency Neurosurgery

Any neurological condition in which the intracranial tension has risen to a level causing a shift of the brain stem from midline, unequal pupil sizes, or a threatened coning of the brain.

Stem calls for an emergency neurosurgery. A severe head injury and hypertension with substantial intracranial hemorrhage are the most common causes. Other such causes are the intracranial tumors, malignant or benign, or recovery from cranial neurosurgical procedures.

In many ways a conservatively manageable hemorrhage even if large enough has better prognosis than a cerebral infarction. In hemorrhage the white matter merely shears apart the white matter, and the actual cell death except around the edge of the hemorrhage is little. As the hemorrhage resolves, the cerebral functions appear again. Oftentimes, considerable age-related cerebral atrophy allows for a large hemorrhage to be accommodated without increase in intracranial tension, as in elderly hypertensive patients.

However, once it becomes apparent that a surgical intervention is imminent, there is hardly any time left for preparing the patient, as can happen in other surgeries like abdominal catastrophes and polytrauma not including the cranial trauma to name a few. Unlike major abdominal surgical conditions, the pain or fluid losses may not be severe. If a patient has uncontrolled diabetes or hypertension, its management has to be real time, as the patient is shifted to the theater as well as intraoperatively. As immediate measures a nitroglycerine puff is helpful in reducing the blood pressure. It works on the principle of large-scale vasodilatation which results in peripheral pooling of the blood, which in turn results in reduced venous return to the right and the left ventricles. These two factors combined result in quick lowering of the blood pressure in such situations.

In such situations a paradoxical situation often arises. Often times such patients are referred to a higher center over long distances. Such patients even now are being infused with 20% concentration of mannitol, every few hours ranging from 6 to 8 to control brain swelling. The effects this practice can produce at times are more disastrous than the condition itself. Invariably it results in significant dehydration and relative hypotension with large losses of electrolytes. Sodium loss in particular adds to the already depressed cognitive levels of the patients as it is intimately related to such cerebral functions. In such situations the operative risk rises further. The center in which the first two authors worked together for long has discontinued mannitol for over three decades now. But mannitol administration is still practiced, and its effects have to be taken into consideration.

7.10.1 Head Injuries

A number of head-injured patients are received in a hyperadrenergic state, i.e., they have an increased cardiac output, tachycardia, and excess of catecholamines in circulation. This state is thought to be central in origin. It serves to create havoc with the blood glucose values and results in hyperglycemia and ketonuria leading to metabolic acidosis which may at times be severe. In addition, the compensatory mechanism, viz., increase in respiratory rate which can remove CO_2 and compensate for the metabolic acidosis, may not be available to the unconscious, head-injured patient due to central respiratory depression and/or mechanical obstruction to the airway. This will lead to a dual acidosis – metabolic, due to diabetes, and respiratory, due to less than adequate respiratory effort.

Postoperatively, the time for which the hyperadrenergic state may last is not immediately predictable. Continued use of mannitol leads to continued depletion of water and electrolytes.[4] Besides, it may not be possible to institute NG feeding in the head-injured patient due to development of gastric bleeds (stress ulceration). This complication is by no means uncommon in neurological emergencies and may, at times, be very severe. That leaves the clinician with the only alternative of infusing glucose which may produce hyperglycemia which can be inappropriate for recovery. Hence, glucose has to be maintained at low levels.

Hypoglycemia maximally affects the brain. It increases the risk of focal neurological deficits, encephalopathy, seizures, and permanent cognitive dysfunction in patients with brain injury. To avoid low glucose levels in the blood supplied to the brain, blood glucose is not to go below 100 mg/dL. French guidelines define hypoglycemia as blood glucose of 3.3 mmol (60 mg/dL). French guidelines consider blood glucose of 2.2 mmol (40 mg/dL) as severe hypoglycemia. In conscious otherwise normal patients, brain stem dysfunction occurs at around 50–55 mg/dL level of glucose. It is likely to lead to more brain stem dysfunction in a patient already having higher intracranial pressure [29].

Ketosis is a rather prominent problem here, because it is dual in origin—one due to the existing diabetes with increased insulin resistance and the other due to starvation with or without hyperadrenergic state. After the first 48 h, GIK infusion can very well serve for the subsequent days before enteral feeding can be established satisfactorily. The daily insulin requirement of the patient as the hyperadrenergic state settles down also declines.

7.10.2 IV Fluid Administration in Neurosurgery

IV fluid administration during emergency neurosurgery follows the standard guidelines according to recommendations of the Brain Trauma Foundation which include the use of crystalloids, hypertonic saline, mannitol, blood, and blood products as required. The blood products in particular do not increase glucose level in any significant manner. This is discussed elsewhere also in the volume.

---

[4]Acetazolamide, 250 mg thrice a day, is used in patients with brain edema instead of mannitol, which once the surgery is over is possibly not required to be given at all. Acetazolamide does contribute in a small way to metabolic acidosis but helps in increasing the respiratory drive reducing the hypercapnia-induced CO_2. It also has a mild diuretic action.

Fluids which are hypo-osmolar to plasma should be avoided. In neurosurgery, if hypo-osmolar fluids are infused, the osmolarity of plasma is lowered. Fluids such as 0.45% saline and 5% dextrose in water are hypo-osmolar. Once the dextrose is metabolized, only free water remains. An osmotic gradient gets established due to reduced serum osmolarity. This leads to water movement across the blood-brain barrier (BBB) into the cerebral tissue. It thereby increases brain water content, that is, cerebral edema. Increase in the intracranial pressure is potentially lethal if brain stem compromise or coning occurs.

In neurosurgery, the enteral feeding may not get established within few days. All the energy required has to come through IV supplementation. Ten percentage fructose dextrose fluids would serve the purpose by reducing the water intake while supplying energy. The resultant hyperglycemia can be controlled with aggressive insulin infusions thereby preventing ketosis as well. However IV fluids with 10% dextrose do not have the saline component. Hence, as the dextrose gets metabolized, only water remains. Salt-free, glucose containing solutions are avoided in both brain and spinal cord injuries as discussed above. Glucose administration can worsen outcome. It causes both local and global ischemia. It increases tissue acidosis which may increase neurologic damage [30].

7.10.3 Intracranial Tumors and Neurosurgery

Neurosurgery, whether routine or emergency, poses a special situation for the diabetic patient. As far as routine neurosurgery is concerned, a sufficiently large tumor in the brain can rarely be considered as "routine," except when it is extremely slow growing. In most cases in India, by the time a brain tumor is diagnosed, it poses, what can best be described, as "semi-emergency." In fact, for the neurosurgeon, the clock starts ticking, the moment he diagnoses a brain tumor. Tumors within the bony cranial cavity get diagnosed due to their property of occupying space and increasing the intracranial tension. The bony cranial cavity does not expand to accommodate the rising intracranial volume and adjust to the pressure therefrom. That leads to the consequent threat of impending "coning" of the brain stem at any time. Hence these lesions must be dealt with as quickly as possible after their diagnosis.

In all the neurological surgical or nonsurgical but critical conditions described above, one constant feature of management is the introduction of steroids often in large doses. If a person is having diabetes, the blood glucose invariably escalates dramatically, and whatever control may have been present prior to starting steroids would be lost. Even in persons without diabetes, there will be unacceptable hyperglycemia in most cases due to other factors present. As a consequence of this, the surgery can wait for just a few days, but not for too long, since "good" metabolic control must be achieved as quickly as possible in people with or without diabetes. In fact, steroids may actually serve to unmask latent diabetes in this situation.

Needless to say, whether these patients have type 1 or type 2 diabetes, in this surgical situation, they have to be treated as insulin-dependent diabetic patients.

Patients requiring steroids should be admitted, a 24 h glucose profile is drawn and appropriate insulin schedule is started. Steroids are administered as needed by an appropriate route. Subsequent to the 24-h profile, more routine and fewer glucose measurements will be required. Control could be obtained rapidly, provided each high reading is acted upon to increase the subsequent insulin dose; the actual methodology of glucose control under steroids will be discussed below.

There are many perioperative conditions in which glucocorticoids are used. High doses are needed in head trauma and intracranial malignancy. Steroids are used in neurosurgical procedures after the operation also. A patient who is already on steroids may need a neurosurgical operation—for example, renal or other organ transplant patients or patients with type 1 diabetes mellitus for pulmonary or rheumatologic diseases. These patients are on maintenance doses of steroids. The dose regime with prednisone greater than 7.5 mg/day, dexamethasone greater than 0.75 mg/day, or hydrocortisone greater than 30 mg/day will require high stress dose short-term corticosteroid treatment preoperatively. These doses should be continued and then tapered to maintenance doses postoperatively. This avoids development of adrenal insufficiency in the intra- and postoperative stages since the adrenal in these patients is suppressed. Inevitably the insulin requirement under steroids could be about two to three times the outpatient dose or even more.

7.11 Glucocorticoids and Hyperglycemia in Surgery

Glucocorticoids primarily increase the insulin resistance native to a patient with diabetes. Soon after initial exposure to corticosteroids, insulin receptor and postreceptor functions on hepatocytes and adipocytes are altered by interfering with the insulin binding to the receptors. Steroids similarly interfere with the binding and uptake of insulin to the adipocytes and the muscle cells. These actions of steroids result in increased hepatic output of glucose, gluconeogenesis, and lipolysis. The net effect is worsening insulin resistance and hyperglycemia.

Steroid-dependent patients could either be on high-dose steroids, or they could be in a phase where the steroids are being tapered. Continuous variable-rate IV insulin infusion is particularly useful in controlling the blood glucose in such patients because of easy upscaling or downscaling of the infusion rate over a large range. Type 1 patients are vulnerable to steroid effects [31]. If this is not possible, subcutaneous insulin may be used safely with monitoring. This helps keep the hyperglycemia attaining high levels. It is also useful in avoiding hypoglycemia due to monitoring. It is also helpful in keeping the blood glucose in a narrow range.

7.11.1 Glucocorticoids and Management of Hyperglycemia

There is a diurnal variation to the steroid effect on plasma. The maximum response of increased blood glucose under the steroid effect is in the postprandial situations, and glucose can rise to very high levels [32].

7.11.2 Single Daily Steroid Administration

If a patient is on a single morning dose steroids, the blood glucose may reach its highest levels by 4–12 h. This level may get much lower later even to a baseline overnight. That means the fasting and post-breakfast rise in blood glucose will be rather low. The plasma insulin level therefore should match the late rise in blood glucose. To achieve this, intermediate-acting insulin given in the morning at breakfast time is effective. It peaks and maintains its level during these 4–12 h after morning steroid dose. To control the post-breakfast and post-lunch rise of glucose can be met with adding rapid-acting insulin to the morning intermediate insulin. Since the patient is in wards, it is highly desirable to use separate doses of both to be mixed in the syringe. This allows large variations in the dose of each with much better and far quicker control. (That is to say, fixed dose combinations should not be used.)

This variable and calibrated dose variation also reduces the need to use insulin to control post-lunch glucose rise. In case if the post lunch is higher, it is possible to use the separate short-acting insulin pre-lunch in doses which can be varied. There are different ways of using insulin and that of monitoring also. More details of it will be found in the Chap. 11.

This regime within a couple of days can also bring the pre-dinner glucose to a reasonable level. Since the hyperglycemic response to steroids during the night is lower, the doses of both intermediate- and rapid-acting insulin can be varied as in the morning, calibrated lower. This will avoid hypoglycemia in the early morning till breakfast is taken. This avoids the Somogyi effect of hyperglycemia after a hypoglycemic episode.

As an alternative to rapid-acting insulin, short-acting insulin like lispro or aspart can be used to control postprandial peaks with intermediate insulin with variable dosing for both. Varying the doses of intermediate- and short-/rapid-acting insulin needs some experience, which should be obtained by those who manage glucose control. The use of short-/rapid-acting insulin independently pre-lunch and in the evening to control pre-dinner glucose levels makes it little more complex. For other physicians, there is another option. It is to use true long-acting insulins like glargine or detemir with three short-acting insulins with each major meal. Long-acting ones can be used not only at bedtime but also in the morning. One can use short-acting aspart with an intermediate-acting aspart in premixed injectable cartridges either twice or thrice with each meal. The use of premixed insulin is already mentioned.

Any regime should be considered on the basis of its ability to control the delayed hyperglycemia in the day and blunted hyperglycemic response in the night. The rapid-acting insulin may have advantage over the short-acting insulin in this situation. The short-acting insulin does not stack in the blood as does the rapid-acting insulin. The use of short-acting insulin therefore may not be able to control the delayed hyperglycemic response. In fact, three doses of regular/rapid insulin stack stay for adequately long in the plasma and would maintain sufficient level in the blood in the evening when the hyperglycemic effect of the steroid is likely to be pronounced, hence may be more effective. (See the details in the Chap. 11.) For the same reason of stacking, rapid-acting insulin at this time may cause midmorning hypoglycemia [31].

That leaves only the intermediate- or long-acting insulin to achieve adequate levels. These insulins do not have a peak level. Hence large doses of truly long-acting insulins are less likely to cause severe of significant hypoglycemia especially in the night [33]. The disadvantage is that the dose can be varied only once in 24 h hence less flexible. Insulin regime has to be adjusted to the Indian food pattern in a hospital when patient is eating fairly well. The patient will usually have a long wait of at least 9–11 h between dinner and breakfast.[5]

If truly long acting insulin is the choice in single-dose steroid regime the quantum needed could be higher than 30 units/24 h.

7.11.3 Multiple Steroid Doses in 1 Day

With multiple steroid doses get established, the impetus to a gluconeogenic process takes place round the clock, and there is a constant high hyperglycemic state. This has to be and can be counterbalanced by the above regimen with aggressive insulin dosing to keep the plasma levels of insulin high throughout the night and most of the day time. The above regime will serve the purpose well.

However, especially when multiple doses of steroids are given and the full continuing dosing is achieved, three more stages need consideration since they are part of the entire perioperative process and call for different strategies to control hyperglycemia and not allow development of severe hypoglycemia. These stages are as follows:

1. Time relation of glucose with its stepwise rise, as the initial steroid doses are administered.
2. Fully established high-dose steroid administration with peak glucose levels achieved.
3. When steroids are tapered with its time relation with the glucose levels coming down.

1. Time relation of stepwise rise of glucose as the initial steroid dose is initiated. The glucose level rises typically 12–24 h after the *initial* steroid administration. In neurosurgery, the long-acting steroids like dexamethasone are used. Steroids after binding with a surface receptor are internalized and then bind to specific nuclear sites to induce their changes. That takes time and explains the time lag between

[5] For the pharmacokinetic and pharmacodynamic properties of these insulins, please see the chapter of the same title in this volume. It will help to make a choice among the many available now. The major differences among them are the frequency and severity of hypoglycemia during the night in particular. This consideration minimizes its importance in the situation of steroid-induced hyperglycemia with or without diabetes.

steroid administration and hyperglycemia. When more steroid doses are given, each one spikes the glucose levels, and high blood glucose level gets established and will not continue to rise further even if steroids are continued. Such glucose levels have to be brought down. This can easily be achieved by anticipatory stepping up of insulin quantum as soon as the steroids are started. The additional units over the basal doses will depend upon the first glucose reading after the steroid is given and the experience the treating physician has acquired in this aspect.

This measure will at its least blunt the high rise of glucose, and subsequent doses of insulin can be stepped up quickly to get the situation under control in shorter period. There is no reason to be apprehensive about the anticipatory increase in insulin when the glucose is not that high. The reason is the high insulin resistance which quickly develops once a substantial dose of steroid is administered. This helps particularly in emergency situations of any kind and semi-emergencies like a pontine meningioma.

2. Fully established high-dose steroid administration with peak/blunted glucose levels achieved is not so much a state of hyperglycemia but a state of high insulin resistance. The only way it can be controlled is to raise the plasma insulin level by aggressively increasing the insulin units. We have used up to or more than 200 U of human regular insulin daily three times with an intermediate-acting insulin generally at dinner in addition routinely. As the experience increases and the residents and nurses get more tuned to this exercise in the wards or in the postoperative ICU, each insulin dose can be increased for as early a control as possible. However it is not as easy and needs efficient communication between the two to keep each subsequent dose changing. By empowering and training our staff, we have been able to control the glucose preoperatively within 72–96 h.[6]
3. Time relation of steroids when they are being tapered with the glucose levels coming down is typically a reverse of the situation described in 1 above. At the first reduction of steroid doses, the glucose does not fall immediately. It has a time lag of about 24–36 h. The corollary is that the insulin doses should be lowered about 24–36 h later when one or more glucose readings tend to a normal or a lesser level. In doing so hypoglycemia is not a concern since the insulin resistance is high and steroids step up the gluconeogenesis.

   Very tight metabolic control is somewhat difficult to achieve under steroid administration though. A minimum fasting blood glucose level around 140 mg% can be considered adequate, if ketonuria is absent. Their electrolyte levels also have to be done repeatedly as potassium loss is twofold—one due to increased osmotic glycosuria and the other due to steroid-induced sodium retention and simultaneous potassium depletion. Electrolyte and fluid losses will be compounded if there is active and significant vomiting due to raised intracranial tension.

In intraoperative management of neurosurgical patient, the general guidelines for management remain the same as for any "major" routine surgery.

[6]One other situation where such or even higher units of insulin are needed is the gestational diabetes or in diabetes with pregnancy since that is also a high insulin resistance state with hyperglycemia which has to be controlled at all costs.

We recommend the use of insulin infusions as the method of choice for glucose control intraoperatively. A syringe pump is not always necessary but recommended and may become mandatory in a very special situation in which severe glucose fluctuations are likely to be encountered. This is the case of a growth hormone-secreting pituitary tumor where preoperative glucose control may sometimes be impossible. *Joslin's Diabetes Mellitus*, 2005 edition, mentions that 25% of these patients develop diabetes. Some of these patients continue to have very high blood glucose levels even with large doses of insulin, and their glucose control can be achieved only after the offending tumor has been removed. Such patients need insulin infusion via syringe pump and a close monitoring of blood glucose levels.

Especially postoperatively, the monitoring may have to be continued for days as once the glucose level starts falling, the insulin requirements will go down, and hypoglycemia may supervene if one is not careful. The other situation in neurosurgery where syringe pump may be required is when multiple drips may run, some may be administered in glucose containing solutions and some may not. Some may run at a faster rate than others and all these variables may change. The net effect of all of them can be computed by the blood glucose monitored and the insulin infusion rate and by changing the latter in either direction, by administering insulin on x number of units per hour basis by syringe pump.

The principles of postoperative management of neurosurgical patients with diabetes do not differ from any major surgery. The only variable would be the time lag in starting the enteral feeding. In those cases where the chances of recovery to an adequate level of consciousness are low, a percutaneous endoscopic gastrostomy may be undertaken to effectively maintain nutrition.

7.12 Surgery in Diabetes with Renal Disease

End-stage renal disease (ESRD) affects up to 40% of diabetic patients [34]. Its full manifestation is dependent on the duration of diabetes and genetic predisposition as well. In ESRD the plasma insulin clearance is reduced considerably leading to higher insulin levels. This is coupled with poor gluconeogenesis which the kidneys routinely contribute to and the poor caloric intake during the uremic phase. Together the risk of developing hypoglycemia increases considerably. Many oral antidiabetic drugs cannot be used in chronic kidney disease patients including biguanides (metformin), sulfonylureas, and alpha-glucosidase inhibitors [35, 36].

The most complex and difficult situation for management of elective/emergency or surgery in life-threatening situations is in the presence of significant renal disease. These patients may or may not be on dialysis. If they are on regular dialysis, the situation is controllable and somewhat better. In type 1 diabetes, since the disorder is more severe than type 2, these patients may develop renal disease far more frequently and much earlier than type 2 patients do. With it come hypertension and involvement of the coronary vasculature and retinopathy. Peripheral as well as autonomic neuropathy is commoner in type 1 diabetes. This may be seen particularly in centers which handle diabetic foot presenting as Charcot's or sepsis with local abscesses. In most such cases, the patient is likely to be in full diabetic ketoacidosis, with an element of uremia adding to the acidotic state. In such cases the management described under Emergency Surgery in all its aspects elsewhere in this volume will have to be undertaken.

Many other considerations place limits on the aggressive management of emergency situations in end-stage renal disease. The fluids and electrolytes and acid-base balance are more difficult to handle. Appropriate reduction in the drug doses including the anesthetics and insulin. In significant renal disease, aggressive fluid therapy has no place. It will have to be moderated with a close and constant watch on circulatory and cardiac fluid overload which can develop quickly. Rehydration is not going to be followed by copious diuresis in such patients, unless the degree of prerenal azotemia is the dominant feature of renal disease as it presents here. In majority of such patients, it is not going to be so. The native renal insufficiency will be what prevails. The presence of chronic edema indicates expansion of the extracellular compartment with low tissue oxygen concentrations as well as hypoalbuminemia. There will also be profound vasoconstriction due to the endothelial factors. The likelihood of hyperkalemia developing quickly even with attempts at low dose potassium infusions is also high.

Emergency peritoneal dialysis is a partially effective remedy. One of its major limitations would be intra-abdominal catastrophe in which case it cannot be used. Urgently undertaken hemofiltration also may not prove to be that enabling. If life is threatened, as in infected diabetic foot, the preservation of life gets the highest priority. The guiding principle would be to remove the surgical cause even under unfavorable situations since if it is not done, the life is at stake. To do the best, the only way is to do what minimum is necessary in a measured way under careful clinical and laboratory monitoring discussed extensively. Taking the patient and her relatives in full confidence without holding back any serious considerations or heightening them unduly would be a prudent approach.

The pathophysiology of significant/end-stage renal disease has a few more features which need to be understood. The main one is the interplay of insulin and kidney disease in diabetes. About 25% of the circulating insulin is degraded by normal kidneys. The tubular cells do not display insulin resistance hence insulin easily enters the cells and gets degraded. Insulin being a small molecule gets easily filtered and internalized by renal tubules which have large number of receptors and singularly lack insulin resistance. Renal disease starts from the stage of hyperfiltration in the initial period of newly detected diabetes and progresses over time. At this stage the blood that circulates through kidney is much higher in volume with higher than normal GFR. Over years as the glomerular lesions develop and the glomerular number rapidly declines, it leads to the reduction of glomerular filtration. It results in progressive decline in the quantities of insulin filtered that is presented to the tubules. At the same time less quanta of insulin are degraded by the tubular cells; therefore higher levels of insulin will continue to circulate. If regular or intermediate-acting insulin is being given as multiple injections, then there will be "stacking" effect and higher levels of plasma insulin leading to hypoglycemia.

In end-stage renal disease, this situation is also complicated by the generally poor intake of the nutrients due to uremic acidosis and depressed storage of glucose in the body, while the insulin sensitivity may go up. These mechanisms will lead to hypoglycemia which could be sudden, severe, or unexpected. This was also the reason why in significant renal disease, the teaching in yesteryears had been to administer only crystalline or regular insulin to avoid hypoglycemia. In the 1990s, this teaching was emphatic about not using intermediate- or long-acting insulin. Once the purified porcine and then recombinant insulins became the norm, the irregular dissociation of bovine porcine insulin combining with insulin autoantibodies causing hypoglycemia was also removed. On the other hand, the insulin resistance in Indian patients appears to be too high even under adverse conditions like uremia. As a result control with regular insulin alone was simply not achievable. Over a few years, it became apparent that intermediate-acting insulin even in the presence of significant renal disease is a must without having to unduly fear hypoglycemia.

However, it is advisable to keep the following guidelines in mind while using insulin in the end-stage renal disease.

1. Watching a patient for hypoglycemia when insulin is being administered is of paramount importance.
2. Adequate intake assured to modify insulin dose before injecting. This is relevant because renal failure predisposes a patient to nausea, vomiting due to uremic acidosis.
3. Sometimes of course, more insulin may be required, and short-acting insulin alone may not control blood glucose adequately. Cautious, gradual increase with even an addition of intermediate-acting insulin will generally be needed more often than not.
4. It will also presuppose some knowledge imparted to the relatives about how to suspect hypoglycemia, what kind of symptoms may arise, the seriousness of those symptoms, and how to treat it.
5. Generally speaking OHAs are contraindicated and can cause profound, prolonged recurrent hypoglycemia. In early stages of renal involvement, repaglinide 1 mg with each meal is safe. If a meal is skipped it should also be skipped.
6. Poor intake by the patients may sometimes require intravenous support and relevant reductions or increases of insulin doses. In investigations using intravenous radio contrast agents, renal status in non transplant surgeries should be checked to detect deterioration if any.
7. In short, repeated blood glucose estimations are necessary in this situation, both intra- and postoperatively. It may have to be extended to 48–72 h postoperatively. Frequent monitoring using low and flexible intravenous insulin regime will be more effective if oral calorie intake is poor and till satisfactory food intake is restored.
8. Anemia is often quite significant despite injections of erythropoietin. The reason for that is the commonly found severe iron deficiency. The serum iron estimation is done only rarely but erythropoietin is regularly given. Oftentimes

even hemoglobin is not checked to see if it is improving. Without replacing iron preferably intravenously, no amount of erythropoietin can correct anemia. In the last several years, the author finds oral iron as having little effect in improving anemia after months of administration. He also finds intravenous iron safe hardly ever producing anything but transient pains. IV administration of iron could be followed by substantial doses of vitamin B12, especially in vegetarian patients.[7]

9. In emergency situations, packed RBCs are the only option.
10. If the iron replacement with erythropoietin is considered cumbersome and costly, PRBCs are certainly a direct cost-effective option.
11. Hypoalbuminemia, a constant accompaniment of significant renal disease, is a high-risk factor for mortality. Parenteral administration of 10% or 20% albumin is costly and has temporary and has short-term effect in the overall fluid status. These patients have all other concomitants of end-stage renal disease like hypocalcemia and hyperphosphatemia which need control by supplemental calcium and vitamin D3. Injectable variety of D2 is of no use since this prodrug cannot be converted to its active form due to the renal insufficiency, since kidneys do the final conversion. The nutrient intake of uremic patients is also poor. It improves once these patients are stabilized on hemodialysis. Multiple vitamin mineral deficiencies should also be corrected.
12. In addition, in patients with diabetic nephropathy, the presence of other diabetic complications may be considered as inevitable. In today's world renal transplant is the only proper answer to this malady.

7.12.1 Renal Transplant in Patients with Diabetes

Diabetes mellitus is now a common cause in adults going for renal transplant due to the development of end-stage kidney disease. The vast majority of patients with diabetes undergoing kidney transplant belong to the type 2 variety. However it is better studied in type 1 diabetes. In a large study of type 1 diabetic patients who received a renal transplant, the recipient and graft survival rates were equivalent to nondiabetic patients as studied in the first 2 years after the renal transplant. The total number of type 1 diabetes thus evaluated was 529. This is undoubtedly attributable to good perioperative management of glucose control. This was undertaken by admitting the patients for few days before the transplant was carried [37].

[7] In Northeastern India, correcting anemia in patients without nephropathy is also a difficult undertaking. Many native populations have widespread prevalence of hemoglobinopathy with characteristic normochromic microcytic RBCs. No matter what one may try, it is not possible to raise Hb beyond 9 g/dL. Similarly, there is widespread prevalence of congenital polycystic kidneys in these and other populations to a lesser extent which over years lead to end-stage nephropathy. The practice of prescribing PPIs (proton pump inhibitors) is almost universal. PPIs may be contributing to B12 deficiency. The water content of heavy metals, particularly arsenic, is high. Whether it interferes in the process of iron absorption leading to correction of anemia or causes it is not clear.

There are two issues which need attention that are relevant to this volume. The first is the survival of the graft in a patient with diabetes. The second is whether new-onset diabetes develops in a patient who did not have diabetes before transplant. These two are briefly discussed here. Immunosuppressive drugs like glucocorticoids, CNIs (tacrolimus and cyclosporine), and mammalian target of rapamycin (mTOR) inhibitors (sirolimus and everolimus) increase insulin resistance and may lead to new development of diabetes. All three mechanisms—insulin resistance, impaired insulin secretion, and beta cell function—are responsible one way or the other when immunosuppressants are used [38–42].

Early renal transplantation allows for a greater survival benefit for all CKD patients whether they have or do not have diabetes. Patients with diabetes generally have lower rate of survival in CKD undergoing transplant [43]. It is observed that the longer survival benefit is seen in a live donor kidney than in dead donor kidney transplants which stands to reason especially in early transplants [44].

It is further observed that in the first year of transplant, patients who did not have diabetes prior develop new-onset diabetes. Roughly 15–30% of these will now develop diabetes. As the transplant years progress, 4–6% of the patients, which is a much smaller number, will develop diabetes every year. This figure is more or less the same in patients who do not undergo transplant in that 1 year and are on supportive treatment as they wait for it [45–47].

Kidney transplant surgery would be a challenge in those patients morbidly obese having type 2 diabetes. The technique and experience of bariatric surgery now available is quite adequate. If undertaken, it may improve the general condition of the patients to undergo renal transplantation. Simultaneous pancreatic and kidney transplant is more difficult. It is equally likely that the posttransplant medicines will affect the new pancreas as well [48].

Insulin requirements after transplant go up and virtually return to pre-disease level. Steroids in posttransplant period will further necessitate stepping up insulin therapy. Monitoring of the drug levels used to prevent graft rejection is an important and expensive part of the management since it reflects on the insulin resistance in the years after transplant. If these levels are low, hypoglycemia would be frequent. If the levels of immunosuppressive drugs is high, there will be hyperglycemia.

The other drugs routinely used in diabetes management are either reduced or stopped in ESRD, whether a patient is on dialysis or without it. Two levels of eGFR are important considerations in reduction of many of these drug doses. eGFR 30–60 mL/min/1.73 m^2 and eGFR is <30 mL/min/1.73 m^2. Metformin is reduced when eGFR is 30–60 mL/min/1.73 m^2. It should be stopped if eGFR is <30 mL/min/1.73 m^2. DPP-4 inhibitors—alogliptin, saxagliptin, sitagliptin, and vildagliptin—start accumulating in the body with eGFR <60 mL/min/1.73 m^2 without creating much toxicity. Saxagliptin cannot be used in end-stage renal failure. Linagliptin has no dose adjustment requirement in renal impairment due to hepatic metabolism. Other DPP 4 inhibitors can be used in reduced doses.

Currently used sulphonylureas are relatively long-acting drugs. They do act for up to 24 h. The half-life of sulphonylureas increases as the renal failure worsens. It thereby raises the risk of severe hypoglycemia due to continued insulin release which is not efficiently degraded. SGLT2i require adequately preserved renal function for their effect. It functions on the basis of causing glucose loss in the urine. The level of eGFR up to which dapagliflozin may be used is more than 60 mL/min/1.73 m^2 but not below. Empagliflozin has a lesser limit of eGFR more than 45 mL/min/1.73 m^2 below which it should be discontinued. Acarbose is stopped if eGFR <25 mL/min/1.73 m^2. There is no data on what happens to pioglitazone in dialysis. Hence it should not be used on patients who have reached the stage of ESRD. If the eGFR is less than 30 mL/min/1.73 m^2 GLP-1 RA, exenatide and liraglutide should be stopped. NSAIDs (non-steroidal anti-inflammatory drugs) and any other nephrotoxic drugs should also be avoided [49].

Hemodialysis and continuous ambulatory peritoneal dialysis (CAPD) are two treatment options to maintain homeostasis to the extent possible if renal transplant is not immediately possible. Hemodialysis, correction of anemia, improving calcium levels and controlling the rise of phosphate with medications, and a well-planned diet will help these patients.

In CAPD the dialysate solution used will differ with various clinical parameters. When icodextrin (Extraneal®) is used, it creates certain difficulties in measuring glucose levels in blood. With icodextrin use, the blood glucose detected is higher, but it is in reality a falsely elevated blood glucose. In all the three ways of testing, that is, with glucose dehydrogenase, pyrroloquinoline quinone, or glucose-dye-oxidoreductase, the pseudo elevation of blood glucose is detected. This may lead to higher insulin dose administration which is not needed. Intravenous immunoglobulin preparation, such as Intragam®, has maltose. Cytomegalovirus (CMV), immunoglobulin, and tetanus immunoglobulin if used intravenously can also interfere with glucose estimation if glucose dehydrogenase strips are used.

7.13 Peripheral Arterial/Vascular Disease (PAD/PVD) in Patients with Diabetes

Peripheral arterial/vascular disease (PAD/PVD) generally means arterial diseases of lower limbs, in people with or without diabetes. Presence of PAD can either cause dry gangrenes or become a major deterrent for infected or uninfected wound from healing or causes loss of limb or life. The presence of PAD is also the single most important indicator of systemic, cardiac, cerebral, and other vascular problems, even if PAD is asymptomatic. Presence of PAD is strongly associated with concomitant coronary and systemic arterial atherosclerosis, but not vice versa.

PAD can be diagnosed by good clinical examination without need for any tests, but awareness about it needs to increase further. The first step in the preoperative assessment is to palpate the following arteries of the lower limbs on both sides—the popliteal, dorsalis pedis, and the posterior tibial arteries. The reason is that PAD in diabetes essentially involves arteries below the popliteal. Symptoms and findings give the level of ischemia in the vascular tree. A third of patients with PAD are asymptomatic but need aggressive medical therapy to prevent future systemic cardiovascular events like myocardial infarction, stroke, injury, and pedal ulcer formation with subsequent limb loss since these patients remain at the highest risk for the rest of their life.

PAD in people with diabetes will generally have several atherosclerotic lesions through the length of the single or multiple arteries. These changes occur at a younger age, progress more rapidly from early critical limb ischemia to gangrene, have a more selective distribution in infrapopliteal arteries, and have higher risk potential for sudden progression from intermittent claudication to limb-threatening ischemia. In India prevalence of it is from 6% to 15% [50]. It is a more aggressive disease in India.

In neurogenic claudication, pain is positional and may start even at the first step, not immediately relieved by rest as in lumbar canal stenosis. In venous claudication, the pain appears later in the day, with leg swelling; it is a bursting type of pain, relieved by limb elevation; it is caused by the iliac vein occlusion and not from varicose veins. Arterial claudication typically occurs after walking at the claudication distance and is relieved by rest. Claudication does not necessarily precede tissue loss or rarely progresses to critical limb-threatening ischemia, in which less than 1% undergoes amputation in a year. But in India, external injury, mostly because of barefoot walking, pushes a patient towards limb and life-threatening ischemia.

The presence of PAD is not an indication for invasive procedures like angiogram or MRA/CTA or coronary workup, unless they have symptoms related to coronary disease. To increase walking distance in PAD cilastazole, exercise program and additional medical therapy is needed with that of diabetes.

Delay in the diagnosis of limb-threatening ischemia is due to late presentation of the patient and lack of awareness/diagnostic skills in the care providers. Debridement without recognizing limb ischemia significantly increases morbidity, mortality, and costs. Thromboangiitis obliterans (TAO) or Buerger's disease has only one risk factor of which is excessive smoking, and the age should be less than 45 years with distal, infrapopliteal disease.

Ankle brachial index (ABI) is the next step in the diagnosis and severity of PAD. First ankle arterial pressure is obtained, and then the brachial arterial pressure is measured. Then the brachial pressure is divided by the pressure of the ankle arteries, namely, dorsalis pedis and posterior tibial on both sides. The ABI of 0.9–1.3 is a good indication that healing of an ulcer will happen without intervention for PAD. ABI of less than 0.9 has high sensitivity, specificity, positive predictive value, and negative predictive value. It has an overall accuracy of 98% to diagnose PAD. ABI of less than 0.8 is seen in patients who suffer from claudication. ABI of less than 0.5 is seen in patients with rest pain. All patients with ABI of less than 0.8 will be at a higher risk to develop cardiovascular events in time to come. They should therefore be treated to avoid these events. Those with ABI under 0.50 have twice the mortality over 5 years. For each decrease in ABI of 0.10, there is an increase in relative risk of major cardiovascular event by 10.2% [51]. Exercise stress testing with measurement of ABI before and after exercise-induced pain can detect or rule out occult PAD.

Within the ambit of perioperative management, surgical intervention is called for in the presence of a wound not healing over 2 weeks due to ischemia as the basic cause with or without infection, where a limb or life is threatened due to PAD or if the claudication seriously limits functional ability and means of livelihood, or sudden worsening of symptoms or critical limb-threatening ischemia. It can occur with complete occlusion of diseased artery. Presence of even a small gangrene should immediately resort to evaluating and treating PAD. There is no known medical therapy, and nearly all patients need revascularization, either surgical, endovascular, or hybrid procedures, i.e., combined surgery + endovascular at one sitting.

As the RBCs pass through the capillary circulation, oxygen diffuses in the tissues; transcutaneous oxygen pressure (TcPO2) measures excess of oxygen diffusion from red blood cells. A TcPO2 pressure of less than 40 mm is considered inadequate for healing. Normal TcPO2 is more than 60 mm. This pressure gives an idea of oxygenation in the tissues of the most peripheral parts of the lower extremities. This in turn gives an idea of the microcirculation and the likely metabolic state of the adjacent interstitial spaces. This is an indication of how advanced the state of arterial occlusion is at rest. It can be assessed after exercise also. TcPO2 has an advantage over the ABI. Patients with diabetes and renal disease often have an ABI of 1.3. It happens because of non-compressible vessels due to sclerosis of the tunica media of the arteries. One may tend to consider this ABI as adequate for arterial blood flow which it may not be. TcPO2 values are not affected in this condition also and may measure values which are far less than the ABI may indicate. TcPO2 values indicate whether Hyperbaric Oxygen Therapy will further help to heal Diabetic Foot Ulcer, strengthening the advice to patients to undergo that.

TcPO2 measurement is done by placing probe heated at a standard 44 degrees Celsius against the skin. That causes vasodilation and a local reactive hyperthermia facilitating oxygen diffusion across the skin. It diffuses towards a cathode and gets reduced. TcPO2 is measured via electrochemical reduction at a cathode. Oxygen defusing across the skin and towards the cathode in the probe is reduced. This reduction is proportional to the number of oxygen molecules and is measured as oxygen pressure. The dorsum of the foot, anteromedial calf approximately 10 cm below the patella, and the thigh 10 cm above the patella are the usual locations for measuring TcPO2. TcPO2 measurement at rest, tissues do not have higher metabolic demands. Hence the TcPO2 will be demonstrably lower only in severe arterial occlusion. In less occluded arteries, it may still be normal. If a patient is asked to exercise the limb, the metabolic demand and the need for the oxygen increase. However the TcPO2 measurement may not proportionately rise due to and depending upon the severity of the arterial occlusion and may be able to pick up less occluded arteries as well. The TcPO2 sensitivity thus increases to 100% following exercise, for reasons mentioned above. However its sensitivity when compared to results of angiography lowers to about 77% at rest [52]. For more details see additional readings at the end of the chapter.

Outcomes of the operative methods of revascularization also depend on the wound burden and extent of infection. Morality is about 5–6% in a competent center with the other surgical and medical backup with which the wounds heal. Open surgical bypass is preferably done with saphenous or other autogenous venous conduit. These veins are the best to save the limbs for longer duration, of over 90% at 1 year. In aortoiliac reconstruction, limb salvage remains above 90% at 5 years and femoral-distal bypass about 70% at 3 years. Since patient population is getting older with multiple comorbidities, in high-risk patients minimally invasive endovascular procedures have replaced many of the surgical procedures because of lower morbidity and mortality. Response is upwards of 80% in patients with femoral-distal occlusive diseases [50].

Extensive revascularization of lower limb arterial tree can be performed with limb salvage. Its efficacy is equal to bypass procedures, but the long-term patency is lower than open bypass procedures. It is about 50–60% for femoropopliteal segments at 1 year and about 50–70% for infrapopliteal interventions at 6 months, and the patency may not remain. But the limb salvage remains high, equal to bypass. The drug-coated balloons (DCB) have better patency up to 2 years but are more expensive. The newer "vascular mimetic" stents, which conform to severe anatomical changes that femoral artery undergoes with various movements, have yielded superior results, up to 2 years but at a markedly increased costs. Long-term results are pending. The mortality of endovascular interventions is about half or even a quarter of "open" surgical procedure [50].

"Hybrid" procedures in multi-segmental limb-threatening/occlusive disease are ones where patients undergo angioplasty and "bypass" at the same sitting, reducing the surgical burden of extensive open procedures. Patient with femoral occlusion and infrapopliteal disease can undergo femoral-popliteal bypass with infrapopliteal angioplasty to increase foot perfusion. Such procedures should be done in specialized centers with access to "hybrid" catheter laboratories and operating theater suites. In diabetic PAD the costs for the procedures which should come down considerably since the stent prices have come down in India significantly.

Unquestionably limb salvage is more cost-effective than amputation in mid- and long-term with superior quality of life of patients. Aggressive control of hypertension and diabetes, antiplatelet drugs, statins, or the lipid lowering agents, even with normal lipid profile, is used to prevent progression of systemic cardiovascular disease and events. The drugs to be avoided are beta-blockers, especially propranolol which have marked effects of peripheral vasoconstriction. If the use of beta-blockers is important, those with the least vasoconstrictive action should be used in as minimal a dose as possible. Stopping of smoking, control of diabetes, and foot care are needed. Cilastazole (100 mg bid) is the only effective drug in diabetic PAD if tolerated.

7.13.1 Peripheral Vascular Surgery and Prophylactic Antibiotic Use

Many authorities recommend using prophylaxis for any procedure involving vascular prosthetic material placement like the hemodialysis access grafts. Antibiotic prophylaxis is not indicated for carotid endarterectomy or upper extremity bypass grafts unless prosthetic material is used. Preoperative administration of a cephalosporin has been shown to decrease the incidence of postoperative wound infection in:

1. Resection of abdominal aorta and a graft placement.
2. Lower extremity bypass grafting where groin incisions are made.
3. Lower extremity amputations for ischemia [26].

References

1. Niles NW, McGrath PD, Malenka D, et al. Survival of patients with diabetes and multivessel coronary artery disease after surgical or percutaneous coronary revascularization: results of a large regional prospective study. Northern New England Cardiovascular Disease Study Group. J Am Coll Cardiol. 2001;37:1008–15.
2. Investigators TBARI. Influence of diabetes on 5-year morbidity and mortality in a randomized trial comparing CABG and PTCA in patients with multivessel disease. Circulation. 1997;96:1761–9.
3. Crock PA, Ley CJ, Martin IK, Alford FP, Best JD. Hormonal and metabolic changes during hypothermic coronary artery bypass surgery in diabetic and non-diabetic subjects. Diabet Med. 1988;5:47–52.
4. Devineni R, Mckinzie FN. Surgery for coronary artery disease in patients with diabetes mellitus. Can J Surg. 1985;28:367–70, cited by Subhankar Chowdhury, Sujoy Ghosh SUPPLEMENT OF JAPI JULY 2007 VOL. 55.
5. Burton D, Nicholson G, Hall G. Endocrine and metabolic response to surgery. Cont Educ Anaesth Crit Care Pain. 2004;4(5):144–7. https://doi.org/10.1093/bjaceaccp/mkh040.
6. Hirsch IB, McGill JB. Role of insulin management of surgical patients with diabetes mellitus. Diabetes Care. 1990;13:980.
7. Baumann H, Gauldie J. The acute phase response. Immunol Today. 1994;15:74–9.
8. Desborough JP. The stress response to surgery. Br J Anaesth. 2000;85:109–17.
9. Wright PD, Johnston IDA. The effect of surgical operation on growth hormone levels in plasma. Surgery. 1975;77(4):479–86.
10. Alberti KG, Marshall SM. Diabetes and surgery. In: Alberti KG, Krall LP, editors. Diabetes annual/4. New York, NY: Elsevier; 1988. p. 248–71.
11. Clutter WE, Rizza RA, Gerich JE, Cryper PE. Regulation of glucose metabolism by sympathochromaffin catecholamines. Diabetes Metab Rev. 1988;4:17–30.
12. Schricker T, Carvalho G. An ounce of prevention worth a pound of cure. Can J Anesth. 2004;51:948–9.
13. McAlister FA, Man J, Bistritz L, et al. Diabetes and coronary artery bypass surgery: an examination of perioperative glycemic control and outcomes. Diabetes Care. 2003;26:1518–24.
14. Simmons D, Morton K, Laughton S, Scott DJ. A comparison of two intravenous insulin regimens among surgical patients with insulin dependent diabetes mellitus. Diabetes Educ. 1994;20:422–7.
15. Bolk J, van der Ploeg T, Cornel JH, et al. Impaired glucose metabolism predicts mortality after a myocardial infarction. Int J Cardiol. 2001;79:207–14.
16. Lawrie GM, Morris GC, Glaeser DH. Influence of diabetes mellitus on the results of coronary artery bypass surgery. JAMA. 1986;256:1967–71.
17. Halkos ME, Lattouf OM, Puskas JD, et al. Elevated preoperative hemoglobin A1c level is associated with reduced long-term survival after coronary artery bypass surgery. Ann Thorac Surg. 2008;86:1431–7.
18. Mangano DT, Layug EL, Wallace A, et al. Effect of atenolol on mortality and cardiovascular morbidity after non cardiac surgery. Multicenter Study of Perioperative Ischemia Research Group. N Engl J Med. 1996;335:1713–20.
19. McAlister FA, Amad H, Man J, Tandon P, Bistriz L. Diabetes and coronary bypass surgery. Diabetes Care. 2003;26:1518–24.
20. Furnary A, Gao G, Grunkeimer GL, et al. Continuous insulin infusion reduces mortality in patients with diabetes undergoing coronary artery bypass grafting. J Thorac Cardiovasc Surg. 2003;125:1007–21.
21. Rady MY, Ryan T, Starr NJ. Perioperative determinants of morbidity and mortality in elderly patients undergoing cardiac surgery. Crit Care Med. 1998;26:225–35.
22. Haga KK, McClymont KL, Clarke S, et al. The effect of tight glycemic control, during and after cardiac surgery, on patient mortality and morbidity: a systematic review and meta analysis. J Cardiothorac Surg. 2011;6(1):Article 3.

23. Carvalho G, Moore A, Qizilbash B, et al. Maintenance of normoglycemia during open cardiac surgery. Anesth Analg. 2004;99:319–24.
24. Parsonage WA, Hetmanski D, Cowley AJ. Beneficial haemodynamic effects of insulin in chronic heart failure. Heart. 2001;85:508–13.
25. Pomposelli J, Baxter J, Babineau T, et al. Early postoperative glucose control predicts nosocomial infection rate in diabetic patients. J Parent Enter Nutr. 1998;22:77–81.
26. Measley RE Jr. Chapter 3: Antimicrobial prophylaxis: prevention of postoperative infections. In: Merli GJ, Weitz HH, editors. Medical management of the surgical patient. 3rd ed. Philadelphia, PA: Saunders; 2008, eBook ISBN: 9781437710588, Paperback ISBN: 9781416023852.
27. Duncan AI, Koch CG, Xu M, et al. Recent metformin ingestion does not increase in-hospital morbidity or mortality after cardiac surgery. Anesth Analg. 2007;104:42–50.
28. UK Prospective Diabetes Study (UKPDS) Group. Intensive blood-glucose control with sulphonylureas or insulin compared with conventional treatment and risk of complications in patients with type 2 diabetes (UKPDS 33). Lancet. 1998;352:837–53.
29. Jacobi J, Bircher N, Krinsley J, et al. Guidelines for the use of an insulin infusion for the management of hyperglycemia in critically ill patients. Crit Care Med. 2012;40:3251–76.
30. Ali Z, Prabhakar H. Fluid Management during Neurosurgical Procedures. J Neuroanaesthesiol Crit Care. 2016;3(Suppl S1):35–40.
31. Glister BC, Vigersky RA. Perioperative management of type 1 diabetes mellitus. Endocrinol Metab Clin N Am. 2003;32:411–36.
32. Greenstone MA, Shaw AB. Alternate day corticosteroid causes alternate day hyperglycaemia. Postgrad Med J. 1987;63:761–4.
33. Ratner RE, Hirsch IB, Neifing JL, et al. Less hypoglycemia with insulin glargine in intensive insulin therapy for type 1 diabetes. US Study Group of Insulin Glargine in type 1 Diabetes. Diabetes Care. 2000;23:639–43.
34. Plantinga LC, Crews DC, Coresh J, et al. Prevalence of chronic kidney disease in US adults with undiagnosed diabetes or prediabetes. Clin J Am Soc Nephrol. 2010;5:673–82.
35. American Association of Clinical Endocrinologists, AACE Diabetes Resource Center. Management of common comorbidities of diabetes. Jacksonville, FL: American Association of Clinical Endocrinologists, AACE Diabetes Resource Center; 2016. http://outpatient.aace.com/type-2-diabetes/managementof-common-comorbidities-of-diabetes. Accessed June 2016.
36. Kroon L. Making sense of medications for diabetes [lecture]. San Francisco, CA: University of California, San Francisco, Osher Center for Integrative Medicine; n.d.
37. Lum CT, Sutherland DER, Goetz FC, et al. Management of the diabetic patient before, during and after surgery with special emphasis on uremic patients and kidney transplant recipients. Minn Med. 1985;68:693–6.
38. Johnston O, Rose CL, Webster AC, Gill JS. Sirolimus is associated with new-onset diabetes in kidney transplant recipients. J Am Soc Nephrol. 2008;19:1411–8.
39. Chakkera HA, Mandarino LJ. Calcineurin inhibition and new-onset diabetes mellitus after transplantation. Transplantation. 2013;95(5):647–52.
40. Soleimanpour SA, Crutchlow MF, Ferrari AM, et al. Calcineurin signaling regulates human islet beta-cell survival. J Biol Chem. 2010;285:40050–9.
41. Tsang CK, Qi H, Liu LF, Zheng XF. Targeting mammalian target of rapamycin (mTOR) for health and diseases. Drug Discov Today. 2007;12:112–24.
42. Yang SB, Lee HY, Young DM, et al. Rapamycin induces glucose intolerance in mice by reducing islet mass, insulin content, and insulin sensitivity. J Mol Med (Berl). 2012;90:575–85.
43. Mange KC, Joffe MM, Feldman HI. Effect of the use or nonuse of long-term dialysis on the subsequent survival of renal transplants from living donors. N Engl J Med. 2001;344:726–31. https://doi.org/10.1056/NEJM200103083441004.
44. Becker BN, Rush SH, Dykstra DM, Becker YT, Port FK. Preemptive transplantation for patients with diabetes-related kidney disease. Arch Intern Med. 2006;166:44–8. https://doi.org/10.1001/archinte.166.1.44.

45. Cosio FG, Pesavento TE, Kim S, Osei K, Henry M, Ferguson RM. Patient survival after renal transplantation: IV. Impact of post-transplant diabetes. Kidney Int. 2002;62:1440–6.
46. Kasiske BL, Snyder JJ, Gilbertson D, Matas AJ. Diabetes mellitus after kidney transplantation in the United States. Am J Transplant. 2003;3:178–85.
47. Woodward RS, Schnitzler MA, Baty J, et al. Incidence and cost of new onset diabetes mellitus among U.S. wait-listed and transplanted renal allograft recipients. Am J Transplant. 2003;3:590–8.
48. Fourtounas C. World J Transplant. 2014;4(2):102–10.
49. Arnouts P, Bolignano D, Nistor I, et al. Glucose-lowering drugs in patients with chronic kidney disease: a narrative review on pharmacokinetic properties. Nephrol Dial Transplant. 2014;29(7):1284–300.
50. Suresh KR. Statistics from a tertiary Institute of Vascular Surgery, JIVAS, Bengaluru, India. Bengaluru: JIVAS; 2018.
51. Crawford F1, Welch K, Andras A, Chappell FM. Ankle brachial index for the diagnosis of lower limb peripheral arterial disease. Cochrane Database Syst Rev. 2016;9:CD010680.
52. Arsenault KA, McDonald J, Devereaux PJ, Thorlund K, Tittley JG, Whitlock RP. The use of transcutaneous oximetry to predict complications of chronic wound healing: a systematic review and meta-analysis. Wound Repair Regen. 2011 Nov;19(6):657–63.

Additional Reading

National Guidelines for Management of Diabetic Foot, published by Diabetic Foot society of India, 2017.
Preoperative Testing and Medication Management The Ohio State University Wexner Medical Center. 2017.

Special Surgical Situations in Diabetes: Part 2

8

Contents

S. Kelkar et al., *Towards Optimal Management of Diabetes in Surgery*,
https://doi.org/10.1007/978-981-13-7705-1_8

8.1 The Elderly Patient with Diabetes

Most frequently such a patient would usually be advanced in years, often with diabetes of long duration and likely to have obvious or ongoing complication of diabetes. There is poor tolerance of hypoglycemia in the elderly. The discussion that follows is relevant not only to the urological surgical patient but to all elderly patients in general. These points were not explained in greater detail earlier. The elderly Indian is not an active individual. Barring some morning walk which is on the increase in Indian cities despite the traffic congested and somewhat hazardous roads, they are sedentary individuals. Hence, exercise intolerance (either angina or dyspnea) may be difficult to assess clinically. It may not always be possible to put them to treadmill to detect exercise-induced angina. A relatively noninvasive procedure like 64-slice CT to detect coronary calcification degree is advisable if the patient is diagnosed to have symptoms of coronary artery disease.

Making an echocardiography evaluation in today's medical situations (with of course an ECG prior to that) is recommended. The most important finding it is likely to reveal is the inability of the left ventricle to adequately relax to accommodate more blood volume. It is called diastolic dysfunction. It is characteristic finding in diabetes. This results into rise in the end diastolic volume and pressure in the left ventricle. The diagnostic label for these findings is diabetic cardiomyopathy. It is so frequently found nowaday. This indicates the possibility of heart failure and caution against intravenous fluids. This should also be a matter discussed and explained to the patient and relatives in a nonthreatening manner. As already indicated, a thorough physical and investigational check is necessary, especially, in the elderly in whom the cardiac involvement would be prominent.

In the first decade of the new millennium couple of trials aimed for a systolic blood pressure of 130 mmHg. Such a tight control led to systolic blood pressures for variable periods during each day to much lower levels. Such lower systolic blood pressure level if it was not causing any discomfort was also probably tacitly acceptable to the trialists. The aim in fact could be to lower it as much as possible. The diastolic blood pressure at this level of systolic blood pressure led to an unacceptably low diastolic pressure to 60 mmHg or less. If we remember our physiology, it is only during the diastolic period and depending on diastolic pressure the cardiac muscle gets perfused. Thus excessively low diastolic blood pressure in the elderly with tachycardia can easily be seen to have detrimental to cardiac outcomes as it reduces the time of diastolic filling of the coronary arteries. The VO_2 Max will not be reached. The state of coronary arteries as described earlier in this volume adds to reduce the oxygenation of the cardiac muscle. If the cerebral autoregulation fails, it could lead to strokes. We as clinicians see no need to lower the blood pressure below 140/90 mmHg. Like too tight a control of glucose in elderly, it is now contraindicated to have a lower systolic blood pressure.[1]

In clinical practice, even in ICUs, tachycardia in diabetes is not dealt with properly in a substantial number of patients. This happens since the sympathetic autonomic system is intact, in fact unopposed by the parasympathetic system which generally is the first to get affected. The association of beta-blockers increasing the insulin resistance and elevation of glucose (which is the point for inaction) is the reason behind it. While this is true, the degree of hyperglycemia resulting from the more selective beta-blocker usage is not alarming; it is marginal. What resistance it may add to the highly insulin-resistant perioperative period is of a much lower degree. The beneficiary effects of beta-blockers on cardiac muscle and its functioning far outweigh the risks of hyperglycemia. It should be noted that beta-blockers are useful drugs even in heart failure and are routinely used. Like any drug, they should be started in low doses and raised under supervision.

An often neglected practice is to measure the blood pressure in sitting position which detects the postural fall/hypotension immediately. A patient with tightly controlled blood pressure is very likely to suffer from postural hypotension which is even more detrimental since sitting and walking time in a day far exceeds the period of lying down. A patient presenting with tachycardia is unlikely to have postural hypotension but may fail to increase the blood pressure in physiological terms. When cardio-selective beta-blockers are used, the chances that the postural hypotension will get pronounced are small.

8.2 The Urological Surgery in Diabetes

The commonest urological procedure in today's day and age would be transurethral resection (TUR) of either prostate or bladder tumor or basket extraction of ureteric stones. All such patients can be satisfactorily undertaken under regional anesthesia either spinal or epidural, and neither the anesthesia nor the surgery would produce undue pain nor too significant a metabolic decompensation. However, in patients *whose sympathetic autonomic nervous system is affected*, it may land the patient up in profound hypotension after spinal anesthesia. Hence it is desirable to omit the blood pressure medication on the morning of surgery. Under epidural anesthesia, the chances of post epidural fall in blood pressure are less.

[1] Dr. George Bakris speaking in the second International Diabetes Expert's Conference in Pune, India, on 26th of May 2018 was highly critical of the trials which demanded such low blood pressures (as well as tight control in the elderly) since the mortality in these trials was unacceptable.

The target levels of glucose control also should not be rigid or stringent. After ACCORD trial in elderly which sought tight control of blood glucose and resulted in many more deaths, there is no place to advise tight control in elderly today, not only during surgery but under normal circumstances as well. The fasting level of blood sugar need not be less than 140 mg/dL [1].

Hyponatremia is likely to develop in transurethral procedures, especially prostatic resection. It may be precipitated should large volumes of distilled water be used for the purpose of irrigation during TUR. It may get diffused in the circulation. With the use of irrigating solutions like glycine, this danger has been minimized, but glycine is an expensive item, and surgeons in government hospitals and medical colleges may still be forced to fall back upon distilled water for their poorer patients postoperatively. The awareness regarding hyponatremia becomes important as it would lead to drowsiness confusion and rarely convulsions or coma. In a person with diabetes, these same symptoms may be mimicked by hypoglycemia, and the adrenergic responses to hypoglycemia may sometimes be blunted—one, due to continued effect of the spinal or epidural blockade, and two, due to diabetic autonomic neuropathy. It becomes mandatory, therefore, to ascertain blood glucose level along with electrolytes immediately postoperatively and subsequently also at least once.

As some of these patients may have been administered OHA on the night prior to surgery, excluding hypoglycemia in the postoperative period becomes mandatory. Hence, blood glucose estimation is much more important in the postoperative period than is generally believed. It is especially important that the elderly patient should *not* have a blood glucose level less than 120 mg at any time. There is no need to be in a hurry to restart OHAs in these elderly patients until adequate food intake has been very well established. Any hyperglycemic episodes may be treated with small doses of subcutaneous insulin. Essentially, this would entail a necessity to monitor blood glucose at the bed side at least 4–6 hourly by the surgical residents. To add a last line of caution, no patient with diabetes should be treated as a day care surgery. He must be admitted and retained in hospital for at least 24 h postoperatively.

8.3 Ophthalmic Surgery

The diabetic ophthalmic patient for surgery may have retinopathy and will often be accompanied by other microvascular involvements, especially renal disease, and every effort should be made to ascertain the presence and severity of renal disease. There is, ordinarily, no need to shift to insulin from OHAs except if significant renal disease is present. Often, the patient may have no complaints with regard to renal insufficiency, the existence of which may be detected only on a preoperative laboratory check. As already detailed in a previous chapter, OHAs are not recommended for glycemic control in a patient with established renal disease. These patients should, therefore, "ideally" be shifted to insulin a few days earlier, controlled, and then operated if any ophthalmic procedure of considerable duration under GA is contemplated.

If an ophthalmic procedure is done under GA and would last long enough to cause some intraoperative glycemic disturbances and definitely some amount of postoperative nausea and vomiting necessitating administration of intravenous fluids for variable periods of time postoperatively, there is no need to discontinue OHAs for the surgery, except on the day of surgery they may be withheld. Any hyperglycemia may be treated, either intra- or postoperatively, with subcutaneous insulin. Should prolonged intravenous administration become necessary postoperatively, insulin will have to be continued depending on blood glucose levels.

Blood glucose sampling should be done for fasting values and then at least once intraoperatively once the surgery is well under way and action if necessary be initiated. Depending on this the second value, repeat estimations may become necessary. Postoperatively at least one glucose estimation is required to determine if insulin administration would be helpful. Any blood glucose level between 150 and 200 mg/dL is acceptable. After any short procedure, patients should be on slow glucose infusion to void hypoglycemia from the effects of the OHAs taken till the day before surgery. Without this precaution, hypoglycemia is a real danger.

8.4 Gynecological and Obstetric Surgery in Diabetes

Clearly the patients in the first category are likely to be older and may have diabetes as well as other comorbidities. These patients are either postmenopausal or are being operated for severe menstrual disorders. Physiologically a premenopausal woman is protected from myocardial disease. This protection is lost when diabetes develops. The postmenopausal woman has no protection for myocardial disease with or without diabetes. The myocardial affliction in women is believed to be more serious with poorer outcomes. For the diabetic women undergoing gynecologic minor surgery, the pre-, intra-, and postoperative considerations are similar to those for urologic surgery. It is only rare that they have to be shifted to insulin if their control on OHAs is satisfactory, since these patients resume oral intake within a few hours and glucose control is not an issue. The women who are past the stage of conception can be managed easily either on OHAs if they are well controlled on OHAs prior to surgery. Intraoperatively small dose of subcutaneous or IV insulin may be required. If these women are controlled with only insulin or a combination of OHAs and insulin, the same doses have to continue till the night prior to surgery. The management of the glycemia if the surgery is in the morning or afternoon should be as discussed in Chap. 6.

The women with diabetes undergoing obstetric surgery related to pregnancy could be older. In India those with gestational diabetes are more likely to be younger. The risk for myocardial disease would be less compared to the postmenopausal women if the exposure to diabetes is short, prior to surgery, but it is there. The mother having gestational diabetes is likely to develop diabetes later. The risk for it is 50% in the next 5 years. It will increase if weight and physical activity are not maintained.

8.4.1 Gestational Diabetes Mellitus (GDM)

The scenario of gestational diabetes in India and the Developed World of the Western are strikingly different in terms of age—early and late. The pregnancy in a known diabetic state, with much higher age, is the concern in the West. The 1940 risk classification made by Priscilla White hence is far more relevant in the West. The prevalence of GDM in India has been shown to be 12–17%. The prevalence of impaired glucose tolerance (IGT) in urban India in the age group of 29–39 years has been shown to be 11–12%. The diagnostic criteria for gestational diabetes are closer to those of IGT. This group is more likely to move in GDM category with the added high insulin resistance of pregnancy [2].

8.4.2 Prevalence of GDM in the South Eastern Populations

Prevalence of GDM will vary in different ethnically related communities. One leveler could be a setting of a particular nation in which many communities will share the common environment and economic level, but will not obliterate the differences fully. In South Western Sydney, Australia, multiple Southeast Asian populations were studied. The total number investigated was 850. The diagnostic tool used was oral glucose tolerance test (OGTT) after 75 g of glucose was consumed orally. Southeast Asian women migrating to Sydney had the lowest fasting glucose levels but the highest 2 h glucose level among various groups. In contrast, women who had come from the Islands of South Pacific Ocean had the highest fasting levels but the lowest 2 h levels. There are several other trials listed below which show a composite picture of Southeast Asian and Afro-American women in the USA with respect to GDM. Averaging these trials, the prevalence can be stated as Indians 11.7%, Chinese 10.17%, Vietnamese 6.25%, Afro-Americans 14.5%, Southeast Asian and Pacific Islanders 10.25%, Filipinos 6.9%, South Koreans 3.9%, and American Indians 6.09%. The drawback of all these studies is that these populations have been studied in highly developed countries. These studies also do not give us the native population statistics in their native land [3–11].

The prevalence of gestational diabetes mellitus (GDM) in India in different parts of the country has varied. Different methods for making a diagnosis have been used in India. The variance is wide—from 3.8% to 21%. GDM as might be expected was found more frequently in urban areas than in rural areas [12–19].

8.4.3 Diagnostic Criteria for GDM

There have been many criteria for diagnosing GDM since 1960. These have been discussed by Mohan et al., in 2016 in a detailed review article [20]. Two of these criteria seem most relevant to India. One recommendation is a one-step 75 g of glucose tolerance. If the fasting glucose is more than 92 mg/dL (5.1 mmol/L), 1 h 180 mg/dL (10.0 mmol/L), and 2 h 153 mg (8.5 mmol/L), it is considered diagnostic of GDM. International Association of Diabetes and Pregnancy Study (IADPS) recommend this method [20]. Diabetes in Pregnancy Study Group India (DIPSI) undertakes one-step 75 g of glucose irrespective of fasting or fed state. If the 2 hr. blood glucose is more than 140 mg, it recommends making diagnosis of GDM. Sensitivity and specificity of the DIPSI criteria increase significantly if the threshold is lowered to 110 mg/dL [20]. This is not a definitive or prescriptive statement to be followed by all. Within the scope of this volume, the readers are further referred to this article, as additional reading, and make their own decision in choosing their criteria to diagnose GDM.

8.4.4 The Time for First Testing for GDM

This has also been debated for long. Traditionally the time was 24–28 weeks of pregnancy. The prevalence is likely to be higher, and GDM is likely to start earlier. This requires consensus to veer to the time of first prenatal visit for registration. Prof Seshiah in personal communication has suggested as early as possible for Indian females since the prevalence is high and insulin protection can be offered since the period of organogenesis is in the first trimester. If thus diagnosed, better protection to the fetus can be offered in this important period. Any pregnant woman with parental or family history of diabetes or has had GDM in one or more previous pregnancies should receive earliest possible *diagnosis*. Earliest diagnosis of GDM becomes important if factors like bad obstetric history, pregnancy in elderly female, if the babies born earlier had large birth weight, were present singly or in combination. In fact in any lady, planning for pregnancy should receive a *preconception preparation* even if she does not have diabetes at the planning time (see below.) In elderly females who may be undiagnosed for diabetes at the time of pregnancy, an HbA1c of more than 6.5 or 7 is an acceptable criterion along with fasting glucose more than 126 mg/dL or a random glucose more than 200 mg/dL, with or without symptoms [20]. Since there is a noticeable rise in late pregnancies even in India, this criterion may be considered good precautionary measure. It is also advisable to test such cases for retinopathy, hypertension, neuropathy, and urinary albumin. Logically if the first testing does not establish GDM, the next occasion to test would likely be at 24–28 weeks.

8.4.5 The Pathophysiology of GDM

The gestational diabetes is a high/very high insulin-resistant state albeit temporary, as long as pregnancy lasts, where the beta cell response to keep glucose less than the diagnostic criteria is inadequate. The cause of this resistance is the high levels of placental hormones like beta HCG and others which continue to rise as the placenta grows. Most young women can respond to this challenge by secreting larger quanta of insulin and maintain the glucose milieu. GDM occurs when this compensation fails. In type 2 diabetes, the putative condition is high insulin resistance, uncompensated by the hyperinsulinemic response initially. Many believe that GDM is type 2 diabetes unmasked because of pregnancy. This idea derives its support from the development of diabetes in 50% or more women who have had GDM in the next 5–10 years.

8.4.6 The Management of GDM

The management of the 9 months of pregnancy is out of the purview of the book. We would however like to make a few important points with respect to GDM which need emphasis for all concerned.

1. Women with GDM will rarely have symptoms. It is all about the fetus developing normally. That does not mean they may not have other complications.
2. The insulin requirements in GDM can be high or very high. There is no limit to raise the insulin doses during the entire period of pregnancy. Any insulin regimen and any type of insulin, human, or analogue that works can be used.
3. The fasting should be less than 95 mg/dL or even lower to about 80 mg/dL. In GDM women rarely will feel hypoglycemic even with such low readings.
4. All postprandial readings should be less than 120 mg/dL. For it to be achieved, the preprandial levels should be low enough.
5. Dietary regimens are tailored according to the trimester requirements. Timely food and insulin injections are necessary. Late-night snacks/milk is essential and early small snack in the morning to avoid ketonemia which is detrimental to the fetus. Ketone testing is important to detect diabetic ketoacidosis (DKA) in its earliest stages in females with type 1 diabetes. DKA is more likely to occur in type 1 DM ladies in general and in pregnancies as well. Ketones should be checked when a patient of GDM is sick or the RBS is more than 180 mg/dL. Diabetes as such and DKA in particular leads to high death rate in fetuses. In addition ketonemia more likely to be detected in the morning fasting state either due to in poorly controlled DM or due to prolonged intervals between meals, particularly overnight. It is shown to be associated with subnormal intelligence and reduced fine motor skills in newborn babies of GDM mothers [21].
6. Even occasional glucose shoot ups are toxic to the fetus. Spontaneous fetal loss towards the term is known in GDM, and fetal monitoring is essential, often with admission.
7. The total weight gain should be appropriately decided by the obstetrician.

8.4.7 Preparation of the GDM Mother for the Ongoing Pregnancy

8. In case of established diabetes or gestational diabetes pre conception counselling started well before pregnancy actually occurs is necessary for a healthy and fruitful result at delivery. The GDM mother has to face a complicated course

involving many daily situations and organ systems resulting in an altered physiological condition. It affects both mother and the fetus. Hence it is essential to make the mother aware about challenges she will be facing in this situation. The chronological sequence of it is given below.

(a) Preplanning counselling prior to conception especially in earlier GDM or mothers with established diabetes.
(b) Clear explanations to both parents about the risk of congenital anomalies, spontaneous abortions, and the relation of glucose control with and for the better outcome, both for mother and the fetus/neonate.
(c) Mother's fitness assessment with special attention to retinopathy, nephropathy, neuropathy, hypertension, and ischemic heart disease.
(d) The parents of preferably both spouses should have a genetic counselling. It is more important in elderly ladies who want to or have become pregnant.
(e) Counselling should also cover advice regarding good diet, hygiene, and proper treatment of other medical illnesses if any. This should include the advice to keep the drugs taken to a minimum and that such medicines should be checked with the doctors to know if they are contraindicated in pregnancy. A striking example is of ACE inhibitors commonly used in diabetic hypertension which are *an absolute contraindication* in pregnancy-induced hypertension.
(f) Total stoppage of alcohol and tobacco, presence of which can enhance the risks to both.

9. With previous history of GDM assessment of glucose level, HbA1c should be undertaken at the first visit. The 60–70% higher risk of developing diabetes in the next 5–10 years should be explained with the advice to do blood glucose yearly after delivery. Evaluating weight, with advice for weight reduction where necessary, is desirable.
10. Stress relief in GDM: The very diagnosis of GDM creates a chain of reactions in Indian society within the household and our myriad relational circles. The stress in GDM can be analyzed and understood if the details below are conveyed to all concerned. Pregnancy is one of the most coveted expectations after marriage by most couples. When the pregnancy test is positive, the first reaction is of course happiness of having achieved the goal. But later on either by herself and/or people around her by their instructions or experiences, the stress begins.

    If she is working, the travelling difficulties and the work stress get added. All these stresses get magnified if she has any additional medical ailment. The addition of a freshly diagnosed GDM adds a new dimension to this stress. Here the role of an obstetrician and the diabetologist is very important. Here the open communication from both the obstetrician and diabetologist with the couple and their immediate family circle alone will establish faith, honesty, and cooperation in frequent visits as will be needed during the gestational period. The open communication between these three parties about facing the situation builds clarity and faith, and the honesty of the explanations is properly received.

The last measure is to inject a confidence in achieving the final goal of getting a near normal baby. Thus, active involvement of mother is vital in making final decision. An attempt to find out and satisfy her needs is also a part of the counselling. A positive encouragement and reduction in fear complex will help the mother to give better results. Making a priority list of expectations and actions in these patients will help. For example, a working woman with GDM against one not working will have different priorities. Explaining what GDM is only one aspect of this endeavor. The family and the mother should be prepared to accept healthy denial of expectations against her priorities whenever necessary, without losing the balance of care to have better life and end results. This will reduce stress in coping and complying with the situation.

Stress of hospitalization: In all situations, hospital admission right through till discharge is a stress to a patient and to the family. Staying away from home adds to it and may alter glucose levels. Thus the role of the team of treating doctors is important. The role of physician lies in allowing some acceptable physical activities to the patient including handling permissible work on laptop along with reading, listening to music, meeting non-troublesome friends and relatives. Last but not the least is to discharge the patient earliest with optimal stay in the hospital.

11. In Self-Monitoring of Blood Glucose (SMBG) the onus of checking blood glucose by a rapid assay glucose meter is on the pregnant woman; it has to be checked more frequently as compared to other times. This short period of gestational diabetes however is most rewarding in response to this expectation since the patient and the family are prepared to undertake all measures for a healthy baby. SMBG is technically easy, minimally, or only slightly painful and is of tremendous help for the patient to self-adjust her diet and even insulin once she is familiar with it. In pregnancies with bad obstetric history and GDM, continuous glucose monitoring (CGM) systems are also available.
12. Risks during pregnancy: These risks and complications are common to all pregnancies but are more frequent and difficult to manage in a gestational diabetic mother as well as a person with already existing diabetes who becomes pregnant. There is no doubt that even milder degree of higher glucose levels is a risk for the development of abnormalities to the fetus. But the death rate is low. As in diabetes, there is no cutoff level of glucose level that can differentiate between low-risk and high-risk pregnancies. The general rule is lower the glucose level better. Applied to cutoffs for control to prevent complications again, there is no fixed threshold in diabetes [22].
13. Maternal complications of diabetes mellitus:
    (a) Hypoglycemia and hyperglycemia, rarely hyperosmolar state.
    (b) Urinary tract infections—the incidence is around 20%.
    (c) Pregnancy-induced hypertension—the incidence is around 25%.
    (d) Preeclampsia and eclampsia.
    (e) Ketoacidosis.
    (f) Polyhydramnios.
    (g) Development of type 1 or 2 diabetes mellitus.

14. Indications of hospitalization are specific medical and surgical indications for admission. The hospital stay should also be made optimal in duration. The indications are:
    (a) Inability to control glucose tightly.
    (b) Diabetic ketoacidosis, rarely hyperosmolar hyperglycemic state.
    (c) First trimester vomiting excessive over 8–12 h.
    (d) Spontaneous or threatened miscarriage.
    (e) Any other severe infection which is causing hyperglycemia and DKA.
    (f) Evacuation of fetus for nonviable abnormalities (listed below later).
15. Diagnostic testing and fetal surveillance are essential in today's era as fewer pregnancies occur and each becomes precious. In patients with DM/GDM, vigilance must be greater to detect as early as possible the maternal complications and the fetal anomalies to reduce the complication ratio and to improve final result. The tools to be used and the findings to look for are:
    - Ultrasonography (USG) as early as 4–6 weeks shows the sac and fetal pole and by 12–24 weeks measures the biparietal diameter of the fetal head and fetal femur length. The structural abnormalities like neural tube defects, macrosomia, intrauterine growth restriction (IUGR), and/or polyhydramnios can be detected by 28 weeks. Increased monitoring for fetal activity during 32–40 weeks by USG is important on account of increased stillbirths during this period in GDM.
    - Alpha-fetoproteins, genetic amniocentesis, genetic testing for sickle cell anemia, and thalassemia also should be undertaken by the 16th week, during this period.
16. Following euglycemic diet appropriate to the gestational period and the present pregnancy weight insulin should be started if the fasting is above 90 mg by capillary testing or 95 mg by venous plasma method. Similarly if the 1 h postprandial is higher than 120 mg by capillary testing and 140 mg by venous plasma, insulin should be started. There are algorithm for initiation and optimization of glucose control by insulin. The treating physician/obstetrician must keep in mind that this is like type 2 diabetes with excessive insulin resistance. Hence the insulin doses would be higher and will go on increasing as the pregnancy progresses. Hence one need not be concerned with really high doses but administer them and monitor carefully. At times between 36 and 40 weeks, the insulin requirements may go down as the fetal growth accelerates, and it takes away much more glucose than earlier [23, 24].
17. Preoperative/predelivery/preinduction management: Steroids are administered routinely four times a day for 1 day for fetal maturation near term. Women without GDM may not show any hyperglycemic response to the first two or any doses. It is advisable to do blood glucose estimation before each dose in all pregnant women. Before the non-GDM patient is discharged, glucose estimation may be done to be sure that there is no delayed hyperglycemia as is likely with steroids as explained elsewhere. In case of a non-GDM patient, if there is concern over an elevated blood glucose level, an appropriate dose of regular insulin may be given, but most of the time it will not be necessary.

Table 8.1 IV Insulin guidelines during labor and delivery in GDM

BG mg/dL	Adjustments
<60	D10% at 100 mL/h, recheck in 1 h
60–100	DNS at 100 mL/h
100–120	DNS (100 mL/h) + 4 U regular insulin IV
120–140	DNS (100 mL/h) + 5 U regular insulin IV
140–180	DNS (100 mL/h) + 6 U regular insulin IV

The GDM will show a rise in the blood glucose level. As discussed above (see the discussion on neurosurgery in intracranial tumors), an anticipatory increase in the insulin doses she may already be taking even before the steroid is given will control the hyperglycemia. It can be increased to 30% or 50% as a standing order under monitoring, or it could be individually raised and continued for 12 more hours before the patient returns to her pre-steroid dose.

18. Management of labor and delivery: The long- or intermediate-acting insulin is discontinued in GDM once the labor starts. Once the labor sets in, the interval at which blood glucose is tested should be every 2/3 hourly. The blood glucose level maintained between 60 and 100 mg/dL is adequate. Table 8.1 is a rough guideline to start glucose control under different blood glucose levels. Insulin can be increased ad libitum to maintain the glycemic goals.
19. Role of anesthesiologist in GDM: As mentioned earlier, the anesthesiologist will come in picture whenever surgical intervention is necessary. Besides clinical examination and glycemic control, he is or should be involved with the following:
    (a) Management of vomiting, with the administration of antiemetic like inj. Ondansetron and inj. Pantoprazole to counteract the hyperacidity. If there is accompanying/consequent dehydration, fluid and electrolyte imbalance should also be restored. This is achieved by administering adequate quantity of ringer lactate and normal saline because in such situations the blood glucose is usually high. This has to be brought to euglycemic levels with insulin administration.
    (b) In pregnancy, the tone of GI sphincter is altered or reduced in normal as well as perioperative period. The affected autonomic nervous system also reduces the stomach tone resulting in delayed stomach emptying. These two conditions would lead to regurgitation or vomiting with the attendant danger of aspiration during conduction of anesthesia, induction, and postoperative recovery period. Attempts at prevention of aspiration of stomach contents are a must. It is for this reason that the spinal/epidural anesthesia is preferred in cesarean section with or without GDM.
    (c) Pregnancy-induced postural hypotension: This is due to fall of the gravid uterus on the inferior vena cava in supine position reducing venous return resulting in hypotension. The IVC is a right-sided paraspinal vein. For the prevention, patient should be told to lie in left lateral position. On the surgical table, the right side is elevated to remove the pressure of gravid uterus over the inferior vena cava.

(d) Delivery: Due to the availability of multiple modes of assessment of maternal and neonatal monitoring, it is not really necessary to have an early intervention in delivering the baby. Early intervention may have been necessary in the bygone era to reduce the fetal morbidity and mortality. Here the role of regional anesthesia plays an important role.
(e) Neonatologist: As one anticipates on delivery, the neonate may have complications arising from hypoglycemia, hypothermia, convulsions, and congenital anomalies. Hyperbilirubinemia, hypocalcemia, respiratory infections, and few others mentioned elsewhere necessitate a good teamwork between the anesthesiologist and neonatologist.

20. Anesthesia in labor has a major role in regional anesthesia due to various reasons explained earlier. Still there are a few definite indications for general anesthesia in labor like:
    (a) Skin lesions on the lumbosacral region.
    (b) Operative urgency due to maternal or neonatal cause.
    (c) Spinal abnormalities.
    (d) Medical illness including cardiac disease, preeclampsia or eclampsia with convulsions.
    (e) Allergy or sensitivity to local anesthetic agents.

    Preoperative assessment should cover preoperative history, examination, and investigations as usual. The additional common factors that pose very high risk in this group are hypertension, preeclampsia, sepsis, and renal dysfunction. These should be investigated and controlled. Evaluation of end organ damage is also important and should be done.

    Tight glycemic control is vital over the perioperative period. It should be achieved by using short-acting insulin infusion. The insulin dose as discussed at many places before in this volume is adjusted to the hourly plasma glucose measurement. It is mandatory in most if not all cases. The parturient whose diabetes in diet controlled may not need IV insulin. In cases where the glucose fluctuations are wider, intraoperative blood glucose monitoring could be half-hourly also.

    In pregnancy the esophageal sphincter tends to be lax, and aspiration should be actively avoided during surgery. Metoclopramide (10 mg) can be administered 30–40 min before anesthesia. It enhances forward gastric emptying and increases lower esophageal sphincter tone. A liquid antacid should be given immediately before surgery.

    Early labor pains are generally mild. With low tolerance of patient, analgesia for labor and vaginal delivery may have to be given. Pain relief can be achieved with small doses of narcotic drugs like butorphanol or nalbuphine. Larger doses of systemic medication as above carry the risk of respiratory depression for both the mother and the newborn.

    Epidural anesthesia is a preferred mode of labor analgesia as well as labor anesthesia. It is associated with a few obvious advantages:

- It blocks the sympathetic outflow, thereby reducing the catecholamine release.
- It may indirectly increase placental blood flow.
- Maternal lactic acid production is reduced, and as a consequence, it also reduces fetal acidosis.

The preferred drug is 0.25% bupivacaine for the induction of epidural analgesia. The maintenance analgesia is obtained with a continuous infusion of 0.0625–0.125% bupivacaine with 8–10 mL of 2 μg/mL of fentanyl hourly. In an alternate method, the epidural test dose of 1.5% lidocaine with 1:200,000 dilution of epinephrine effectively results in analgesia during labor. Thoracic 10 vertebral sensory level can be achieved with 15 mL of 0.04% bupivacaine with 1.66 μg/mL fentanyl. The same mixture infused at 15 mL/h achieves continuous analgesia during labor [25]. It provides excellent pain relief during the first as well as the second stage of labor. In a forceps delivery which increases pain, dense perineal anesthesia is necessary; if it becomes necessary, 8–10 mL 3% 2-chloroprocaine or 2% lidocaine with bicarbonate added will achieve durable pain relief of epidural anesthesia. Further if cesarean delivery becomes necessary or desirable, the same indwelling epidural catheter can be used for that also.

Epidural anesthesia has a higher failure rate. It is a little more difficult technique than giving spinal anesthesia. This necessitates early catheter placement, particularly in view of the anticipated difficult labor. It also allows these patients to get accustomed to the initial effect of epidural anesthesia like with tingling, numbness, heaviness, etc. That also gives anesthetist time to make assessment of the situation to decide whether any alternate anesthesia management for airway management might become necessary and prepare for that. Combined spinal-epidural (CSE) technique may be more advantageous in this group of patients. The general anesthesia in this group of patients will be associated with high risk.

If the expertise to administer epidural or equipment like the epidural indwelling catheter is not available, the alternative is spinal anesthesia with hyperbaric bupivacaine with dextrose in sitting position. It provides good perineal anesthesia as well as relaxation. The perineal relaxation facilitates the vaginal delivery and is less likely to cause birth trauma. In GDM the babies are often large. Sitting spinal anesthesia will be important and useful in such deliveries to reduce birth trauma. If the delivery is going to be urgent and operative, it would be a good practice to place an epidural catheter when spinal anesthesia is given. This is the combined spinal-epidural technique.

(f) If it is a practice to do cesarean under spinal anesthesia, a post anesthetic hypotensive shock could be lethal to the fetus.

21. As soon as the placenta is out, there is a precipitous fall in the counter regulatory placental hormones, an equally precipitous fall in insulin resistance and blood glucose, and insulin infusion may have to be stopped, while the glucose continues to be administered (see above for intermediate-acting insulin administration in these cases). A few glucose readings in the day to follow will decide if the insulin requirement has completely disappeared.

In some cases, the blood glucose does not fall in spite of the placenta being completely removed. In such times, appropriate insulin infusion will have to be given, shifting to effective subcutaneous insulin once the patient resumes her diet, as in any surgery discussed beforehand at many places. At times it takes 24 h for the glucose to get normalized. If the blood glucose continues to remain high, there is every possibility that the woman was having undetected diabetes at the times she conceived. In such cases, insulin is continued till the baby weans off from the breast milk. OHAs, particularly glibenclamide, are known to pass through the breast milk and will overstimulate the baby's pancreas and lead to profound hypoglycemia. It may give rise to hypertrophic islets.

22. Postpartum and postoperatively glycemic management consists of checking blood glucose once daily, thereafter PPBG when on regular diet. Usually, the blood glucose returns to normal by 48–96 h in 95% of cases with GDM. The diet should be calibrated to weight reduction postpartum if there was excessive gain or an isocaloric diet to maintain proper weight or a hypercaloric diet with liberal calcium and vitamin D supplement to maintain the calcium content in the breast milk to normal. It may be beneficial to get an OGTT with 75 g of glucose at 6–12 weeks postpartum to assess risk.
23. Many women conceive on metformin. If it is well tolerated, then it should be continued in pregnancy and after delivery. Discontinuing it may give rise to hyperglycemia. It reduces the insulin doses and helps lose some initial weight.
24. In case of persistently elevated blood glucose after delivery, the diets will have to be carefully revised allowing the child to have the elements that are needed but not to allow weight gain; in fact an attempt to lose weight should be started if the woman does not have ideal body weight. The diets should help weight loss or gain as would be the case. If the obesity persists, it has to be addressed appropriately since this would be one of the most potent factors for diabetes to develop in the years to come in at least 50% of these women. Potential to develop type 2 diabetes depends on age of diagnosis, severity of GDM, and other risk factors mentioned earlier and related to garden variety of type 2. In India no attention is paid to losing weight after delivery.
25. Preconception counselling if another pregnancy is planned is highly recommended.
26. Hypoglycemia in GDM: While hyperglycemia is toxic to the fetus, maternal hypoglycemia is known not to have any effect on the fetal maturity as fetus absorbs his requirement irrespective of what the blood glucose level the mother has. Secondly, the time of organogenesis is long past in the first 3 months or 12 weeks. Hence occasional hypoglycemia is unlikely to cause any damage.
27. "Euglycemic diet" for GDM suggested below is about calorific management and the composition. The per kg per day calorie requirements are determined based on the ideal weight. It means that if the body weight is less than ideal, the calorie recommendations will be higher and if the weight is in excess, the calorie consumption per kg will be less.

Table 8.2 Distribution of calories in a day in GDM

Meal	Calorie %
Breakfast	10–15
Snack	5–10
Lunch	20–30
Snack	5–10
Dinner	30–40
Snack	5–10

(a) 30 kcal/kg of ideal body weight/24 h with body weight between 80% and 120% of ideal body weight.
(b) 24 kcal/kg ideal body weight/24 h with body weight more than 120% ideal body weight.
(c) In women whose body weight is less than 80% of ideal body weight, 40 kcal/kg/24 h ideal body weight is used.

The composition should be 40–50% of carbohydrates, 30–40% of fat, and 20% of protein to be divided as shown below (Table 8.2). Compared to usual practice of three meal patterns in diabetes, a pregnant woman with GDM should resort to more frequent small meals to avoid ketosis, especially in the morning [26].

8.4.8 Diabetic Parturient

Pregnancy in a woman who already has diabetes is an altogether different type of situation for the consultants to manage. As is well known, 50% of people at diagnosis of diabetes will have some form of tissue damage. A diabetic parturient is no exception. Excellent diabetes control before conceiving is the single most important factor for optimal development condition for the fetus. It will also help the mother to have a smooth course and lower occurrence of complications. If conception occurs at a time when diabetes is uncontrolled, severe congenital malformations in fetus are likely to occur four to five times higher. Half of fetal deaths in developed countries are due to malformations that are lethal [27]. There is probably a continuum of rising malformations with rising HbA1c levels. With HbA1c less than 8.5, the malformation frequency is 3.4%, but above and continuing it is 22.4% in diabetic parturients [28]. Equally important is the assessment of the complications like maternal age, duration of diabetes and its general state of control, severe retinopathy, diabetic nephropathy, hypertension, and hypoglycemic unawareness that are some of the most important factors which dictate the advisability of the conception or otherwise. The classification developed by Priscilla White provides details of risk stratification.

The following review by Nibedita Pani summarizes most of these issues well.

8.5 Diabetic Ketoacidosis (DKA)

In pregnancy with existing diabetes, DKA is most likely to develop in the second and third trimesters. It is one of the major causes of fetal mortality and morbidity in pregnancy in a diabetic mother. Fetal loss can be as high as 50% [29, 30]. DKA is likely to occur in bacterial infection due to rise of insulin resistance and subsequent insulin inadequacy. In gastroenteritis, anorexia, nausea, and vomiting will decrease food intake, and the attending professional or the relatives or patient is likely to suspend insulin doses for fear of hypoglycemia when the need is to actually step up insulin dose and try to eat as much as possible. For those diabetic women on continuous subcutaneous insulin infusion pump, stoppage of insulin delivery due to pump malfunction will result in hyperglycemia. If the pump runs away speedily, it may cause hypoglycemia and then hyperglycemia. Treatment with β-sympathomimetic agents, with or without glucocorticoid therapy through increased insulin resistance, could also be a cause. Poor medical management resulting in decreased caloric/insulin supplementation or non-compliant patient can similarly precipitate DKA [21, 31]. Pregnant diabetic woman can develop ketoacidosis with blood glucose as low as 200 mg/dL [25].

Hypoglycemia in insulin-treated patients as a whole is far too common. It will be a risk all the time in women with diabetes now pregnant. Development of autonomic neuropathy in diabetes is relatable to severity and duration of diabetes. If it is present to significant extent in pregnant woman with diabetes, there will be blunting of the characteristic adrenergic symptoms of hypoglycemia leading to its unawareness. The counter regulatory responses may also be lower in some pregnant diabetic women [32]. Since the β-adrenergic receptor blocking agents blunt the hypoglycemic adrenergic drive, hence it is better to avoid or use them with judicious caution in diabetic patients [33]. Renal insufficiency and/or associated decreased caloric intake in hospitalized patients with diabetes is a major precipitating factor for hypoglycemia [34]. The elevated progesterone levels of pregnancy are associated with delayed gastric emptying. Delayed and unpredictable gastric emptying causes glycemic swings which are also unpredictable and can move from a hyperglycemic to hypoglycemic value. The glucose control then becomes difficult. Fetal bradycardia, as low as one hundred beats/min in the latter half of pregnancy, could indicate severe maternal hypoglycemia [35–37].

Left ventricular size, stroke volume, and heart rate are reduced in a pregnant woman with already existing diabetes. This could be due to the as yet a symptomatic diabetic cardiomyopathy as well as asymptomatic subclinical autonomic neuropathy. The volume expansion should be under close monitoring to avoid fluid overload. Epidural anesthesia for cesarean section might be a better mode to be administered [38].

Chronic preexisting hypertension in this group is defined as a blood pressure level greater than 140/90 mmHg. It must be treated. Prophylactic antihypertensive therapy may be started for GDM at 130/80 mmHg. Excessive lowering of blood pressure has an association with intrauterine growth retardation (IUGR) [27].

In pregnancies in already existing diabetes, preeclampsia and eclampsia are common. Priscilla White classification F is defined as severe preeclampsia with nephropathy. The latter will lead to low serum albumin levels. It reduces the intravascular colloid oncotic pressure considerably changing the dynamics of fluid movement across various vascular compartments. Very low colloid osmotic pressures in addition lead to hemodynamic instability. That makes them susceptible to develop pulmonary edema if the volume loading preparatory to regional anesthesia is not monitored closely with more sophisticated methods [25].

The anesthetic technique used could lead to placental insufficiency which will directly influence the well-being of the neonate. Even mild, well-controlled gestational diabetes is found to be associated with placental abnormalities [39]. High maternal glucose levels rapidly cross the placenta to reach glucose concentrations in fetal blood that approximates the level in the mother. The fetal pancreatic insulin response is quick and substantial. The effective consumption of glucose under insulin increases fetal oxygen consumption. This is proportional to fetal insulin levels. There is a thereby a fall in both venous and arterial oxygen content. Oxygen supply from the umbilical artery becomes inadequate. It results in progressive rise in the oxygen difference between the umbilical artery and vein. Thus, through several mechanisms, acute and chronic hyperglycemia contributes to fetal hypoxia and acidosis [40].

Management of labor and delivery: Gestational diabetes is the most commonly associated endocrine disorder with pregnancy. The need for frequent daily monitoring of blood glucose and other parameters, alterations in insulin dosing, and treatment of other complications in pregnancy with preexisting diabetes increases the cost and level of care needed. It is also associated with considerably increased adverse outcomes in the fetus and then the neonate and to the outcome of the pregnancy. The maternal risks in the intrapartum period are also fraught with many likely complications and health hazards especially with increasing maternal age and preexisting diabetes. It needs well-coordinated multidisciplinary management and appropriate screening. This is a period in which the patient and the families are likely to be highly motivated. With these three factors, a normal outcome of pregnancy is possible with minimized risks [41].

Diabetic mothers are at a much higher risk than a gestational diabetic mother. They should be delivered in a hospital with the required facilities by a team of consultants who direct, monitor, and treat the patient. The tighter the blood glucose control and longer the periods over which it is sustained, the greater is the chance to avoid neonatal hypoglycemia. Regular blood glucose monitoring and changes in the insulin regimen are needed to achieve that. In a diabetic pregnancy, the intermediate acting insulin dose prior to pregnancy is reduced to one third and given as basal insulin with regular insulin. This is in contrast to the gestational diabetes where short-acting insulin is used [12]. Capillary blood glucose levels are monitored hourly on the labor floor. If the blood glucose goes above 120 mg/dL, an IV infusion of regular insulin in nonglucose containing fluid is used to bring blood glucose level within normal limits. If the blood glucose is lower, then either the insulin infusion rate is reduced or a 5% glucose solution can be added at 125 mL/h (2–3 mL/kg/h through a three way). On the first day after delivery, the insulin levels even in a diabetic mother would come down but may not normalize as in gestational mothers. Roughly half of the dose of intermediate-acting insulin used before pregnancy is given to the patient. If it becomes necessary to control the prandial peaks, regular insulin may be added.

Mothers who have diabetes prior to conception will deliver proportionately larger babies. In such cases, vaginal delivery could be more difficult than in the normal population. This will increase the rate of assisted deliveries. The percentage of such assisted deliveries, more frequently episiotomy, may ultimately need urgent cesarean section in greater number of mothers [41]. If a cesarean delivery become necessary, an indwelling epidural catheter is a better choice for labor analgesia. In view of the serious adverse effects, both the mother and the neonate suffer; in diabetic mother the multidisciplinary care in a protocolized and standard manner should include anesthetists also. It should be carried dynamically and closely.

8.6 Anesthesia for Cesarean Section

Aside from hypertension, renal insufficiency, sepsis, and preeclampsia, pregnancy with existing diabetes has additional risks. The cardiovascular risk is painless MI. The more major risks are with respect to autonomic neuropathic disturbances like orthostatic hypotension and decreased variability of the heart rate. The same causes decreased response to medication. Atropine may fail to increase heart rate, and beta-blocker propranolol may not reduce the heart rate as expected. Tachycardia while resting, neurogenic atonic bladder and diminished threshold of cough reflex may be present singly or combination. The obstructive sleep apnea as well gastroparesis may get accentuated. Regional particularly spinal anesthesia will carry higher risk for hypotension. Hence noninvasive testing of autonomic function should be considered useful. Preclinical diabetic cardiomyopathy, autonomic neuropathy, and low colloid osmotic pressure from renal protein wasting may exacerbate hemodynamic instability and also put the pregnant diabetic patients at risk of developing pulmonary edema with overenthusiastic hydration. Optimization of glycemic control is vital over the perioperative period [42].

8.7 Regional Anesthesia

Regional anesthesia is positively indicated compared to general particularly if there is no contraindication to the spinal over the epidural group. Maternal glycemic control has to be satisfactory if either spinal or epidural anesthesia which is more appropriate is considered for the pregnant diabetic mother. The patient will generally receive aggressive preanesthetic volume expansion with balanced salt solution fluids without dextrose to avoid hypotension which could be lethal to the fetus. Aortic and inferior vena caval compression by the gravid uterus adds to the development of hypotension in addition to other mechanisms by reducing the venous return. If hypotension does develop, it should be treated aggressively by using ephedrine. In a diabetic pregnant, mother with severe autonomic neuropathy in particular additional and quick sympathetic blockade could be risky for hemodynamic adaptation.

In such cases, epidural anesthesia is preferred because of the sympathetic blockade as a result of slower onset.

Proper perioperative positioning and padding of extremities are important to avoid peripheral nerve injuries. The spinal canal infection is an understandable risk, but there is no published data available on it or the CNS infections in his group. However diabetes is definitely a risk factor for development of spontaneous epidural abscess in nonpregnant patients. The importance therefore of strict aseptic technique must be emphasized.

Postoperative analgesia is important for controlling pain and to avoid catecholamine release which may cause hyperglycemic swings after delivery. Morphine can be given intrathecally (0.2 mg) or epidurally (3 mg). It offers excellent analgesia for up to 24 h. It does not cause excessive sedation and may give rise to occasional pruritus. If the analgesic effect of morphine wears off and pain starts again, a nonsteroidal anti-inflammatory drug can be given. Pruritus can be treated with small doses of naloxone or nalbuphine (5 mg IV). Intravenous Dilaudid, hydromorphone or Demerol or meperidine, can be given if general anesthesia has been administered. Giving epidural morphine is obviously not the choice.

Spinal anesthesia is administered with 12 mg of hyperbaric bupivacaine (0.75%) with 10 μg fentanyl added to it. In any urgent operative situation like fetal acidosis, an already present epidural catheter is logically the most preferred [37].

8.8 General Anesthesia (GA)

Pregnant women with diabetes undergo general anesthesia for the same reasons nondiabetic pregnant women may have. Urgent cesarean intervention for whatever reason would be the most frequent. There could also be conditions that make regional anesthesia not advisable to be discussed later below. GA can be problematic because of stiff joint syndrome, limited atlanto-occipital joint extension limiting neck extension making intubation difficult. Thorough aspiration is needed in Gastroparesis to avoid aspiration. Medications and equipment needed for managing a difficult airway, including those for fiber-optic intubation, should be readily available. Variation in response to intubation like heart rates, mean arterial pressure, and vascular resistance in the diabetic group has been noted. Cardiovascular and impaired counter regulatory hormone responses to hypoglycemia may be blunted under GA. In regional anesthesia, patients are able to tell about the sensations hypoglycemia may give rise to. Half hourly blood glucose monitoring for patients undergoing GA is recommended [43, 44].

8.8.1 Special Anesthetic Considerations in Both General and Regional Anesthesia

Diabetic parturients with association of severe preeclampsia and diabetic nephropathy with hypertension could be the worst combination in a pregnant diabetic.

Invasive monitoring to assess the fluid status and cardiovascular function and pulse oximetry and monitoring of urine output are important. Invasive monitoring will be useful when continued in the immediate postpartum period. Coagulation status in particular before regional anesthesia is called for since deranged coagulation may result in hemorrhage in the spinal canal. Determination of whether there is airway edema is necessary before intubation. These patients at a risk for developing edema often do so after delivery [45]. Infection is the important cause of morbidity in this group.

Fetal complications in a pregnant already diabetic woman: intrauterine, during delivery, and in the period following it:

- Acute in utero or postpartum complications are intrauterine/neonatal death in early or sudden fetal death around 37 weeks which is well known in diabetic mothers. Macrosomia is the most common intrauterine finding. The fetus is large for gestational age, is dysmature, and weighs typically over 4 kg. During vaginal delivery, shoulder dystocia and birth injury/trauma may occur more commonly since the baby size is large. Intrauterine growth retardation, abortions, structural malformations in central nervous system like anencephaly and encephalocele, meningomyelocele, holoprosencephaly, and spina bifida are more common. Except for the last, all other findings are indications of termination of pregnancy as soon as they are detected. Earliest institution of folic acid tablets may help to form a normal neural canal.
- Transposition of great vessels, ventricular septal defect, situs inversus, single ventricle, hypoplastic left ventricle, and pulmonary hypoplasia seen in the fetuses of this group of women are lethal in the neonatal stage. The chances of long-term survival in skeletal malformation like caudal regression, agenesis and multicystic dysplasia of the kidneys, gastrointestinal malformations like anal/rectal atresia, and small left colon will be meager.
- In the immediate postpartum period, neonatal respiratory distress syndrome, neonatal hypoglycemia, and neonatal hyperbilirubinemia, fetal complications like possible impairment of cognitive development are also likely [41].

Graphically the neonatal complications can be related to the days of life of the fetus (Fig. 8.1).

8.9 Surgery on Critically Ill Children with Type 1 Diabetes

Taken all the three elements together, it would not be surprising to get rather disappointing results. In hospital mortality, sepsis or seizures did not find any benefit with tight control of glucose. It however reduced the need for new dialysis. The meta-analysis of six such trials with 4000 critically ill type 1 children was reviewed. As expected tight glucose control resulted in significant increase in any and serious hypoglycemia [46].

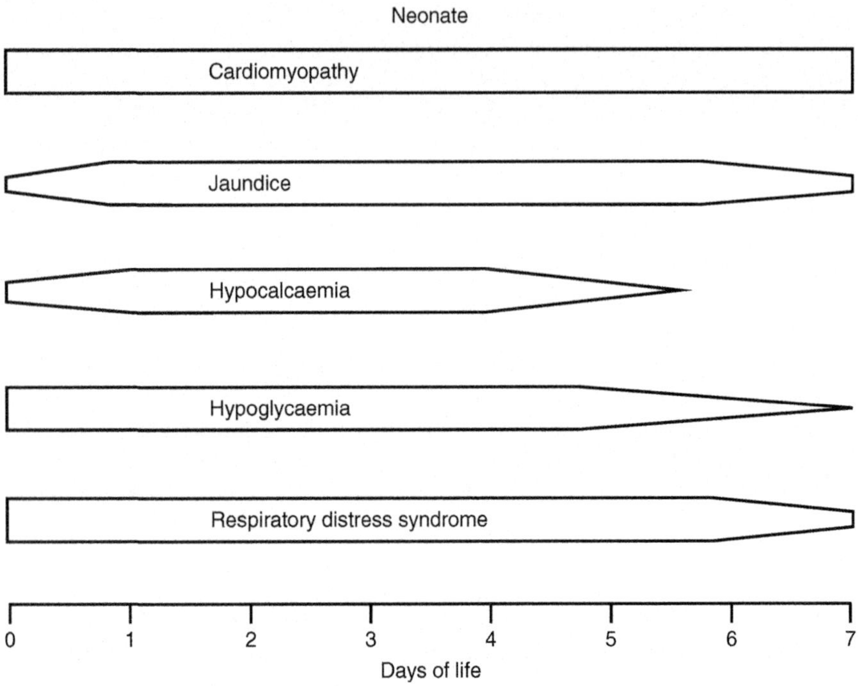

Fig. 8.1 Neonatal complications related to the days after birth

On the contrary, in surgical adult and pediatric intensive care unit, tight glucose control to normal-for-age fasting blood glucose levels reduced mortality. With tight control of blood glucose, 19% more number of patients could be discharged during any time interval from the ICUs. Reduction of T3/rT3 was probably associated with it, while increase in this ratio led to higher mortality [47].

In the section below, a number of issues related to pregnancy and bariatric surgery are also discussed among many other factors.

8.10 Bariatric Surgery with Particular Reference to Diabetes

Let it be clearly understood that bariatric surgery is not a panacea for cure of diabetes in all patients. Post surgery obesity, lipid abnormalities and hypertension may recur in a few years, in fewer patients, are milder and don't push patients to pre surgical levels. It is quite effective for in case of failed attempts to reduce especially morbid obesity. It will also improve the comorbidities such as diabetes which are directly relatable to obesity.

Bariatric surgery falls into two categories. The first one restricts the physical capacity of the stomach to a very small volume so that only little food can be consumed at a time. It may or may not be a permanent reduction. The other one is a combination of permanent restriction of the stomach capacity with a gastric bypass which also causes malabsorption of food contents. These two techniques are briefly described below.

8.10.1 Simple Restrictive Surgeries

The laparoscopic adjustable gastric band (LAGB): It is a restrictive procedure that inserts a band around the proximal stomach; the band is connected to a subcutaneous port. The band can be manipulated to restrict the stomach capacity.

Laparoscopic sleeve gastrectomy also is a restrictive procedure but in contrast to the above is an irreversible change in the gastric capacity. It removes large portion of the greater curvature of the stomach leaving the stomach "sleeve" along the lesser curvature. It can be done as the first part of a duodenal switch (see below) or as a standalone procedure.

8.10.2 Bypass and Malabsorptive Surgeries

Roux-en-Y gastric bypass (RYGB) is a combination of anatomically restrictive and physiologically malabsorptive surgical technique. By separating the proximal and distal stomach, it creates a small gastric pouch. The proximal gastric pouch is anastomosed to a loop of the jejunum, which is called the "Roux limb." The distal stomach is bypassed. The proximal small bowel ("Y limb") is anastomosed distally to the jejunum.

Biliopancreatic diversion (BPD): By a laparoscopic procedure, a sleeve gastrectomy is created. The remaining stomach is attached to lower portion of the smaller intestine, interrupting the normal passage of food through the duodenum and upper jejunum. It thus results in bypassing biliary and pancreatic contribution causing malabsorption. BPD with or without duodenal switch is a similar combination for anatomic restriction creating malabsorption.

Alternatively the remaining stomach is attached to the upper small intestine. It also creates simultaneously a separate biliary loop. Both the loops connect to a common channel of the lower small intestine, the duodenal switch. This is a more mutilating procedure. The anatomical and functional integrity of the GI tract is considerably disturbed. This leads to substantial issues of physiological disturbances resulting in malabsorption. Its causes, effects, and remedies are described below. The management of the deficiencies arising from the malabsorptive nature of the surgery is the real challenge in these surgeries.

8.10.3 Epidemiology

The rising prevalence of noncommunicable disease and its severe complications particularly when morbid obesity develops place a huge economic and life burden on the human beings, where conventional and least mutilating or nondestructive mechanisms do not seem to improve the fate of those afflicted. In addition when diabetes appears on the scene, the risks to life increase exponentially. Out of all patients diagnosed with diabetes up to 55% are obese. Moreover, impaired glucose tolerance and/or fasting hyperglycemia accounts for an additional 10–30% of populations. 15–30% of those undergoing bariatric surgeries have diabetes. Around 225,000 bariatric surgeries are performed per annum.

8.10.4 Criteria for Eligibility for Bariatric Surgery

National Institutes of Health has laid down standard criteria for eligibility for bariatric surgery. In the context of rising prevalence of diabetes, the criteria should be understood in terms of obesity-induced health disasters and obesity when diabetes or any of its comorbidities is present. It also tacitly assumes that there are substantial barriers even after a sustained effort to reduce obesity. Body mass index (BMI) is the ratio of weight of a person divided by the square of the height in meters. This is the primary criterion.

1. BMI $\geq$ 40 kg/m^2 appears to be clearly beyond any conservative measures to reduce it in any substantial way.
2. Or a BMI $\geq$ 35 kg/m^2 with at least one obesity-related comorbidity. This could be considered as the earliest alarm sign, whereas more abnormalities may be detected simultaneously, and allowing progression and later development of diabetes may not stand to reason.
3. Obese patients with T2DM and a BMI lower than 35 clearly have at least an associative coincidence. It should also be considered for bariatric surgery since surgical treatment effectively ameliorates for long periods and may even resolves diabetes once the BMI is brought down.
4. In Asian populations, development of diabetes can jump up as the BMI tips above 24%. Higher BMIs would lead to higher prevalence of diabetes with the risks going up. Hence the BMI could be lowered by 2.5 kg/m^2 especially if the associated cardiovascular risks are higher. This criterion is according to the recommendation of International Diabetes Federation (IDF) position statement.

Adverse factors associated with candidates for bariatric surgery are:

- Conglomerate 1: Age more than 45 years; super-obesity, i.e., BMI $\geq$50 kg/m^2; T2DM, hypertension, and hyperlipidemia; and male gender.
- Conglomerate 2: Nonalcoholic fatty liver disease (NAFLD) or nonalcoholic steatohepatitis (NASH) (see above for the difficulties caused by the enlarged left lobe of liver during bariatric surgery) and gastroesophageal reflux disease (GERD).
- Conglomerate 3: Consumption of alcohol and drug abuse in morbid obesity is commoner, and dependence is more prevalent. This is bound to lead to difficulty

and will pose postoperative complications. Alcohol withheld after surgery is a big issue because of its grossly altered metabolism.

- Conglomerate 4: Presence of pseudotumor cerebri, venous stasis disease which is likely to lead to pulmonary embolism postoperatively, asthma, severe urinary incontinence, debilitating arthritis, or considerably impaired quality of life indicate far serious destruction of the bodily systems managing which is not a simple matter [48, 49].

8.10.5 Psychological Issues of Importance in Bariatric Surgery

Perioperatively the tendency and actual attempts at suicides are in excess of other population. 30% of the suicides occur within the first 2 years postoperatively. Almost 70% of all suicides occur in 3 years after surgery [50]. There is a lifetime history of suicide attempts at 10%, a rate higher than general population [51]. Other serious adverse factors are obstructive sleep apnea (OSA), or the obstructive hypoventilation syndrome caused by obesity, or a combination of OSA and OHS. Roughly one third of patients for bariatric surgery may have moderate to severe OSA with apnea hypopnea index ≥15/h [52].

8.10.6 Preoperative Measures

As discussed above, an effort to lose as much weight as possible preoperatively as possible is advised by many bariatric centers. Very low-calorie diet, popularly called VLCD, consists of 600–800 kcal/day. Depending upon the weight loss, it can be continued from 3 weeks to 3 months. Moreover, in patients prescribed a preoperative VLCD period, any glucose-lowering drugs will most likely need reduction in dose.

Aside of weight loss VLCD may reduce the liver size. Patients with morbid obesity who invariably suffer from a certain degree of hepatosteatosis or even nonalcoholic steatohepatitis have much enlarged size. Intraoperatively along with obesity, the enlarged liver interferes with the technique of bariatric surgery. To facilitate the surgery and to get access to the stomach, the left lobe of the liver needs to be displaced by retractors. VLCD is likely to help in this aspect of surgery by reducing liver size.

The following are guidelines recommended based on current experience regarding antidiabetic management for patients undergoing bariatric surgery.

1. It is desirable if the preoperative optimal glycemic control can be established by diet, physical activity, and antidiabetic drugs. How successful the efforts may be is not adequately studied in this group of patients.
2. HbA1c less than 6.5%: Preoperatively in patients with type 2 diabetes, HbA1c more than 6.5% correlated with unsatisfactory postoperative glucose control. The weight loss in this group was less compared with another group with lower HbA1c.

3. Familiarity with self-blood glucose monitoring and dose adjustment with insulin or insulin secretagogues is highly desirable. These skills are likely required over a prolonged period after bariatric surgery, and continuous dependence of care providers is not possible. However in more problematic situations, ready access to consultation with a diabetes nurse, general physician, or diabetologist should be available and is of great importance.
4. In patients prescribed VLCD before surgery, often during a period of 2 weeks, insulin secretagogues may have to be/should be discontinued depending upon the glucose readings.
5. If the drugs are stopped, fasting blood should be tested for glucose intermittently. If it is found to be above 180 mg/dL, again and again the drugs should be reintroduced. They should be given as half of previous dose.
6. In VLCD the prandial peaks are going to be lower since the calorie intake is restricted. That logically suggests 50% reduction in premixed or rapid-acting analogues. Doses of long-acting analogues or neutral protamine hagedorn (NPH) insulin should be decreased by 30%.
7. Patients on multiple doses of insulin should monitor glucose at least twice a day with a goal of plasma glucose 110–180 mg/dL. Further adjustments of the insulin doses should be considered if this level is not achieved.
8. Patients are instructed how to reduce the insulin doses if hypoglycemia or repeated plasma glucose <90 mg/dL occur. The decrease in insulin dose preceding the hypoglycemia would be around by 50%.
9. All other antidiabetic drugs are retained until the day before surgery. i.e., metformin, GLP-1 analogues, inhibitors of dipeptidyl peptidase 4 (DPP 4 inhibitors), glitazones, and acarbose.
10. On the day of surgery, it is recommended not to give any antidiabetic medication, and glucose is monitored and regulated by intravenous insulin infusion or repeated doses of rapid-acting insulin.

8.10.7 Intraoperative Control

Needless to say that frequent blood glucose estimations and correspondingly fixed insulin administration would be required for glycemic control. Insulin alone should be used intraoperatively, preferably by the IV infusion route. As with any major surgery, better preoperative control is associated with better intraoperative controls.

8.10.8 Diabetes Management in Postoperative Period (Day 0–3)

1. In the immediate postoperative period, the doses of insulin and/or oral hypoglycemic agents are likely to be minimalistic since the oral intake is substantially reduced.
2. With Roux-en-Y or billiopancreatic diversion, blood glucose could become normal within days of surgery, quite rapidly. This will happen well before any significant weight loss is registered.

3. Oral intake is increased over the first few days as per the practices of the center or the surgeons. Most diets will begin as clear liquids. Over days full liquid or high-protein, low-fat, and low-carbohydrate pureed foods are given.
4. In any hospitalized patients, best insulin regimen is the basal bolus that too if the individual components are varied as per glucose levels and the time. Recommended level of fasting blood glucose is between 80 and 110 mg/dL. Postprandial glucose levels should be maintained below 180 mg/dL.
5. Irregular intake is not uncommon in the initial days postoperatively. In such cases only short-acting insulin with food may maintain the glucose limits mentioned above.
6. Insulin secretagogues should be discontinued in the immediate postoperative period. Other oral agent doses should be withheld or adjusted in patients who did not require insulin preoperatively.

8.10.9 Optimization of the Postoperative Care

Postoperatively the surgeons will look after the issues related to surgical procedures like anastomotic leaks, revision procedures that may be needed in the immediate postoperative period, if there are issues of regurgitation, intolerance to food, etc. But the major responsibility of looking after the multiple factors arising from the surgical procedures is the responsibility of the bariatric physicians, who should be adequately trained and are an integral part of the team that manages it. The following is a brief description of what needs to be done in this area [53].

In the first few days after surgery, avoidance or minimization of regurgitation and vomiting is desirable. Both these events can threaten the integrity and safety of the recent surgical procedure. This can be achieved by avoiding solid food in the first few days and changing the food consistency to solids over weeks. It may also lead to severe vitamin B1 (thiamine) deficiency [54].

Usually, there will be food intolerances which tend to diminish over time. In particular in the first year after surgery, protein intake tends to remain lower than recommended. It is in the first year after surgery that majority weight loss takes place. Protein intake may/can increase later. Keeping these likely variations in mind, the dieticians should take care in minimizing the low protein intake issue in the first couple of months and a couple of years after surgery. The recommended protein intake is 60 g/day at its minimum. Better would be if tolerated 1.5 g/kg ideal body weight per day. Much bigger protein intake of 2.1 g/kg ideal body weight per day may be required in individual cases [55].

High protein intake aimed at is to reduce the loss of lean body mass in the operated patient. Protein intake may be variable, but 80–90 g/day protein intakes are associated with reduced loss of lean body mass [56–58]. The lower protein intake immediately postoperatively can be made up by the use of protein supplements [59]. Possibility of protein deficiency is also dependent on the length of the Roux-en Y gastric bypass (RYGB). If the distal Roux limb is more than or equal to 150 cm, the protein deficiency could be as high as 13%. If the Roux limb is less than 150 cm, it is likely to be much less, about or less than 5% [60, 61]. Biliopancreatic diversion is much more malabsorptive, and protein malnutrition may range from 3% to 18% [62].

8.10.10 Vitamin and Mineral Supplements Immediate Postoperatively and to Continue

It is possible to start clear liquids with low sugar content within 24 h after surgery. The recommended intakes of vitamin and mineral supplementations are two adult multivitamin plus mineral supplements containing iron 45–60 mg, folic acid, and thiamine in large doses of elemental calcium (1200–1500 mg in divided doses); at least 3000 IU of vitamin D, zinc, copper 2 mg/day, and selenium are important for routine replacement instead of waiting for the corresponding deficiency syndromes to develop (see below). Vitamin B12 should be given parenterally to maintain B12 levels [53].

Zinc deficiency: Hair loss, pica meaning eating inedible matter like soil, significant distortion of the sense of taste, and in male patients with hypogonadism or erectile dysfunction.

Copper deficiency: Anemia, neutropenia, myeloneuropathy, and impaired wound healing.

Selenium deficiency: Associated with malabsorptive bariatric surgery developing unexplained anemia, fatigue, persistent diarrhea, cardiomyopathy, or metabolic bone disease.

Thiamine deficiency: Rapid weight loss, protracted vomiting, prolonged parenteral nutrition, excessive alcohol use, manifest neuropathy or severe encephalopathy, peripheral edema, and heart failure. Such patients should be treated with intravenous thiamine, 500 mg/day, for 3–5 days, followed by 250 mg/day for 3–5 days or until resolution of symptoms and then with 100 mg/day, orally lifelong [53].

8.10.11 Other Postoperative Events: Diarrhea and Steatorrhea

Disordered bowel habits, increased frequency of loose stools with urgency, bloating, and smelling flatulence are related to fat and carbohydrate malabsorption and to bacterial overgrowth. These symptoms were common in the era of bypasses due to gastroduodenal ulceration. These features may become troublesome in malabsorptive bariatric surgery like biliopancreatic diversion. It may interfere with social functioning. Dietary manipulation, with the avoidance of high-fat and high-starch food, and the regular or intermittent use of intestinal antibiotics like rifamixin 200–400 mg/bid for 7 days every month may help [63].

8.10.12 Dumping Syndrome and Hypoglycemia

It occurs because of the quick passage of calorie-rich food from the stomach to small bowel. The symptoms are of hypoglycemia and fainting; these could be non-specific.

Sigstad's score index higher than seven points is suggestive of dumping [64]. After surgery there is alteration in the secretion of Glucagon Like Peptide, (GLP-1). Lately it has been suggested that the alterations in the secretion of GLP-1 after bariatric surgery may also contribute to the development of this syndrome [65].

8.10.13 Bariatric Surgery, Diabetes, and Comorbidities Related to Diabetes

Intolerable obesity which is found to be extremely difficult to reduce has become a common problem. Bariatric surgery is the answer in the short term. It is fairly efficient for reducing weight considerably and quickly. Amelioration of type 2 diabetes for years to come is commonly achieved with reduction or amelioration of co morbidities like hypertension, dyslipidemia, and CAD and associated risks also for many years. The restrictive procedures are the sleeve gastrectomy and laparoscopic adjustable gastric band ligation or plication of the stomach. These are less efficient in reducing weight and ameliorating type 2 diabetes over a longer period of time. All the other malabsorptive types of surgeries like RYGB are also restrictive and give more satisfactory long-term results in sustained weight reduction and remission of type 2 diabetes. These however are likely to lead to more complex nutrient deficiency and management.

8.10.14 Immediate Postoperative Management of Diabetes

In the immediate postoperative period in bariatric surgery, insulin in different forms may be needed. The basal insulin dosage may be calculated as 0.3 U/kg of body weight and given under monitoring. The glucose levels recommended is less than 140 mg/dL. If necessary, short-acting insulin can also be used. For every 40 mg rise of glucose above 140 mg/dL, 1 U of insulin may be increased in whatever dose frequency [66].

Postoperatively intermittent blood glucose monitoring will guide about the antidiabetic medications. Most of the antidiabetic medications have to be withheld as these will cause hypoglycemic episodes. Metformin properties and effects are employable here first to aid the weight loss and then to prevent diabetes from recurring again. It should be continued postoperatively until prolonged diabetes remission gets established. Metformin can safely be administered in submaximal doses of 850 mg once or twice a day depending upon the tolerance. It can be started from the third day after surgery. The only precondition would be to ascertain that the renal function allows the use of it (see Chap. 6). After gastric bypass surgery, biological availability of metformin increases by 50%. It would be prudent to start with lower doses titrated up to maximal permissible limit [66]. If diabetes continues and/or declines over a period, a suitable insulin regime (discussed in Chap. 11) should be instituted to achieve glycemic targets in nonintensive care unit hospitalized patients.

In the intensive care unit, as part of a prophylaxis against deep venous thrombosis (DVT) low-molecular-weight heparin is recommended for all patients in the first

24 h itself. It also includes modern compression devices for the calves after bariatric surgery. Early mobilization from the bed and walking is encouraged immediately after surgery and long-term DVT prophylaxis after hospital discharge if there is a past history of DVT. They are the high-risk patients. Even if there is a previous history of pulmonary embolism, an inferior vena caval (IVC) filter is *not* recommended since its hazards outweigh the risks [53].

The effect of weight loss on dyslipidemia and hypertension are variable and/or incomplete, even short-lived. Lipid lowering and antihypertensive medications should not be stopped unless clearly indicated. Intermittent monitoring of lipid and blood pressure levels and control by treatment for the same are the same as in metabolic disorders (see below). The drugs which cause edema as a side effect are not used since they will show a falsely elevated status against the actual loss of weight. In the first week after surgery, blood pressure tends to go down due to dehydration. Therefore diuretics should be withheld, and IV fluids as required should be used [67].

8.11 Long-Term Postoperative Diabetes Management

8.11.1 Diabetes Mellitus

Patients who go in complete diabetes remission will have to be checked for recurrence of diabetes with a frequency determined by the patient parameters and lab results. The screening for other comorbidities, microvascular complications, and the treatment thereof will also follow the same routine, and medications as required should be adjusted. Screening schedules could be distanced considerably if diabetes remains in remission for more than 5 years (see below as well) [68].

In bariatric surgery, the weight loss continues over several years often steadily. Longitudinal follow-up of those undergoing surgery has shown these percentage weight losses to be −23%, −17%, −16%, and −18% in 2, 10, 15, and 20 years. In control group, these changes varied from no change to −1% at 20 years. Bariatric surgery is beneficial as there is a long-term reduction in overall mortality, decreased incidence of (new) diabetes as such, myocardial infarction, stroke, and cancer in women. The diabetes remission rate can increase several fold at 2 and 10 years. In those with high levels of basal insulin and raised glucose levels, the results are predictably better. This state would be indicative of high resistance to insulin with massive or morbid obesity as the cause and decreasing occurrence of (new) diabetes as obesity reduces are predictable. High level of BMI at baseline does not predict the same outcome [69].This would indicate greater relevance of bariatric surgery in diabetes and not necessarily as a definitive treatment for obesity reduction, (authors).

In the same study quoted above, total resolution of type 2 diabetes was defined as fasting glucose less than 6.1 mmol/L without the use of glucose-lowering medication. After 2 years, 72% were reported to have gone in remission. There is a continuum of time with massive obesity causing insulin resistance which will result in pancreatic insulin insufficiency resulting in a diabetic state. When the offending obesity is continuously reduced by bariatric intervention, the number of patients with newly diagnosed diabetes during follow-up will decrease. It was found on follow-up that new diabetes developed in only 1% at 2 years and 7% at 10 years. In the control group conventionally treated, it was 8% at 2 years and 24% at the end of 10 years. Among the bariatric techniques, Roux-en-Y gastric bypass, in particular, can result in the resolution of type 2 diabetes in 42–75% at up to 2 years after surgery. Diabetes-related mortality and all-cause mortality are also reduced significantly after gastric bypass [69].

8.11.2 Surveillance and Treatment of Hypertension After Bariatric Surgery

Nearly a third of those who come for bariatric surgery will have hypertension. On the short term, weight loss and considerable improvement in the blood pressure status follows [70]. Diuretics are avoided in this phase [71]. Some patients over the longer time distance do develop blood pressure again [69]. Those who continue to remain normotensive should be judiciously monitored as specific for the age group [62].

8.11.3 Bariatric Surgery and Lipid Abnormalities

It would not be surprising to find the lipid abnormalities normal or without the need for anti-lipid agents in the first year. The combined procedures—restrictive and malabsorptive—will have a better or more striking effect. The number of patients receiving lipid-lowering agents prior to surgery dropped from 86% to 27% in the first year after RYGB [72]. Lowering of LDL cholesterol and triglyceride levels and the period of maximum weight loss in the first 1–2 years were the same time intervals. Both the weight and lipid levels stabilized after that. HDL cholesterol increased (partly as other lipids went down) from 6 weeks to 1–2 years above the baseline level [73, 74]. Total cardiovascular risk determines the maintenance level of LDL cholesterol. It is fixed as less than 2.6 mmol/L in people with high risk and less than 3.0 mmol/L in people with moderate risk [75]. Such patients using any anti-lipid medication should be monitored closely for both the control levels and adverse events during the first years [76].

Hormonal and metabolic changes, surgical failure, nutritional vagaries, mental health issues, and physical inactivity are the factors responsible for weight gain after the initial losses [77]. Fifty percent of patients in 2 years after the postsurgical period regain 5% of their body weight [78]. Composition of diet determines long time reduction in the weight after bariatric surgery. Calorie dense foods with adequate lean protein mass are the chief requirements. Substantial quantities of fruits and vegetables increase the volume of food, adding fibers. These elements are responsible for not gaining weight again. The volume needs minus the calories become necessary after a long follow-up period after surgery. It is in this period that the capacity of the stomach slowly, but imperatively, expands and appetite begins to increase [56].

In RYGB and adjustable gastric banding patients' weight loss reaches a plateau for the weight loss. To continue weight loss, one reasonable option is to use appetite suppressants like phentermine alone or a phentermine-topiramate combination. This comes as added measures to other ongoing ones like diet, calorie management, physical activity, etc. [79]. Liraglutide is an excellent satiety inducing drug. It may also be used as an alternate/added medical treatment in patient whose weight loss turns out to be poor after surgery [80].

Bariatric surgery patients tend to develop gallstones. Hence, drugs like gemfibrozil or octreotide which increase the likelihood of formation of gallstones should be avoided [81]. Carbamazepine, phenytoin, and selegiline need acidic environment for normal absorption. Attention for adequately dosing it for full effect is necessary [82].

8.11.4 Bariatric Surgery and Pregnancy

Obese women may be infertile or their cycles could be anovulatory. Weight loss and its quantum, higher the better, are the key to increased fertility. The type of procedure does not matter [83]. Various procedures tested for this against weight loss and fertility measures are intragastric balloon, gastric banding, sleeve gastrectomy, and RYGB [84]. Fetal and maternal outcomes in untreated obesity are suboptimal compared with those with pregnancy after bariatric surgery [85, 86]. It appears desirable that pregnancy should be avoided in the first 1 or 2 years. This period is characterized by rapid weight loss, metabolic fluxes, and nutritional deficiencies. This period has also been reported to have higher obstetric complications like stillbirths. Guidelines recommend delaying pregnancy for at least 12 months [87, 88].

It is but logical that GDM rates and hypertension are less during mothers after bariatric surgery [85, 89, 90]. In mothers conceiving after they undergone bariatric surgery, a reduced incidence of macrosomia has been shown in neonates [89]. Miscarriage rates are high in women with untreated obesity. This number may go down after bariatric surgery [91–93].

(Higher) age, number of deliveries (parity), (possibly a delayed) date of delivery, and smoking status certainly pose as detrimental to the outcome of pregnancy as a normal fetus after bariatric surgery [94]. Contrarily, the decrease in the (frequency) of preeclampsia, GDM and hypertension in mother, and macrosomia or congenital malformations are regularly reported after bariatric surgery [95]. Biliopancreatic diversion has more malabsorptive potential over RYGB. The number of babies small for gestational age is found to be higher in women undergoing billiopancreatic diversion than RYGB. Higher rates of SGA infants have been reported following billiopancreatic diversion as compared to RYGB [88]. There is a similar gradient between RYGB and gastric banding or sleeve gastrectomy. Intrauterine growth retardation (IUGR) was more common in RYGB [96].

8.11.5 Couple of Obesity-Related Issues

Type 1 diabetes with obesity may not be as striking as in type 2. If there are patients with type 1 diabetes and morbid obesity, they might also be in need of bariatric surgery. In type 1 diabetes, there is a continuous irreplaceable need for insulin for survival even if obesity is corrected. If this is forgotten, ketoacidosis will set in, in less than 24 h. Those patients are more difficult to control and should be monitored carefully. Involvement and frequent interaction/guidance from a diabetologist in such situation are recommended. While meal-related insulin (rapid-acting) can often be reduced substantially as the meal size decreases after bariatric surgery. Type 1 diabetes could also have an element of insulin resistance of which only one cause—obesity has been removed/reduced. It means that the need for basal insulin may not reduce significantly. Hence the reduction in basal long-acting analogues or NPH insulin if at all should be gradual.

Over the last 10 years, prevalence of type 2 diabetes in teen agers has caught the attention of the medical profession in India as well. Typically these are the "couch potatoes," children with zero physical activities and large quantities of junk food consumption, who gain enormous weight and are later detected to have diabetes. In the initial period, they are treated with insulin since many of them present with high levels of blood glucose. Later when the glucose levels come down, it may be possible in most to be treated by diet and OHAs. Bariatric surgery as an option and experience about it in this age group is still anecdotal in India. A news was published that in the third week of September 2018, one such teen was so heavy that he could not even walk on his own and had urinary incontinence. He was operated after a VLCD diet over 2 months causing a weight reduction of some 10%. At this point, we need to remember that this adolescent type 2 diabetes is significant and rising, with all options including the prevention open.

References

1. The ACCORD Study Group. Effects of intensive blood-pressure control in type 2 diabetes mellitus. N Engl J Med. 2010;362:17.
2. Ramachandran A, Snehalatha C, Kapur A, Vijay V, Mohan V, Das AK, Rao PV, Yajnik CS, Prasanna Kumar KM, Nair JD. the Diabetes Epidemiology Study Group in India (DESI): high prevalence of diabetes and impaired glucose tolerance in India: National Urban Diabetes Survey (NUDS). Diabetologia. 2001;414:1094–101.
3. Beischer NA, Oats JN, Henry OA, Sheedy MT, Walstab JE. Incidence and severity of gestational diabetes mellitus according to country of birth in women living in Australia. Diabetes. 1991;40(Suppl 2):35–8. PMID: 1748263.
4. Savitz DA, Janevic TM, Engel SM, Kaufman JS, Herring AH. World J Diabet. 2015;6(8). www.wjgnet.com.
5. Yuen L, et al. GDM: ethnic differences ethnicity and gestational diabetes in New York City, 1995–2003. BJOG. 2008;115:969–78. https://doi.org/10.1111/j.1471-0528.2008.01763.x. PMID: 18651880.
6. Chu SY, Abe K, Hall LR, Kim SY, Njoroge T, Qin C. Gestational diabetes mellitus: all Asians are not alike. Prev Med. 2009;49:265–8. https://doi.org/10.1016/j.ypmed.2009.07.001. PMID: 19596364.
7. Henry OA, Beischer NA, Sheedy MT, Walstab JE. Gestational diabetes and follow-up among immigrant Vietnam-born women. Aust N Z J Obstet Gynaecol. 1993;33:109–14. PMID: 8216103.
8. Shah A, Stotland NE, Cheng YW, Ramos GA, Caughey AB. The association between body mass index and gestational diabetes mellitus varies by race/ethnicity. Am J Perinatol. 2011;28:515–20. https://doi.org/10.1055/s-0031-1272968. PMID: 21404165.

9. Kim SY, Saraiva C, Curtis M, Wilson HG, Troyan J, Sharma AJ. Fraction of gestational diabetes mellitus attributable to overweight and obesity by race/ethnicity, California, 2007–2009. Am J Public Health. 2013;103:e65–72. https://doi.org/10.2105/AJPH.2013.301469. PMID: 23947320.
10. Radesky JS, Oken E, Rifas-Shiman SL, Kleinman KP, Rich-Edwards JW, Gillman MW. Diet during early pregnancy and development of gestational diabetes. Paediatr Perinat Epidemiol. 2008;22:47–59. https://doi.org/10.1111/j.1365-3016.2007.00899.x. PMID: 18173784.
11. Hedderson M, Ehrlich S, Sridhar S, Darbinian J, Moore S, Ferrara A. Racial/ethnic disparities in the prevalence of gestational diabetes mellitus by BMI. Diabetes Care. 2012;35:1492–8. https://doi.org/10.2337/dc11-2267. PMID: 22619080.
12. Seshiah V, Balaji V, Balaji MS, Panneerselvam A, Kapur A. Pregnancy and diabetes scenario around the world: India. Int J Gynaecol Obstet. 2009;104:S35–8. PubMed: 19154999.
13. Seshiah V, Balaji V, Balaji MS, Panneerselvam A, Arthi T, Thamizharasi M, et al. Prevalence of GDM in South India (Tamil Nadu) – a community based study. JAPI. 2008;56:329–33. PubMed: 18700640.
14. Zargar AH, Sheikh MI, Bashir MI, Masoodi SR, Laway BA, Wani AI, et al. Prevalence of gestational diabetes mellitus in Kashmiri women from the Indian subcontinent. Diabetes Res Clin Pract. 2004;66:139–45. PubMed: 15533581.
15. Grewal E, Kansra S, Khadgawat R, Kachhawa G, Ammini AC, Kriplani A, et al. Prevalence of GDM among women attending a Tertiary Care Hospital AIIMS. Sorrento: Presented at DIPSI 2009 and 5th DIP Symposium; 2009.
16. Singh DI, Devi BT, Devi IK, Singh PT. Scientific presentation volume of the first national conference of the DIPSI, Chennai, Feb 2006.
17. Yuvaraj MG. Data presented at the first national conference of DIPSI, Chennai, Feb 2006.
18. Swami SR, Mehetre R, Shivane V, Bandgar TR, Menon PS, Shah NS. Prevalence of carbohydrate intolerance of varying degrees in pregnant females in Western India (Maharashtra) – a hospital-based study. J Indian Med Assoc. 2008;106:712–4. PubMed: 19368095.
19. Divakar H, Tyagi S, Hosmani P, Manyonda IT. Diagnostic criteria influence prevalence rates for gestational diabetes: implications for interventions in an Indian pregnant population. Perinatology. 2008;10:155–61.
20. Bhavadharini B, Uma R, Saravanan P, Mohan V. Screening and diagnosis of gestational diabetes mellitus – relevance to low and middle income countries. Clin Diabet Endocrinol. 2016;2:13. https://doi.org/10.1186/s40842-016-0031.
21. Rodgers BD, Rodgers DE. Clinical variables associated with diabetic ketoacidosis during pregnancy. J Reprod Med. 1991;36:797–800. PubMed: 1684993.
22. Leibowitz H. Joslin's textbook of diabetes mellitus. 14th (special Indian) ed. Boston, MA: Joslin Diabetes Center; 2005. p. 678.
23. Constant DR, Imarah J. prophylactic insulin treatment of gestational diabetes reduces the incidence of macrosomia, operative delivery and birth trauma. Am J Obstet Gynecol. 1984;150:836.
24. Friedel N, Hadden D. Summery and recommendations of the second international workshop—conference on gestational diabetes mellitus. Diabetes. 1985;34:123.
25. Datta S III. Anesthetic and obstetric management of high risk pregnancy. Philadelphia, PA: Mosby; 1996. p. 334–6.
26. file:///storage/emulated/0/Android/data/com.hancom.office.hword.editor.hword_apk/files/clipData/clip_image.png.
27. Joslin EP. Joslin's textbook of diabetes mellitus. 14th ed. Boston, MA: Joslin Diabetes Center; 2005. p. 1036–8.
28. Miller E, Hare JW, Cloherty JP, et al. Elevated maternal hemoglobin A1c in early pregnancy and major congenital anomalies in infants of diabetic mothers. N Engl J Med. 1981;304: 1331–4.
29. Cousins L. Pregnancy complications among diabetic women: review 1965–1985. Obstet Gynecol Surv. 1987;42:140–9. PubMed: 3104845.
30. White P. Pregnancy complicating diabetes. Am J Med. 1949;7:609–16. PubMed: 15396063.

31. Cullen MT, Reece EA, Homko CJ, Sivan E. The changing presentations of diabetic ketoacidosis during pregnancy. Am J Perinatol. 1996;13:432–49.
32. Hoeldtke RD, Boden G, Shuman CR, Owen OE. Reduced epinephrine secretion and hypoglycemia unawareness in diabetic autonomic neuropathy. Ann Intern Med. 1982;96:459–62. PubMed: 7065562.
33. Popp DA, Tse TF, Shah SD, Clutter WE, Cryer PE. Oral propranolol and metoprolol both impair glucose recovery from insulin-induced hypoglycemia in insulin-dependent diabetes mellitus. Diabetes Care. 1984;7:243–7. PubMed: 6376017.
34. Fisher K, Lees JA, Newman JH. Hypoglycemia in hospitalized patients: causes and outcomes. N Engl J Med. 1986;315:1245–50. PubMed: 3534567.
35. ter Braak EW, Evers IM, Willem Erkelens D, Visser GH. Maternal hypoglycemia during pregnancy in type I diabetes: maternal and fetal consequences. Diabetes Metab Res Rev. 2002;18:96–105. PubMed: 11994900.
36. Lankford HV, Bartholomew SP. Severe hypoglycemia in diabetic pregnancy. Va Med Q. 1992;119:172–4. PubMed: 1643123.
37. Kimmerle R, Heinemann L, Delecki A, Berger M. Severe hypoglycemia incidence and predisposing factors in 85 pregnancies of type I diabetic women. Diabetes Care. 1992;15:1034–7. PubMed: 1505305.
38. Airaksinen KE, Ikäheimo MJ, Salmela PI, Kirkinen P, Linnaluoto MK, Takkunen JT. Impaired cardiac adjustment to pregnancy in type I diabetes. Diabetes Care. 1986;9:376–83. PubMed: 3527613.
39. Nylund L, Lunell NO, Lewander R, Persson B, Sarby B. Uteroplacental blood flow in diabetic pregnancy: measurements with indium-I 13m and a computer linked gamma camera. Am J Obstet Gynecol. 1982;144:298–302. PubMed: 7124844.
40. Madsen H, Ditzel J. Changes in red blood cell oxygen transport in diabetic pregnancy. Am J Obstet Gynecol. 1982;143:421–4. PubMed: 7091207.
41. Pani N, Mishra SB, Rath SK. Diabetic parturient – anesthetic implications. Indian J Anaesth. 2010;54(5):387–93. PMCID: PMC2991647 PMID: 21189875.
42. Hall GM, Hunter JM, Hall GM, Cooper MS. Core topics in endocrinology in anesthesia and critical care. New York, NY: Cambridge University Press; 2010. p. 104.
43. Vohra A, Kumar S, Charlton AJ, Olukoga AO, Boulton AJ, McLeod D. Effect of diabetes mellitus on the cardiovascular responses to induction of anesthesia and tracheal intubation. Br J Anaesth. 1993;71:258–61. PubMed: 8123403.
44. Lev-Ran A. Sharp temporary drop in insulin requirement after caesarean section in diabetic patients. Am J Obstet Gynecol. 1974;120:905–8. PubMed: 4429109.
45. Sibai BM, Mabie BC, Harvey CJ, Gonzalez AR. Pulmonary edema in severe preeclampsia/eclampsia: analysis of thirty-seven consecutive cases. Am J Obstet Gynecol. 1987;156:1174–9. PubMed: 3578433.
46. Chen L, Li T, Fang F, Zhang Y, Faramand A. Tight glycemic control in critically ill pediatric patients: a systematic review and metaanalysis. Crit Care. 2018;22:57.
47. M G, Mesotten D, Wouters PJ, Desmet L, Vlasselaers D, Vanhorebeek I, Langouche L, Van den Berghe G. Effect of tight glucose control with insulin on the thyroid axis of critically ill children and its relation with outcome. J Clin Endocrinol Metab. 2012 Oct;97(10):3569–76. https://doi.org/10.1210/jc.2012-2240.
48. DeMaria EJ, Murr M, Byrne TK. Validation of the obesity surgery mortality risk score in a multicenter study proves it stratifies mortality risk in patients undergoing gastric bypass for morbid obesity. Ann Surg. 2007;246:578–82. PubMed: 17893494.
49. DeMaria EJ, Portenier D, Wolfe L. Obesity surgery mortality risk score: proposal for a clinically useful score to predict mortality risk in patients undergoing gastric bypass. Surg Obes Relat Dis. 2007;3:134–40.. EL 3, SS. PubMed: 17386394.
50. Tindle HA, Omalu B, Courcoulas A, Marcus M, Hammers J, Kuller LH. Risk of suicide after long-term follow-up from bariatric surgery. Am J Med. 2010;123:1036–42.
51. Chen EY, Fettich KC, McCloskey MS. Correlates of suicidal ideation and/or behavior in bariatric-surgery seeking individuals with severe obesity. Crisis. 2012;33:137–43.

52. de Raaff CA, Pierik AS, Coblijn UK, de Vries N, Bonjer HJ, van Wagensveld BA. Value of routine polysomnography in bariatric surgery. Surg Endosc. 2017;31:245–8.
53. Mechanick JI, Youdim A, Jones DB, Garvey T, Hurley DL, McMahon M, Heinberg LJ, Kushner R, Adams TD, Shikora S, Dixon JB, Brethauer S. Clinical practice guidelines for the perioperative nutritional, metabolic, and nonsurgical support of the bariatric surgery patient. Obesity. 2013;21(1):S1–27. https://doi.org/10.1002/oby.20461.
54. Aills L, Blankenship J, Buffington C, Furtado M, Parrott J, Allied Health Sciences Section Ad Hoc Nutrition Committee. ASMBS allied health nutritional guidelines for the surgical weight loss patient. Surg Obes Relat Dis. 2008;4(Suppl):S73–S108.
55. Mechanick JI, Youdim A, Jones DB, Garvey WT, Hurley DL, MM MM, Heinberg LJ, Kushner R, Adams TD, Shikora S, Dixon JB, Brethauer S. Clinical practice guidelines for the perioperative nutritional, metabolic, and nonsurgical support of the bariatric surgery patient-2013. Obesity. 2013;21(Suppl 1):S1–S27.. Recommendations for protein intake are variable but higher protein levels of 80–90 g/d) are associated with reduced loss of lean body mass. Recommendations for protein intake are variable but higher protein levels of 80–90 g/d) are associated with reduced loss of lean body mass
56. Faria SL. Dietary protein intake and bariatric surgery. Obes Surg. 2011;21:1798–805. PubMed: 21590346.
57. Raftopoulos I. Protein intake compliance with morbidly obese patients undergoing bariatric surgery and its effect on weight loss and biochemical parameters. Surg Obes Relat Dis. 2011;7:733–42. PubMed: 21925961.
58. Billy, H., Okerson, T. Changes in body composition following gastric bypass or gastric banding. Abstract #1315. AACE 21st annual scientific and clinical congress; May 23–27, 2012, Philadelphia, PA.
59. Bavaresco M, Paganini S, Pereira Lima T, et al. Nutritional course of patients submitted to bariatric surgery. Obes Surg. 2010;20:716–21. PubMed: 18931884.
60. Faintuch J, Matsuda M, Cruz ME, Silva MM, Teivelis MP, Garrido AB Jr, Gama-Rodrigues JJ. Severe protein calorie malnutrition after bariatric procedures. Obes Surg. 2004;14:175–81.
61. Byrne TK. Complications of surgery for obesity. Surg Clin North Am. 2001;81:1181–93.
62. Mechanick JI, Kushner RF, Sugerman HJ, Gonzalez-Campoy JM, Collazo-Clavell ML, Guven S, Spitz AF, Apovian CM, Livingston EH, Brolin R, Sarwer DB, Anderson WA, Dixon J. Medical guidelines for clinical practice for the perioperative nutritional, metabolic, and nonsurgical support of the bariatric surgery patient. Endocr Pract. 2008;14(Suppl 1):1–83.
63. Potoczna N, Harfmann S, Steffen R, Briggs R, Bieri N, Horber FF. Bowel habits after bariatric surgery. Obes Surg. 2008;18:1287–96.
64. Sigstad H. A clinical diagnostic index in the diagnosis of the dumping syndrome. Changes in plasma volume and blood sugar after a test meal. Acta Med Scand. 1970;479–486(8):188.
65. Yamamoto H, Mori T, Tsuchihashi H, Akabori H, Naito H, Tani T. A possible role of GLP-1 in the pathophysiology of early dumping syndrome. Dig Dis Sci. 2005;50:2263–7.
66. Rometo D, Korytkowski M. Perioperative glycemic management of patients undergoing bariatric surgery. Curr Diab Rep. 2016;16:23.
67. Busetto L, Dicker D, Azran C, Batterham RL, Farpour-Lambert N, Fried M, Hjelmesæth J, Kinzl J, Leitner DR, Makaronidis JM, Schindler K, Toplak H, Yumuk V. Practical recommendations of the obesity management task force of the European Association for the Study of Obesity for the Post-bariatric Surgery Medical Management. Obes Facts. 2017;10:597–632. https://doi.org/10.1159/000481825.
68. Buse JB, Caprio S, Cefalu WT, Ceriello A, Del Prato S, Inzucchi SE, McLaughlin S, Phillips GL II, Robertson RP, Rubino F, Kahn R, Kirkman MS. How do we define cure of diabetes? Diabetes Care. 2009;32:2133–5.
69. Sjöström L. Review of the key results from the Swedish Obese Subjects (SOS) trial – a prospective controlled intervention study of bariatric surgery. J Intern Med. 2013;273(3):219–34. https://doi.org/10.1111/joim.12012.
70. Buchwald H, Avidor Y, Braunwald E, Jensen MD, Pories W, Fahrbach K, Schoelles K. Bariatric surgery: a systematic review and meta-analysis. JAMA. 2004;292:1724–37.

71. Jordan J, Yumuk V, Schlaich M, Nilsson PM, Zahorska-Markiewicz B, Grassi G, Schmieder RE, Engeli S, Finer N. Joint statement of the European Association for the Study of Obesity and the European Society of Hypertension: obesity and difficult to treat arterial hypertension. J Hypertens. 2012;30:1047–55.
72. Schauer PR, Kashyap SR, Wolski K, Brethauer SA, Kirwan JP, Pothier CE, Thomas S, Abood B, Nissen SE, Bhatt DL. Bariatric surgery versus intensive medical therapy in obese patients with diabetes. N Engl J Med. 2012;366:1567–76.
73. Bays HE, Jones PH, Jacobson TA, Cohen DE, Orringer CE, Kothari S, Azagury DE, Morton J, Nguyen NT, Westman EC, Horn DB, Scinta W, Primack C. Lipids and bariatric procedures part 1 of 2: scientific statement from the National Lipid Association, American Society for Metabolic and Bariatric Surgery, and Obesity Medicine Association. J Clin Lipidol. 2016;10:33–57.
74. Risstad H, Svanevik M, Kristinsson JA, Hjelmesæth J, Aasheim ET, Hofsø D, Søvik TT, Karlsen TI, Fagerland MW, Sandbu R, Mala T. Standard vs. distal Roux-en-Y gastric bypass in patients with body mass index 50 to 60: a double-blind, randomized clinical trial. JAMA Surg. 2016;151:1146–55.
75. Catapano AL, Graham I, De Backer G, Wiklund O, Chapman MJ, Drexel H, Hoes AW, Jennings CS, Landmesser U, Pedersen TR, Reiner Ž, Riccardi G, Taskinen MR, Tokgozoglu L, Verschuren WM, Vlachopoulos C, Wood DA, Zamorano JL. 2016 ESC/EAS guidelines for the management of dyslipidaemias. Eur Heart J. 2016;37:2999–3058.
76. Jakobsen GS, Skottheim IB, Sandbu R, Christensen H, Røislien J, Asberg A, Hjelmesæth J. Long-term effects of gastric bypass and duodenal switch on systemic exposure of atorvastatin. Surg Endosc. 2013;27:2094–101.
77. Kushner RF, Sorensen KW. Prevention of weight regain following bariatric surgery. Curr Obes Rep. 2015;4:198–206.
78. ASMBS Professional Resource Center. https://asmbs.org/resources/. Accessed 22 Nov 2017.
79. Schwartz J, Chaudhry UI, Suzo A, Durkin N, Wehr AM, Foreman KS, Tychonievich K, Mikami DJ, Needleman BJ, Noria SF. Pharmacotherapy in conjunction with a diet and exercise program for the treatment of weight recidivism or weight loss plateau post-bariatric surgery: a retrospective review. Obes Surg. 2016;26:452–8.
80. Pajecki D, Halpern A, Cercato C, Mancini M, de Cleva R, Santo MA. Short-term use of liraglutide in the management of patients with weight regain after bariatric surgery. Rev Col Bras Cir. 2013;40:191–5.
81. Sardo P, Walker J. Bariatric surgery: impact on medication management. Hosp Pharm. 2008;43:113–20.
82. Azran C, Wolk O, Zur M, Fine-Shamir N, Shaked G, Czeiger D, Sebbag G, Kister O, Langguth P, Dahan A. Oral drug therapy following bariatric surgery: an overview of fundamentals, literature and clinical recommendations. Obes Rev. 2016;17:1050–66.
83. Teitelman M, Grotegut CA, Williams NN, Lewis JD. The impact of bariatric surgery on menstrual patterns. Obes Surg. 2006;16:1457–63.
84. Musella M, Milone M, Bellini M, Sosa Fernandez LM, Leongito M, Milone F. Effect of bariatric surgery on obesity-related infertility. Surg Obes Relat Dis. 2012;8:445–9.
85. Maggard MA, Yermilov I, Li Z, Maglione M, Newberry S, Suttorp M, Hilton L, Santry HP, Morton JM, Livingston EH, Shekelle PG. Pregnancy and fertility following bariatric surgery: a systematic review. JAMA. 2008;300:2286–96.
86. Guelinckx I, Devlieger R, Vansant G. Reproductive outcome after bariatric surgery: a critical review. Hum Reprod Update. 2009;15:189–201.
87. Parent B, Martopullo I, Weiss NS, Khandelwal S, Fay EE, Rowhani-Rahbar A. Bariatric surgery in women of childbearing age, timing between an operation and birth, and associated perinatal complications. JAMA Surg. 2017;152:1–8.
88. Gonzalez I, Rubio MA, Cordido F, Breton I, Morales MJ, Vilarrasa N, Monereo S, Lecube A, Caixas A, Vinagre I, Goday A, Garcia-Luna PP. Maternal and perinatal outcomes after bariatric surgery: a Spanish multicenter study. Obes Surg. 2015;25:436–42.

89. Willis K, Lieberman N, Sheiner E. Pregnancy and neonatal outcome after bariatric surgery. Best Pract Res Clin Obstet Gynaecol. 2015;29:133–44.
90. Kominiarek MA. Preparing for and managing a pregnancy after bariatric surgery. Semin Perinatol. 2011;35:356–61.
91. Boots C, Stephenson MD. Does obesity increase the risk of miscarriage in spontaneous conception: a systematic review. Semin Reprod Med. 2011;29:507–13.
92. Whyte M, Pring C, Cooke D, Hart K, McGowan BM, Subramanian D, Shave J. Pregnancy after diabetes obesity surgery (PADOS): incidence and outcomes. Pregnancy Hypertens. 2014;4:239.
93. Alatishe A, Ammori BJ, New JP, Syed AA. Bariatric surgery in women of childbearing age. QJM. 2013;106:717–20.
94. Kjaer MM, Lauenborg J, Breum BM, Nilas L. The risk of adverse pregnancy outcome after bariatric surgery: a nationwide register-based matched cohort study. Am J Obstet Gynecol. 2013;208:464.e1–5.
95. Belogolovkin V, Salihu HM, Weldeselasse H, Biroscak BJ, August EM, Mbah AK, Alio AP. Impact of prior bariatric surgery on maternal and fetal outcomes among obese and non-obese mothers. Arch Gynecol Obstet. 2012;285:1211–8.
96. Chevrot A, Kayem G, Coupaye M, Lesage N, Msika S, Mandelbrot L. Impact of bariatric surgery on fetal growth restriction: experience of a perinatal and bariatric surgery center. Am J Obstet Gynecol. 2016;214:655.e1–7.

Additional Reading

Busetto L. Practical recommendations of the Obesity Management Task Force of the European Association for the Study of Obesity for the Post-Bariatric Surgery Medical Management. Obes Facts. 2017;10:597–632. https://doi.org/10.1159/000481825.

Dixon JB, Zimmet P, Alberti KG, Rubino F, on Behalf of the International Diabetes Federation Taskforce on Epidemiology and Prevention. Bariatric surgery: an IDF statement for obese type 2 diabetes. Diabet Med. 2011;28:628–42. https://doi.org/10.1111/j.1464-5491.2011.03306.

Local/Regional Anesthesia for Diabetic Foot Surgery

9

Contents

S. Kelkar et al., *Towards Optimal Management of Diabetes in Surgery*,
https://doi.org/10.1007/978-981-13-7705-1_9

9.1 Historical Evolution of Regional Anesthesia

In 1986, in Mumbai, then Bombay, the real work on diabetic foot began in the equally premier All-India Institute of Diabetes (AIID), SL Raheja Hospital, now Fortis Raheja. AIID had started having concentrated diabetic foot work. All the cases were taken up under general anesthesia with tremendous risk, a practice which continues in large part of the country even now, giving rise to myriad issues discussed in Emergency Surgery and Perioperative Diabetic Emergencies in this volume. In the historic days learning about diabetic foot, assessing it, and the patient, monitoring him before and intraoperatively could be done with few diagnostic/treatment modalities available then; those modalities are now sparingly used.

The instinctive choice was general anesthesia endowed with many and unnecessary serious risks avoided in regional anesthesia now. That was not "the best" to the patients. Today medical profession has a much better developed understanding of the pathophysiology of the diabetic foot, about how to medically evaluate diabetic patients, evaluation of the diabetic foot itself surgically, and how to make the patient with diabetic foot sepsis safer for surgery by preoperative management.

9.1.1 Development in Anesthesia Management in Diabetic Foot Patients

In 1986, there was a lack of monitoring equipment—invasive and noninvasive—both which today have become commonplace. The blood pressure monitoring was manual with ECG running. Pulse oximeter was not available. Often the surgeon signaled the outpouring of dark blood in the operative foot due to congested limb and vascular shunts. The oxygen saturation was judged by the tongue color, and the surgeons were reassured. By the time in a few months, as the pulse oximeter became available, thinking on migrating away from general anesthesia to regional anesthesia had begun. The serious requirement to get away from the major scary problems of desaturated blood and the likes under GA were poignantly realized. Initially it started with simple ankle block. However if the swelling of the foot was well above ankle, the choice then was either spinal or general anesthesia.

The high risks of general anesthesia could be avoided only by the practice of leg blocks. It was based on anatomy since the Peripheral Nerve Stimulator (PNS) or Ultrasonography came later. With some intuition and more daring, the high leg, mid leg, and low leg blocks were attempted on a learning curve. Today with improved availability of PNS/USG machines, high and mid leg blocks have disappeared. Today the sciatic, femoral, and, if necessary, obturator nerve blocks are used by the coauthor PA, for surgery in thigh. Other alternatives are lumber plexus block, fascia iliaca block, or even a three in one block in upper thigh. An easier version of the sciatic block is to block it as it passes through the popliteal fossa and/or simply block the saphenous nerve; later the lower leg block (LLB) was also mastered.

These blocks were superior to mere ankle block in many ways. They worked even if the swelling due to infective or noninfective causes was well above the ankle. As discovered by PA, the calcaneal branch supplying the heel is given proximally in 25–30% of individuals which escapes these blocks which can be easily blocked in LLB. This technique is now routinely incorporated.

9.1.2 Development of Better Local Anesthetics

Today a large number of patients are on various blood thinners, platelet inhibitors, or anticoagulants. The diagnosis of Charcot's foot despite the missed cases has increased. Charcot's is characterized by arteriovenous shunts. In addition to that today far greater numbers of angioplasty procedures are undertaken which increase blood supply to the lower limbs. All such patients presenting with urgent diabetic foot surgery may have one, two, or all the three factors described above, and as a result of which there will be profuse bleeding or blood oozing during and after surgery. It cannot be controlled unless adequate but not excessive vasoconstriction is achieved during the diabetic foot surgery. The addition of 0.5% Xylocaine with one in eight lakh concentration of adrenaline is a recent tool to the present regional anesthesia therapy which can control the bleeding quite effectively from all these causes. By using such low concentration of adrenaline, we have succeeded in reducing the blood loss so much that blood transfusions used earlier in some cases have become extinct. This diluted adrenaline has no effect either on blood pressure or heart rate. Instead post block, both the blood pressure and heart rate start coming down probably due to pain relief and reduction in anxiety.

The advances described above to better assess the risks lead to more definitive explanation of the same to the relatives prior to surgery which has become, and rightly so, mandatory. Regional anesthesia techniques minimize the risks with a better outcome. It has changed the treatment scenario in these patients.

9.2 Spectrum of Foot Complications in Diabetes

For many years India had the highest number of people with diabetes than any other country in the world. In the recent estimates published by the International Diabetes Foundation, China now has the highest numbers of people with diabetes, and till recently [1], more than 62 million Indians have diabetes [1]. The average age on onset in India has consistently been coming down and stands at 42.5 years presently [1]. Diabetes every year is responsible for the deaths of one million Indians approximately [1]. It is well established that diabetes control in individuals worsens as the duration of diabetes increases. The commonest complication ranging from 16% to 66% in different observations and settings is diabetic neuropathy [2, 3]. Cardiovascular complications (23.6%), renal issues (21.1%), retinopathy (16.6%), and foot ulcers (5.5%) are the complications seen in decreasing frequency after neuropathy [2, 3]. The results are quite similar to the results of studies in South Indian population. Foot ulceration in diabetes affects approximately 15% of patients once in their lifetime [3]. Today, in India, 50,000 amputations from among the

60 million people with diabetes are carried out every year. Diabetic neuropathy results in insensate foot and the inability to feel pain, heat, and cold, all of which are noxious stimuli that can lead to foot ulceration. In fewer numbers poor circulation contributes to ulceration.

9.3 The Spectrum of Foot and Ankle Surgeries in Patients with Diabetes

Thus, foot surgery in diabetes mellitus in India is most frequently occasioned by (generally severe) infection in diabetic foot as in deep-seated abscess, widely spreading necrotizing fasciitis, osteomyelitis, etc. The more severe the affliction, the greater it will be life or limb threatening and will lead to major amputations. Neglect of the foot care and of understanding or of education about foot care on part of the patient, irrespective of education level or economic condition, is commonly seen. In the infective foot surgery group, ulcer is always present as the entry point followed by the resultant sepsis. Cellulitis was found in 97.73% of cases. In a couple of large series, the limb-threatening ulcers in patients taken up for surgery were 56.70%. Non-limb-threatening ulcers were found to be 43.29%, and already gangrenous foot was at 14.43%.

Reconstructive foot surgery in diabetes is another common reason for foot surgery in diabetes. These are planned procedures and give time to optimize the patient's condition to the best possible level. Surgeries which may involve any part of the foot and ankle will be most commonly encountered in Charcot's osteoarthropathy. Surgical factors like skill, experience, operative time, and frequency of carrying out such operations will vary, but in general the demands for these factors are high. The type and severity of deformity as a result of neuropathic/vascular changes would also be responsible for the outcomes of surgery.

Skin grafting and other procedures of plastic surgery are required especially to cover large ulcers after acute infective elements have been effectively removed. This facilitates the much faster healing compared to conservative management.

9.4 Risk Factors in Dealing with Severely Infected Diabetic Foot

Serious diabetic foot infections have an extremely high rate of mortality in itself. Hyperglycemia leads to immune response failure leading to anatomical spread of infection and far too commonly septicemia, leading to multiple organ failure. A few additional factors listed below push the mortality percentage even higher. These situations are almost always accompanied by septicemia.

Metabolic instability is characterized by mounting acidosis, dehydration and electrolyte imbalance, and hypotension often leading to cerebral dysfunction or coma. The hemodynamic instability is characterized by abnormal vascular responses leading to shock.

Cardiac dysfunctions are common in long-standing diabetes. These are already discussed in detail in Chap. 3 along with pathologies of other organ systems.

Perioperative period can worsen the recovery or outcome or both due to such multiorgan involvement, aside from the surgical procedural inadequacies if any. High risks of adverse cardiac outcomes are further complimented by metabolic abnormalities given below.

The additional confounding factor is the concomitant, emergency, and restorative medical intervention especially in severely infected diabetic foot that keeps the clinical picture dynamically changing every few hours. Managing that leading to a continuous improvement despite no surgical intervention needs far more infrastructural support and clinical experience as well as acumen.

Above all high levels of glucose are the universal risk factors present, and poor lower limb ischemia leads to delayed control of infection and poor wound healing.

9.4.1 Clinical Implications in Intervening Surgically Early in Such Conditions

In addition to the above factors contributing to mortality is the delay in surgical intervention. There is a lack of the basic understanding that diabetic foot sepsis is the cause of all the factors leading to high mortality. Unless there is adequate, aggressive, and effective surgical intervention, these factors will never improve even to a level barely safe for nonregional anesthesia. These patients are going to be always at high risk. Poor renal function is a fair predictor of poor outcomes of surgery. Any delay in intervening will cause further deterioration of it and will delay and worsen the recovery.

The other basic lacuna in comprehending the situation is the high level of glucose as the most important deterrent to take the patient up for anesthesia both by the anesthetist and the surgeon. In point of the fact, all other factors mentioned above and not the blood glucose level are far more significant for two reasons: one—the risk of these complications the patients carry while the surgical and nonlocal anesthetic intervention is being undertaken. The second is their correction. These factors can be improved over a few hours of aggressive but well-calibrated medical management. This makes the patient's condition much safer for local anesthetic intervention with or without the blood glucose normalizing, the latter being the case more often. During this aggressive correction, the physician should frequently keep attention on the electrolytes.

To achieve such a complex task, a coordinated approach between the anesthetists, physicians tackling the metabolic and hemodynamic instability and lowering glucose, and the operating surgeon is a must. It is a fact that all these three specialties do not coordinate and cooperate in a professional manner in majority setups in India. Safety for anesthesia becomes the major reason for denying taking up the case for the same, more particularly since local anesthesia is not considered as the most appropriate route for the intervention. Mostly it is because of lack of training to administer it or unwillingness. Taking it up here means that general anesthesia will be administered.

At times the surgeons may refuse to take it up for many different reasons. That leaves the physician with an unenviable task of controlling the patient parameters with partial to fair success. However well he may try to achieve the targets which he will not succeed in most of the times. The targets set by the surgeon anesthetist duo may still not be satisfactory to either the anesthetists or the surgeons or both. Such delays merely add to an unsuccessful intervention and higher mortality. Thus, with high risk explained to the patient as a team with a good team understanding, a quick but a complete or near complete job preferably under regional anesthesia should give better chances for the patient's recovery.

9.4.2 The Parameters of Minimum Clinical, Metabolic, and Hemodynamic Achievements

Clinically improved sensorium, decreasing pulse rate towards normalization, decreased respiratory rate, and the depth of each breath, a minimum of 50 mL/h urine output, should be considered adequately safe. All these indicate a far better balanced milieu interior.

The laboratory parameters indicating safety would be a fairly established downward trend of progression of glucose levels with more than 10%/h, or a glucose level around 250 mg/dL is adequate since at this level the immune function returns. Potassium around 3.5 mmol/L and a pH of 7.3 with 15 meq/L of bicarbonates is reasonably safe. When the levels of high blood glucose continue to fall, maintaining potassium level to 3.5 or above, with or without adequate urinary output, is not easy, thereby continuing the high risk if the patient has to be taken up under general anesthesia. Hyponatremia is common and should get corrected with normal saline/hypertonic saline infusions for rehydration. It may cause an extra potassium loss which should be monitored and corrected.

9.5 General Anesthesia: Difficulties Particularly Encountered in Diabetes

Difficult intubations due to glycosylation of the ligaments of the atlanto-occipital joints and cervical spine will limit extension of the neck; about one third of long-term type 1 persons with diabetes present laryngoscopic difficulties characterized by short stature; joint rigidity; tight, waxy skin; and obesity. All these pathologies present preoperatively can worsen during pre-induction period or on induction of general anesthesia. Sudden substantial rise or fall of systolic blood pressure in both hypertensive and nonhypertensive persons during the induction may result in postponing the surgery for hours or a day.

9.6 Disadvantages of Spinal and Epidural Anesthesia

Prevention and management of hypotension is not easy in diabetes in particular, due to high association of sympathetic autonomic nerve degeneration. Resistant hypotension that may last for longer in these patients is detrimental to the organ perfusion.

Central neuraxial blocks produce major upsets in the autonomic nervous system. The success of neuraxial block lies in restricting to the blockage of required spinal segments—excess blockage will worsen the cardiorespiratory stability while less will not give total pain relief. The balance of two is the job of the skillful anesthetist.

Spinal and epidural anesthesia cannot be repeated frequently especially for small but painful procedures like dressing or desloughing. In continuous epidural analgesia, these two procedures can be done over daily gaps.

Regional or local anesthesia is the answer. It is here the interventions can be made safer by administering local or regional anesthesia than taking a patient under general anesthesia. In regional or local blocks, there are hardly any autonomic upsets. This is valuable for high-risk patients with severe disease involving many of the major bodies. These patients are also on a large number of drugs. Secondly, the demands for general anesthesia like a fasting patient, atropinization, or pre-anesthetic sedation or use of anxiolytic drugs if needed are a distinct disadvantage since it alters the hemodynamics as well as the level of sensorium. This could also lead to delayed recognition of hypoglycemia in particular and monitoring the vitals.

9.6.1 Logistics of the Delay in Surgery

If surgery is delayed, monitoring the critically sick patient in the interim period becomes difficult for the already occupied surgeons and the anesthetists once the patient is in the operating theater. The patient may not remain accessible to the treating physicians, and the immediate pre-operative and pre-anesthetic check on blood glucose yielding high values could turn the patient away from being taken up for surgery causing delay of many hours or a day without a guarantee that things will change for better. In fact they may change for worse, causing high level of anxiety to the patients and their relatives leading to acrimonious exchange which are common nowadays. The regional anesthesia removes these difficulties since the patient can be treated till late in the wards.

In the ward, patient's diet continues till only couple of hours before surgery under regional anesthesia. Glucose monitoring under intravenous insulin can be modified till the very last before shifting the patient to surgery. The physician can continue his task almost till the time the patient is shifted to the operation theater. It improves the metabolic as well as hemodynamic abnormalities further, and patient certainly is in a much more stable and improved condition at the time of surgery, if not in a very low-risk category still. These are added advantages.

9.6.2 Some More Advantages of the Nerve Blocks/Field Blocks

1. The patients whose general condition is good, blood glucose is in reasonable control do not need admission. They are ideal for day care. Such patients can be discharged the same evening. The number of operations required on these patients is at times quite frequent; by treating them on day care basis, their expenses are also brought down.

2. They are far safer in high-risk patients. This is the biggest advantage especially in those patients, with various weakened body systems. The risk involved with administration of multiple anesthesia drugs with their potential side effects as in general anesthesia is eliminated in regional anesthesia.
3. There is no intraoperative regurgitation, eliminating the possibility of aspiration and all its consequences. Since the patient is not anesthetized, his/her protective pharyngolaryngeal reflexes are intact virtually eliminating the possibility of aspiration.
4. There is practically no nausea or vomiting postoperatively since no other drug has been administered except the local anesthetics; hence one does not expect these side effects.
5. In fact, if nausea or vomiting starts after the procedure, it could be indicative of deteriorating renal function.
6. The alteration in the drug schedule is minimal since in patients with diabetes which is an especial advantage. That is because they are usually not long starved since only local anesthesia is used. Postoperatively they are given oral liquid feeds practically immediately. Of course a few hours of pre-operative starvation is mandatory, but depending on the patient's general condition, it can be altered (see a related question below).
7. Field block—This is useful in dealing small localized pathologies like corn excision, small infected cysts, abscess, carbuncles, etc., anywhere on the body.
8. There is minimum effect on vital parameters which remain unaltered. At times pre-operatively, if there is a rise in blood pressure and heart rate, it usually comes down as the regional anesthesia reduces local pain and related anxiety.
9. It can be given in an emergency situation with much more safety. Due to regional anesthesia as patient does not lose his protective reflexes along with altering his consciousness, hence it is safe to take the patient for unavoidable emergency operation.
10. To have a fully cooperative, conscious easily arousable patient sliding himself from operation table to the trolley along with no pain, at the end of surgery is the biggest advantage of regional anesthesia. It also leads to restoration to normalcy of routine protocol immediately. The pain-free duration can vary from 4 to 24 h. The most important is the reduction in the morbidity and mortality related to anesthesia.
11. It is highly cost-effective since the patient saves/minimizes on admission and on drugs. If he is one of those unfortunate ones requiring multiple surgeries, saving on cost will be welcomed by him and everybody.
12. The regional anesthesia can be repeated frequently without any hesitation if frequent operations or dressing under anesthesia is required, whereas extending general anesthesia if the surgery gets prolonged is not exactly a simple issue. Giving regional or local anesthesia or field blocks on one more occasion after a few days if second surgery or extensive debridement is needed is easier, whereas a second general anesthesia will continue to have its own risks even if the other risk factors that existed on the first occasion may have ameliorated to a large extent.

9.6.3 Additional Advantages of Regional Anesthesia in Postoperative Period

13. Local anesthesia used singly will largely reduce the risk of postoperative nausea and vomiting. As part of the multimodal technique in general anesthesia, it reduces the need to use opioid drugs. It thus reduces the opioid drugs' side effects also postoperatively. Local anesthetics also have opioid-sparing actions, with resultant reduction of opioid-related side effects. Epidural anesthesia in patients with diabetes is more likely to develop in to an abscess. If gross autonomic neuropathy is present, central neuraxial blockade is also likely to develop in to hemodynamic instability due to its sympathetic blockade. It is believed that there is a tell-tale increase in neuropathy after peripheral nerve blocks.
14. With regional or local anesthesia or field blocks, the patient can be taken up much earlier with more guarantee of surgery taking place than it would be with the general anesthesia. This alone answers the principal key issue that the cause of all the risks and hyperglycemia is the infection to be tackled by surgery, *which is the cause* of septicemia. Once the abscesses are drained or the infective tissues are removed, early control of septicemia can be achieved. This in its turn will lead to accelerated reversal of all the metabolic, hemodynamic, and septic abnormalities to the baseline level where the patient was before developing the sepsis along with reduced demand of insulin.
15. Often when the patient is wheeled to the operating theater, his sympathetic overactivity due to anxiety pushes the blood pressure and heart rates to much higher levels. Under these circumstances administering general anesthesia can carry high risk resulting in postponement of the surgery. But proper counselling with regional anesthesia can be a better alternative to conduct a surgical procedure in this situation.

9.6.4 Eco-friendly Regional Anesthesia

Many agencies in the world are concerned about the increasing global warming and how to prevent or reduce it. Worldwide, anesthesiologists are contributing to reduction of it by various alterations in the anesthesia techniques—to mention a few, (1) using air-oxygen instead of nitrous oxide—oxygen wherein nitrous oxide is a harmful agent, (2) reduction in the use of various fluorinated hydrocarbon-containing inhalational agents, (3) low-flow anesthesia technique, and so on. The important indubitable addition is the increasing use of various local anesthetic agents for giving regional analgesia and anesthesia. That more than 95% operations in diabetic foot are successfully done under regional anesthesia, and probably we can reach close to 100% in coming days and thus become significant.

9.7 Pre-block Preparation

Counselling the patient about safety of the procedure with very low complication rate assures the patient and reduces his anxiety to a greater extent. Reassurance about the success of the block, more so if they have experienced failure earlier, is necessary. The details of the type of block to be administered should also be shared with the patient and the relatives.

Paresthesias may be experienced in local blocks. An adequate anticipatory explanation regarding its likely occurrence will help in clarifying the expectation and doubts of the patient. Reassuring the patient of adequate sedation if required, especially in anxious patients concerned about the comfort and amnesia during the surgical procedure, is of great help.

Edema is quasi universal in diabetes. Application of elastocrepe bandage 2–3 days before (if time permits) or as long as possible prior to regional anesthesia makes the limb soft and supple, improves limb circulation, and improves the success rate of block.

Described below are the details of various blocks given routinely. The local anesthetic preferred for short procedures is 2% Xylocaine. If the procedure is going to last longer, then bupivacaine is used.

9.7.1 Femoral Nerve Block

The basic nerve block is femoral. The technique that is quite easy to master carries a low risk for complications. It has good clinical applications to produce anesthesia during surgery and analgesia postoperatively. The largest branch of the lumbar plexus is the femoral nerve. The anterior divisions of the second, third, and fourth lumbar nerves finally form it. It then descends through the fibers of the psoas muscle and lastly emerges below the inguinal ligament. At the femoral crease, the nerve is covered by the fascia iliaca and separated from the femoral artery and vein by part of the psoas muscle and the ligament of the iliopectineus. From there it descends into the thigh where it again divides into anterior and posterior branches. Careful aspiration to rule out accidental insertion in the femoral vein and artery is of utmost importance during peripheral nerve block injection.

Positioning: The patient is given a supine position with both legs extended. If a patient is obese, femoral arterial palpation is difficult. If a pillow is pushed below the hips, it may make palpation of the femoral artery easier, and the block could be more properly placed.

Procedure: The only anatomic landmark necessary for the femoral nerve block is the femoral crease to identify and properly feel the femoral artery pulse near the femoral crease. This is the important step. The needle is inserted immediately lateral to the femoral artery, in the sagittal plane. The needle is tilted a little headward. As the needle hits the nerve, the quadriceps muscle contracts. Its stimulation is indicated by patellar movement. The quantity needed for effective block is about 10 mL of local anesthetic solution.

Sciatic Nerve: The sciatic nerve is formed by the nerve roots from lumbars 4 and 5 and sacral S1 to S3 nerve roots. It is nearly 2 cm thick and is the largest nerve in the body. The sciatic nerve innervates the posterior thigh. The medial aspect of the leg is innervated by the saphenous nerve. Rest of the leg is innervated by the sciatic.

9.7.2 Sciatic Block at the Hip Level

It can be blocked by multiple approaches. Posterior or the trans-gluteal approach is easy to perform and has a high success rate when properly performed. It is described below.

9.7.3 Positioning for Trans-gluteal Block

The patient is placed in the lateral decubitus position tilted slightly forward, with the hip flexed. The foot on the side to be blocked should be positioned over the dependent leg so that twitches of the foot or toes can be easily observed. This is a modified Sims position. To maintain this position, one more person is needed to help the patient do so. It is very important to ensure that the position should not be changed till the end of the procedure (see below).

9.7.4 Procedure

Anatomical landmarks for the posterior approach to a sciatic block to be identified are (1) the greater trochanter and (2) posterior superior iliac spine (PSIS). These can be easily identified in most patients. Midpoint between these two landmarks is then identified and may be marked. The needle is then inserted at a point 4 cm distal to this midpoint. Stimulation 0.2 to with 0.5 mA electrical current once applied should result in the twitching of the foot or toes before the local anesthetic is injected. This is a must step. Nearly 30 mL of local anesthetic solution is required to get an effective block.

9.7.5 Sciatic Nerve Block at the Level of the Popliteal Fossa

The sciatic nerve consists of posterior tibial and the common peroneal nerves as two separate trunks. The sciatic nerve descends towards the knee. At 5 and 7 cm proximal to the popliteal fossa crease, it separates in two trunks, as posterior tibial and the common peroneal nerves. The components of the sciatic nerve may be blocked at the level of the popliteal fossa by a posterior or a lateral approach.

9.7.6 Positioning for the Posterior Approach

It is given with the patient in the prone position. The three landmarks are the popliteal fossa crease; tendons of the semitendinosus and semimembranosus muscles medially and the tendon of the biceps femoris muscle laterally are located. The needle insertion point is marked at 7 cm above the popliteal fossa crease at the midpoint between the two tendons.

Procedure: Twitches of the foot or toes at 0.2–0.5 mA are induced before the local anesthetic injection. 15–20 mL of local anesthetic solution is required to get an effective block.

9.7.7 Popliteal Block: Lateral Approach

Positioning: It is supine. This position is used if a patient is unable to turn prone for any reason for the post-popliteal approach. The moment the leg is flexed, the tendinous landmarks described below in the procedure become evident. The foot should form a 90° angle to the horizontal plane of the table.

Procedure: The landmarks for the block are as follows: vastus lateralis muscle, biceps femoris muscle, and the popliteal fossa crease. The needle insertion site is marked in the groove between the vastus lateralis and biceps femoris muscles 7–8 cm above the popliteal fossa crease. The needle is inserted in a horizontal plane and perpendicular to the long axis of the leg between the vastus lateralis and biceps femoris muscles and advanced to contact the femur. After femur contact, the needle is then withdrawn to skin level, redirected 30° posteriorly to the angle at which the femur was contacted, and advanced towards the nerve. The depth of the sciatic nerve is typically 1–2 cm beyond the skin-femur distance. 15–20 mL of local anesthetic solution will give an effective block.

9.7.8 Lower Leg Block

This is a modified high ankle block. It has an edge over ankle block since it can be administered even if there is swelling at or above the ankle joint. The four distal branches of the sciatic nerve, namely, the deep and superficial peroneal nerves, the tibial, and sural nerves, are the main ones to be blocked, in addition to the saphenous nerve and lateral cutaneous branches (Fig. 9.1).

Posterior tibial nerve is blocked by injecting local anesthetic just behind the medial malleolus. This point falls one third medially of the distance between medial malleolus and calcaneal end on medial side of ankle. This is given in fan shape technique as described for the deep peroneal nerve (Fig. 9.2).

Deep peroneal nerve is anesthetized using the landmark, immediately lateral to the tendon of the extensor hallucis longus muscle on the lateral side if the shin. The needle is advanced through the skin until bone is contacted. Then the needle is withdrawn back 1–2 mm, and 2–3 mL of local anesthetic is injected (see Fig. 9.3 below).

Sural nerve can be easily blocked in the lateral gutter behind tendoachilles superficial to the fascia with 2–3 mL of local anesthetic agent (Fig. 9.4).

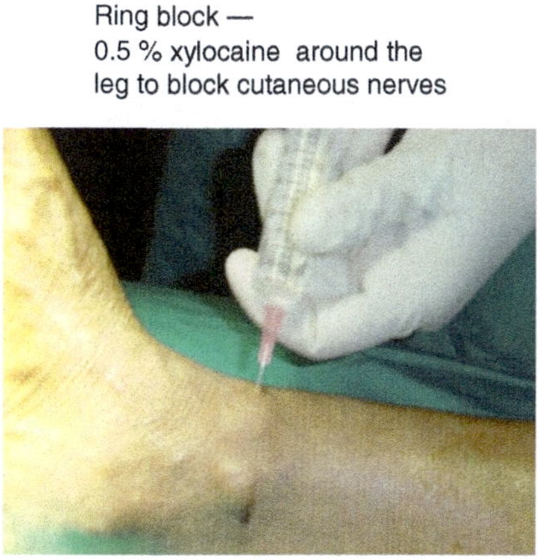

Fig. 9.1 Lower leg or modified ankle ring block

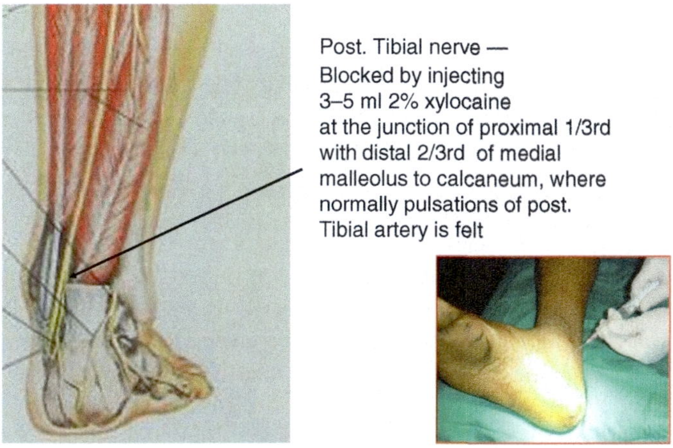

Fig. 9.2 Lower leg block or modified ankle block posterior tibial nerve

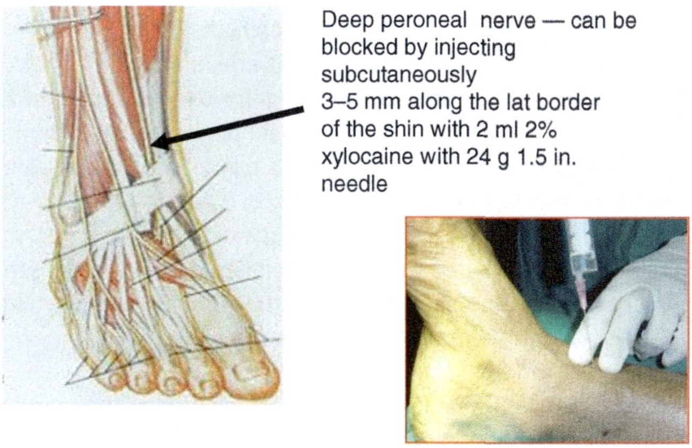

Fig. 9.3 Lower leg block or modified ankle block, posterior view deep peroneal nerve

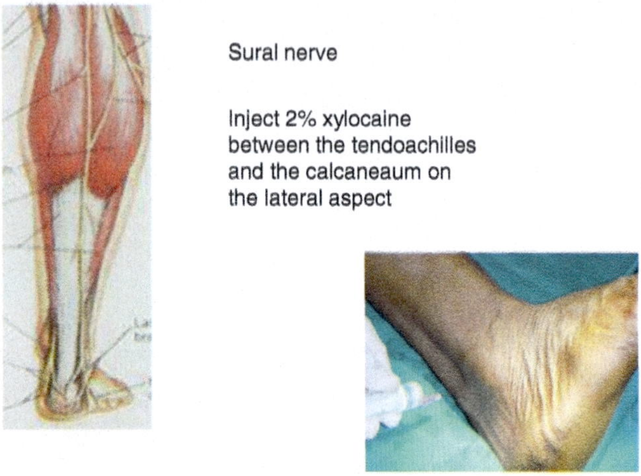

Fig. 9.4 Lower leg block sural nerve

Superficial peroneal, lateral cutaneous nerves of the calf and saphenous nerve blocks—These three nerves are superficial cutaneous extensions of the sciatic and femoral nerves. A block of all three nerves is accomplished using a simple circumferential injection of local anesthetic subcutaneously at the level of 2–3 in. above ankle joint.

9.7.9 Other Anesthesia Modalities

General, spinal, and epidural anesthesia can be given alternatively when there are limitations in using above mentioned regional anesthesia techniques in certain situations detailed below.

1. Patient's unwillingness—This can invariably be tackled by counselling and explaining the patient and the relative safety over other techniques along with the use of awake sedation.
2. Patient's hypersensitivity/allergy to local anesthetic agents.
3. Unsatisfactory condition of skin at the site of injection.
4. These patients are often on platelet inhibitors for one reason or the other; anesthetist should stop these drugs for an adequate period before planning of spinal and epidural anesthesia. For that the patient has to be in stable condition, and surgical intervention can wait.
5. If a patient is on hemodialysis and if he needs one prior to surgery, the patient should be given a heparin-free dialysis. Also coagulation profile, serum electrolytes and serum creatinine should be checked prior to surgery, and corrective measures to the extent possible should be undertaken.

Utmost precautions should be taken while administering either general anesthesia or spinal and epidural anesthesia by overall assessment of the patient. Special care should be taken in:

1. Airway management with difficult intubations.
2. Accidental fall in blood pressure either due to cardiomyopathy or abnormal autonomic nervous system response.
3. Abnormal rhythm with various types of arrhythmias.
4. Perioperative occurrence of ischemic cardiac event.
5. Immediate postoperative obstructive sleep apnoea especially in patients already so diagnosed and on C PAP or those with obesity or short neck etc.
6. Availability of postoperative ICU facility especially in high-risk patients.

9.8 The Commonly Asked Questions About Regional Anesthesia by Our Colleagues

Q1. Why are you required to give anesthesia regionally to a person with already decreased sensations?

The loss of sensations in diabetic neuropathy is rather patchy which will give some pain during surgery. The deep sensations may still be intact. It necessitates effective regional anesthesia. Every effort should be made to avoid the pain during surgery by ensuring complete local analgesia. This helps to have a better control over other systems during surgery.

Q2. If local anesthesia is to be given, do we still need to starve the patient? If yes, why and how long should it be?

In case of any adverse event, it is much easier to manage it in a starved patient. The duration of starving may not be long or overnight. A starvation of 6 h for light solid and 2–3 h of clear liquids prior to surgery is adequate. This is especially useful if conversion of a regional anesthesia to sedation-cum-general anesthesia is needed.

Q3. For some reasons, if surgical procedure has extended beyond the anesthesia time how should it be managed?

Usually analgesia under block lasts for 2–3 h which is normally adequate for the surgical procedure. If it goes beyond this period, the surgeon should inform the anesthesiologist earlier so that it can be managed by the anesthesiologist. The procedure should continue only after the pain relief.

Q4. With the administration of regional anesthesia, can patient be given postoperative analgesia?

Certainly! Use of injection bupivacaine can extend the postoperative analgesia for 5–8 h. The addition of injection clonidine at 1 μg/kg and/or 4 mg of injection dexamethasone to the local anesthetic solutions gives analgesia for more than 24 h. This is being used routinely for all major blocks and also in field blocks.

Q5. As the patient is monitored regularly with a diabetologist why are you asking for such a battery of investigations before surgery?

It is necessary to look at the present status of *all* the systems of the patient preoperatively. The monitoring patient may carry could be older than a week or more.

The parameters are likely to change in a significant manner especially in septic cases, cardiac cases, and patients with nephropathy. The monitoring may not be comprehensive since it would often be done in more stable conditions compared to the one who presents with severe sepsis.

This helps to spell out the actual risk at the point of taking up the patient for surgery. It helps to point out the deterioration of many parameters which could have been better in the previous monitoring. It is worthwhile to remember that glycemic parameter control is just one of the many other parameters.

Q6. What are the different types of nerve blocks/field blocks practiced?

Types of blocks in the leg:

(a) Low leg covers lower 1/3 of leg above the ankle.
(b) Sciatic nerve block in the posterior lower third of thigh.
(c) Sciatic nerve block in the hip region.
(d) Femoral nerve block in the groin.
(e) Field block—This is useful in dealing with localized pathologies like corn excision, infected cysts, abscess, and carbuncles anywhere in the body. The solution usually used is 0.5% lignocaine with one in eight lakh dilution of adrenaline. The surgeon has to wait for at least ten minutes after the injection to have a good dry field.

Q7. Whether and how in the presence of infection the local anesthetic drug will act?

There are two facts to be understood. The injection of local anesthetic drug starts in the relatively normal peripheral zone of the swelling where the pH is close to normal values. This will lead to analgesia in the central area of the pathology and surgery.

Q8. Is there reliable available statistics about the regional anesthesia in diabetic foot surgery?

Yes.

Total No. of patients: 2757. Number of patients who received Leg Blocks: 2425–87.95%.

High Sciatic/Femoral Block No.: 44 or [1.81%].

Mid Sciatic No.: 313 [12.90%].

Low Leg Block No.: 2027 [83.58%].

Failure of the Block: 41 [1.69%].

Remaining 332 patients were given either spinal or epidural or general anesthesia. Nowadays with better technology and more practice, the failure rate of local anesthesia is less than 1%. The success rate achieved is close to 100% in foot surgeries under lower limb blocks. About the sciatico-femoral blocks, the success rate can be improved with application of better methods with the help of peripheral nerve stimulator and sonography machine. A combination of nerve block with field block will create highly satisfactory conditions for the surgeon and the patient [4].

Q9. What advice would you give in cases where local blocks fail?

Total intravenous anesthesia [TIVA] should be given in all patients where local blocks failed, of course after assessing all the necessary prerequisites.

Q10. Are there any particular cautions that need to be exercised for patients given field or local anesthesia?

Since the patient is conscious and aware, the whole team should be extremely cautious about what they talk, comment, or do on the patient's condition and/or any other matter or persons.

The towel clips should be applied on anesthetized part only; resting the forearm or the elbow or keeping the surgical instruments on the unanesthetized part reflexly should be avoided.

Q11. Cox-2 inhibitors and antiplatelet agents are given in majority of long-standing diabetes and are prone to cause excessive bleeding. How do we control this situation?

In addition to above Charcot's osteoarthropathy with its arteriovenous shunts and traumatic coagulopathy, patients can bleed profusely to go in to hypovolemic shock. Such patients will require blood transfusion. A unit or two could be kept in reserve in such cases. Recently the author has started the use of 0.5% lignocaine with one in eight lakh of adrenaline in the subcutaneous tissues where surgical incision is anticipated. This results in diminished bleeding/oozing from the surgical wound, and this also reduces surgical time. The need of transfusion is also reduced and at times averted. This also contributes to postoperative analgesia.

After doing a good number of cases, one learns to where and how much to inject in which direction like extension of a septic pocket or where proximal tendon needs to be excised.

Care should be taken to avoid digital vessels which are lying deep in between the metatarsals.

Q12. What is the role of regional anesthesia in patients who have recently undergone therapeutic peripheral lower limb angioplasties in particular?

Such a patient requiring diabetic foot surgery is at a very high risk for administering general anesthesia due to cardiac and renal involvement, septicemia, and other medical problems. The administration of spinal and/or epidural analgesia is contraindicated due to worry of internal vascular injury and hematoma with risk of developing neurological deficit. Thus, the author feels the safest mode is to administer nerve blocks in these patients.

Q13. How to improve the successful administration of regional/local anesthesia and nerve blocks?

Below the text there are pictorial representations of how to give leg blocks which will be helpful. These pictures are based on surface anatomy landmark which are more or less the same for all and the nerves as well. Yet, the accuracy and certainty of the blocks can be further increased by using a peripheral nerve locator/stimulator

[PNS and/or USG guided] as shown below. The peripheral nerve stimulation evokes motor response with a current up to 0.5–1 mili amperes. Nowadays use of U S G probe is used in combination with/without PNS for better accuracy.

Anatomy text books show the nerve pathways in lower limb. In addition if that is followed by working on the blocks on the amputated legs in one's own place using hypodermic injection needles to locate the nerves and confirm its position by cutting with the knife up to the tip of the needle, it will be immensely helpful to acquire this skill (especially when the abovementioned localizing facilities are not available). This will not only shorten the latency of the nerve block taking up but enhance the duration of the postoperative analgesia. It is affordable and more than useful to improve the results of the regional anesthesia in diabetic and other foot surgeries.

Q14. Does skin grafting on a diabetic foot ulcer need any other anesthesia, analgesia?

The commonly done surgical procedure in recovery rooms in diabetic foot is skin grafting. Nowadays it can be done under combination of topical anesthesia and nerve block.

Application of ointment Prilox, a combination of lignocaine and prilocaine to the donor site and covering it with a plastic sheet and then bandaged for a period of 3–4 h prior to surgery is a useful technique. The patient is then brought to the operation theater. First lower leg block is given. If necessary, 0.5% lignocaine with one in eight lakh of adrenaline is injected. Prilox dressing is removed and the area is surgically cleaned. After testing for pain, the skin graft is removed and applied on the recipient site.

Q15. What should be the important message if a team wants to start practicing this technique?

The important step to success with regional anesthesia in diabetic foot is to practice regularly and learn the course of the nerves before planning any small or a large nerve block. After blocking the limb, the sensations are tested to confirm that it is adequately blocked and then only one should hand over the patient to the surgical team.

For this to be achieved, the patience of the anesthetist, the surgeon, and the patient is very essential. The first most important thing is to keep the patient comfortable, if necessary with awake sedation. This will lead to patient's comfort, the surgeons comfort, and the anesthetists comfort which will finally lead to increased safety.

Pictorial representation of how different blocks are given below. Most relevant today are the lower leg blocks. All the pictures are with permission by Dr. Prakash Ambardekar DA, MD Anesthesiology and coauthor of this volume.

9.9 Cost Consequence Analysis

The patient with only non-complicated surgical diabetic foot can be managed their surgical treatment in an outdoor basis or day care basis treatment which will certainly reduce the effective cost to the patient.

In complicated surgical diabetic foot patient who needs an admission, greatest cost-saving is by taking up the patient as early by achieving early control of the various parameters especially blood glucoses, electrolytes in infective pathologies, thereby reducing the overall time of recovery and subsequent reduction in corrections of parameters. The cost of complications arising out of having to take the patient under general anesthesia are much higher than under regional anesthesia or block with the other costs mentioned earlier just above.

Thus, making use of this mode to help the patient is one of the most cost-effective ways to bring the patient out of the most serious of the diabetic foot complication.

References

1. IDF Atlas 7th edition. 2017. p. 80.
2. Boulton AJ, Vileikyte L, Ragnarson-Tennvall G, et al. The global burden of diabetic foot disease. Lancet. 2005;366:1719–24. https://doi.org/10.1016/S0140-6736(05)67698-2.
3. Boulton AJM, Armstrong DG, Albert SF, et al. Comprehensive foot examination and risk assessment. Diabetes Care. 2008;31:1679–85. https://doi.org/10.2337/dc08-9021.
4. Statistics from SL Raheja Hospital (now Fortis) from Mumbai from 2002 to 2010.

Additional Reading

Handbook of diabetic foot care. 2004. http://www.diabeticfootsocietyofindia.org
http://www.diabeticfootsocietyofindia.org
Kelkar S, editor. National guidelines for management of diabetic foot. 2nd ed. Chennai: Diabetic Foot Society of India; 2017.

Physiology of Insulin

10

Contents

S. Kelkar et al., *Towards Optimal Management of Diabetes in Surgery*,
https://doi.org/10.1007/978-981-13-7705-1_10

10.1 The Physiology of Insulin

It is important to understand the insulin physiology, to comprehend in full the changes that occur in insulin deficiency state, and to facilitate the attempts to bring up the insulin levels to an effective state. In particular the differences in the metabolism between the portal insulin levels and the pharmacodynamics of the exogenously administered insulin should also be understood. In the same section, we will also describe some nonmetabolic actions of insulin underscoring the significance of insulin. Unless these actions and the scope of insulin physiology are precisely understood, the insulin and diabetes management will become a mechanistic unintelligent centered only on glucose control. Sadly this is the state of care in this area across the subcontinent and possibly other less developed countries as well.

10.1.1 The Fed State, Fasting State, and the Postabsorptive State

Insulin and the counter regulatory hormone physiology and actions differ in these three phases. Beginning the discussion with dinner, the absorption of the nutrients goes on for about 5 h, i.e., from say 9 PM it will go on till about 2 AM in the night. As the food intake starts, insulin is secreted from the beta cells depending upon the composition of food and its rate of absorption. One immediate mechanism that kicks in is the secretion of incretins even before the food is gulped called the "cephalic phase." Incretins are peptides secreted by the distal ileal L cells and proximal jejunal K cells in response to meals. The glucagon-like peptide 1 (GLP-1) in particular stimulates the beta cell to secrete insulin.

The rise in blood glucose level after ingestion of meal also stimulates the insulin secretion in the portal vein. First the nutrients absorbed pass through the liver via portal vein and get deposited in the liver under the process of glycogenesis. Fifty percent of the portal insulin will be degraded in the liver in the process of glycogen synthesis. This is called the first pass insulin phase. Glycogen is synthesized in the liver from the circulating glucose under the influence of portal venous insulin levels. The level of insulin in the hepatic veins to the systemic circulation will thus be lower than the portal vein as these veins join the inferior vena cava and go into systemic circulation. Portal vein glucose generally does not exceed 180 mg/dL in both normal and diabetic state [1]. Increased FFAs in portal vein due to excessive consumption of fats reduce the insulin clearance by the liver leading to hyperinsulinemia ([1], p. 3). In normal circumstances adequate insulin will be available in hepatic veins to enhance the tissue glucose uptake particularly in muscles and keep blood glucose within normal range.

The extra glucose which cannot be converted to glycogen passes on to the circulation, and the beta cells are exposed to the increased levels of 4–6 mmol of glucose in nondiabetic state. The glucose enters the beta cells through the GLUT 1 receptors found on the beta cell surface and further metabolized by the Hexokinase IV, the active enzyme, also called Glucokinase. The Hexokinase IV affinity to glucose becomes operative when the blood glucose is above 5 mmol, i.e., 90 mg/dL.

Intracellular glucose is metabolized and produces ATP (energy) that causes calcium influx and secretion of insulin. Two additional mechanisms for the secretion of insulin include the closure of the K^+ ATP channels and an increase in the intracellular calcium released from the endoplasmic reticulum. The secreted insulin continues to pass through portal vein along with digested nutrients to the liver and continuing the action of glycogenesis till all the nutrients are metabolized which normally takes about 5 h. Once the circulating glucose declines to normal levels or slightly below, the insulin secretion is switched off. There are many other factors which affect this process which will be discussed further below.

When the concentration of glucose in blood reaches 10–12 mmol of glucose, there is maximum (pro)insulin synthesis which reaches its peak by 60 min and then declines ([1], p. 66). Such chronically high blood glucose levels in diagnosed or undiagnosed diabetes will lead to exhaustion of the (pro)insulin synthesis. This may also release insulin all the time again to the point of exhaustion which is also discussed below.

When the blood glucose levels drop to 2–4 mmol, the (pro)insulin synthesis starts intracellularly. Such low levels of 2–4 mmol will be rarely reached in circulation, except when there is a drug, diet, and exercise/activity mismatch. This will reflect on the low glucose content of the beta cells in some way to stimulate insulin synthesis. In low glucose setting, the enzyme Hexokinase IV affinity to glucose declines. It results in further decline in the glucose levels in beta cells.

The postabsorptive phase after dinner begins at 1 or 2 AM in the night, the decline of insulin levels due to declining level of glucose. It will cause glucagon release from the alpha cells of the islets of Langerhans. Low levels of circulating insulin during fasting stimulating the secretion of glucagon are facilitated by the liberal exposure of plasma through the fenestrated, i.e., wide windows capillary bed in the islets. The same circulatory feature is also seen in the hypothalamus. As the blood flow continues and comes back through systemic circulation, the glucose and other products go to the intercellular spaces through fenestrations and exert its actions on all the cells of islets of Langerhans. Alpha cells having sensed the normal or the low levels of both insulin and glucose secret glucagon. It is now carried in the portal venous circulation. The singular action of glucagon is to stimulate the hepatic glucose output during the postabsorptive phases when the gut-absorbed glucose is no longer available ([1], p. 45). High levels of portal venous glucagon will then directly cause an increase in the fasting hepatic glucose output in order to keep the blood glucose normal in a fasting state. Once the intestinal supply of glucose stops, the period of postabsorptive state starts and lasts for about 5 h.

The hepatic glucose output under normal or steady state, i.e., neither exercising nor high level of physical activity, can continue to supply the body's glucose requirements for 6–8 h. An element of glucose level increase is also carried out by the secretion of growth hormone in the early hours of the night (see below). After this, the longer fasting state begins. Glucagon also causes and continues the release of fatty acids from the adipose tissues which give free fatty acids and glycerol. If the fasting is prolonged further, the glucose use declines, and the gluconeogenesis from these and other substrates maintains the glucose levels (see below).

10.1.2 The Enteroinsular Axis

In fasting state there is no gastric stimulation, and GLP-1 is not secreted, and there is no absorption of glucose from the gut. That is the reason why insulin secretion is suppressed. The stimulation of insulin secretion due to food ingestion and gut hormone release is called as the enteroinsular axis.[1] This seasaw between the finely tuned mechanisms between the alpha and beta cell secretion under two opposite stimulants maintains the blood glucose balance. This balance is not only dynamic but fluctuates within minutes. The arterial blood supply to pancreatic beta cells is the key factor in activating the insulin secretion. Islets of Langerhans containing beta and alpha cells constitute 1–2% mass of the pancreas but receive 15–20% of the pancreatic blood supply. This underlines the importance of exposing both alpha and beta cells to the full metabolic milieu for proper secretion of insulin and consequently of glucagon as well ([1], p. 48).

In diabetes fasting state as described above results in low levels of portal insulin. This also happens additionally due to beta cell defects in secreting or responding to glucose demand which will be discussed below. These levels are inadequate to effectively cause glycogenesis or suppress or regulate effectively the hepatic glucose output. The longer the fasting state lasts, the more relentless the hepatic glucose output will be through the gluconeogenesis described above (also see below). The glucose will get into the extracellular space in the liver and will be carried to the systemic circulation by the hepatic veins causing a rise in the levels of systemic blood glucose. This is the reason why early morning breakfast is considered essential as it will release insulin and reduce the excessive hepatic output. For the same reason, late night snack or a glass of milk is advised since it reduces the interval between food intakes and helps in optimizing hepatic glucose output. This excessive fasting hepatic glucose output is considered to be a putative feature in the development of type 2 diabetes. In nondiabetic persons the quantum of glucose output in fasting conditions is 1 g/h. However in persons with diabetes, it may exceed 10 g/h, in turn contributing to hyperglycemia.

10.1.3 Neural Regulation of Insulin Secretion

Pancreatic beta cells have a rich vagal nerve supply in addition to the alpha 2 nerve supply. In normal persons small bursts of insulin release occur with a regular frequency from 8 to 16 min. These oscillations seem to be under control of a vagal pacemaker. Epinephrine inhibits glucose-induced insulin synthesis through the stimulation of the alpha 2 sympathetic nerve endings. Importance of neural

[1] In normal persons as well as those with diabetes, the quantum, duration, and the peak of insulin response are less, when stimulated by intravenous glucose infusion compared to oral ingestion. Intravenous glucose stimulation does not invoke the action of enteroinsular axis as no food enters the stomach. In addition to it, there is believed to be a cephalic phase in food intake, which strengthens the enteroinsular axis.

regulation can be judged by the fact that pancreatic transplant recipients have no functioning nerve innervation of the islets leading to a flattened and delayed first-phase insulin release. It may also suggest the additional cephalic contribution to the whole process ([1], p. 118).

10.1.4 Fasting Overnight, Longer Duration of Fasting, or Catabolic States

In longer durations of fasting (or the more severe catabolic or stress states), many more physiological actions related to the substrate utilization in the body tissues occur. The first is characterized by low insulin levels and an increase in glucagon. Glucagon has potent lipolytic actions resulting in an increase in circulating free fatty acids levels. These FFAs when in high concentration tend to further suppress insulin secretion and defects in insulin actions contributing to insulin resistance ([1], p. 265). This reduces the glucose uptake by the muscles leading to less glucose utilization by muscles also referred to as "lipotoxicity." FFAs also become a source of gluconeogenesis in the liver giving rise to higher blood glucose.

The other two alterations in the substrate utilization are characterized by high insulin resistance with or without adequate levels of insulin, leading to less glucose utilization by the cells. The compensation comes from the oxidation of free fatty acids up to 50% of all fuels required by muscle in such states. The muscle glycogen initially depletes to 33% and remains stable at that level. Alanine loss from the muscles, initially high, declines in prolonged fasting. Catecholamines are released in the latter two states in particular; norepinephrine has the maximum lipolytic effect, followed by epinephrine. Cortisol and acidosis interfere with the insulin binding to the insulin receptors, thereby further inhibiting glucose transport in the cells, increasing the glucose levels. Cortisol and growth hormones both also suppress the insulin secretion. Glucagon also rises, facilitating glycogenolysis increasing the blood glucose in circulation and lipolysis further increasing the gluconeogenesis. Glucagon however also increases amino acid uptake in muscles and hence is anabolic to some extent ([1], p. 132). Growth hormone under these circumstances increases insulin resistance but has other anabolic actions.

These mechanisms have evolved with a single purpose of making adequate glucose available to the brain under these conditions to remain optimally functioning to protect the organism. The primary fuel for energy for the brain is glucose only in normal circumstances. Like other organs it cannot use other alternative fuels available in the body. Nor can the brain store any fuels like other tissues. An average human consumes (metabolically and not as food) about 160 g of glucose every day. The brain alone consumes 120 g of it, at 6 g/h constantly.

Even during prolonged fasting, low levels of insulin ketosis may not be significant enough to cause DKA. This can happen in individuals trained in long fasting which can extend to 60–70 days. This could be partly due to the increased insulin sensitivity during fasting. It could also be because of the pulsatile bursts of insulin which keeps the alternate FFA metabolism effective as stated elsewhere. This however is not the case in high catabolic states like generalized sepsis from any cause. In these conditions insulin resistance is extremely high and so are the counter regulatory hormones, which results in both suppression of insulin and its ineffective actions. That leads to DKA.

10.1.5 Glucose Toxicity and Beta Cell Exhaustion

In chronic hyperglycemia by intravenous infusion of glucose over 48 h or high-fat diets, both have been used on a variety of animals in experimental research laboratories. Obese mice, animals with streptozotocin-induced destruction of the pancreas resulting in type 1 diabetes, or diabetic animals without streptozotocin use and many such models have elucidated a variety of mechanisms, many of which are also operative in type 2 diabetes patients. A state of chronic hyperglycemia is present in persons whose diabetes has not been detected. It comes to light when the diagnosis of diabetes is made. A diabetic state is supposed to be present for 5–7 years before a routine diagnosis is made. It was seen in the UKPDS trial, which enrolled newly diagnosed persons with diabetes, 50% of whom had some evidence of tissue damage at diagnosis which indicates a long undetected presence of diabetes to cause it [2].

The elevated levels of glucose sometimes causes the beta cells to become unresponsive to these higher levels of blood glucose, which results in suppression or inadequate secretion of insulin from beta cells. The unresponsive stage continues as glycogenesis is not effective causing a spiraling increase of glucose over days without ketosis. This phenomenon should be called by a twin nomenclature of glucose toxicity[2] and exhaustion of beta cells. In beta cells, this defect is attributed directly to hyperglycemia. Without going in the complexity of experimental research, it may be said that so far, nine different metabolic abnormalities have been considered to be present to cause this unresponsiveness. Long-chain fatty acids in the beta cells increase the acetyl CoA/CoA ratio which leads to increased fatty acid oxidation. Several and complex metabolic reactions finally lead to decreased Hexokinase IV activity resulting diminished glucose metabolism in beta cells and insensitivity in beta cells to respond to glucose challenges. Any treatment or intervention that tends to normalize/reduce glucose reverses this state of unresponsiveness.

Simultaneously, the other direct effect of chronic hyperglycemia that is notable is the beta cell exhaustion in trying to continuously respond to it. It must be remembered that there is an instantly ready pool of insulin just below the beta cell membrane. In store is more packaged insulin in its cytoplasm which is later brought to

[2]This is a commonly met situation in routine clinical practice as well. In newly diagnosed type 2 diabetes, the blood glucose can often be as high as 400 mg/dL. Yet the symptom profile is mild. Hence it is unnecessary to be alarmed by it. Simple measures like significant diet control and primary medication with oral drugs cause a quick reversal of glucotoxicity, and the blood glucose falls rapidly often with small quantities of drugs. It can then be brought under control with little intensification of treatment.

the ready pool below the cell membrane. Prior to this is the proinsulin to insulin conversion followed by its transport to the cell membrane for releasing it under glucose stimulation. Proinsulin to insulin conversion and its packaging need time. Under chronic hyperglycemia when all of these are exhausted, the most basic mechanism of production of preproinsulin must start. It is to be later converted to proinsulin to insulin as store and insulin below the cell membrane ready for release. This chain reaction leads to the depletion of intracellular insulin availability leading to the beta cells unable to respond.

It should become clear by these observations that the enzymatic protein turnover in the cytoplasm of the cells is rapid, whereas the protein synthesis to happen on mRNA takes much longer time (this is a simplified schema of beta cell dysfunction) ([1], p. 67). Chronic hyperglycemia in addition also destabilizes the mRNA for preproinsulin hampering its production ([1], p. 67).

10.2 Insulin Resistance

The concept of insulin resistance needs a little clarification. Insulin resistance is a necessary condition for the development of type 2 diabetes. It is native in those who develop type 2 diabetes. It varies from person to person and is also dependent upon many other factors like obesity and physical activity. It can be reduced to a certain extent by undertaking various measures but not below it. Resistance is said to have developed when higher than the physiological levels otherwise effective in those who do not have type 2 diabetes of insulin are required to be able to act upon the three principle tissues—the liver, muscles, and adipose tissue—to achieve glucose homeostasis. In other words, *hyperinsulinemia and high blood glucose despite it are a state of insulin resistance.* It worsens greatly in acute illnesses. In infective inflammatory conditions, interleukin 1 is released which reduces the biosynthesis of insulin ([1], p. 113).

Below is a simplified schema of biochemical reactions which if abnormal will result in Insulin resistance and result in hyperglycemia by reducing intracellular glucose disposal even in the absence of significantly elevated stress factors or the catabolic state.

10.2.1 Post Receptor Signaling Defects as the Cause of Insulin Resistance

Insulin first binds to its receptor. This binding then signals the insulin receptor substrates 1 and 2 having mitogenic potential and metabolic actions, respectively; it also signals phosphoinositide PI3, and G-protein pathways are activated for all intracellular actions of insulin. Any disturbance in these pathways leads to increase in glucose, diacylglycerol (DAG), and protein kinase C (PKC), causing reduced insulin-dependent glucose disposal. The binding of insulin to insulin receptor is reduced particularly in presence of hyperglycemia.

In incomplete conversion from proinsulin to insulin, raising the proinsulin to insulin ratio, a condition noted in type 2 diabetes results in the inability to bind insulin receptor due to low affinity of proinsulin to it.

Insulin autoantibodies combined with insulin or insulin receptor autoantibodies will also interfere with insulin binding to its receptor. Any one or more of the above situations will lead to post receptor signaling abnormalities.

10.2.2 Glucose Transporter (GLUT)-Related Issues as the Cause of Insulin Resistance

GLUT 4 found ubiquitously to have a low capacity to bind glucose; if the blood glucose exceeds 180 mg/dL, GLUT 4 will be downregulated. Translocation of GLUT 4 on cell membrane is dependent on insulin—IRS—1 axis. If insulin is deficient or unable to act, this process will not take place. Increased flux of gluconeogenic substances—alanine and glutamine amino acids as is commonly found in all stress situations—will also reduce the membrane translocation of GLUT. Translocation to cell membrane is reduced in elevated levels of counter regulatory hormones, particularly steroids. Steroids drive GLUT 4 away from membrane. All these actions finally lead to reduced intracellular transport of glucose and hyperglycemia.

Central obesity, increased waist-hip ratio, and physical inactivity also are the causes of insulin resistance. Adipocytes in diabetic subjects are more resistant to insulin action. GLUT 4 is reduced by 40% in obesity and 85% in type 2 diabetic adipose tissues. Muscle training on the other hand increases its surface translocation and leads to glucose uptake in insulin-independent fashion. Noncellular mechanisms for insulin resistance (less insulin-dependent glucose disposal at a given level of insulin and glucose) can be caused by reduced capillary density which increases as shown in muscles if trained for exercise. Impaired transcapillary passage of insulin could also be a factor.

The factors that increase insulin resistance in septic/catabolic conditions are interference of insulin binding to insulin receptor because of high levels of cortisol which are present in catabolic situations. High levels of counter regulatory hormones cause either inhibition of insulin secretion or its actions since they are insulin antagonists. In release of tumor necrosis factor alpha (TNF alpha) in septic/infective/inflammatory conditions singly or in combination with counter regulatory hormones, other cytokines increase insulin resistance.

Some unusual and infrequent causes of insulin resistance are:

1. Pituitary tumors secreting growth hormone is associated with 25% of the patients developing diabetes and around 30–40 developing impaired glucose tolerance.
2. If there is abnormally mutated insulin receptor, insulin cannot bind with it.
3. Or insulin may bind to inactive receptors, but no activation of post receptor triggering happens. This will work as a negative modulator. Insulin receptor defects cause a conformational change which does not allow insulin to bind with its receptors.

4. In the past, insulin autoantibodies binding with insulin could not bind insulin to its receptors. With modern insulin this is no longer a concern.
5. In conditions called leprechaunism, there is extreme insulin resistance due to lack of surface receptors for insulin to bind.

10.2.3 Dawn Phenomenon and the Somogyi Effect

In humans the circadian rhythm of growth hormone is such that there is always a surge in its secretion at 2 or 3 AM in the night. Growth hormone is a powerful insulin antagonist. This results in reducing the action of the insulin administered at night, either at bedtime or before dinner. If there is a concomitant hypoglycemia during night, this surge will be enhanced since it is a strong stimulant to growth hormone secretion. It results in high level of fasting glucose in the morning, while the other glucose estimations may be within normal or near normal limits. This is called the Dawn phenomenon. This may get confused with the idea that the night doses are not working enough to fix the fasting and may result in administration of a larger does which will enhance this cycle and the other glucose estimations may start going haywire.

Similar to this is a situation, where in spite of continued increase in all doses of insulin to fairly high levels, most blood glucose estimations would be out of control range. This may happen due to transient hypoglycemia on several occasions in a day which gets overcorrected by the body's defense mechanisms against hypoglycemia leading to a paradoxical hyperglycemia. This is called the Somogyi effect. There are several ways to correct this. One is a 24 h glucose profile discussed elsewhere. Continuous glucose monitoring systems (CGMS) can very well detect several hypoglycemic episodes in 24 h. CGMS can be extended to few more days. This however is costly. In both these situations, the problematic doses have to be continued during monitoring to detect hypoglycemia. The third way is to lower substantially all the doses of insulin and subject the patients after a few days to a 24 h glucose profiling and readjust/upscale or downscale the doses.

Besides the stimulator responsive roles of glucose and insulin, there is an important diurnal variation in insulin secretion. In late evening and night, the insulin secretion starts declining, probably to avoid nighttime hypoglycemia which may go unnoticed due to sleep ([1], p. 113). This is supported by the long known prevalence of 3% of all deaths in bed being on account of hypoglycemia [3]. More evidence has shown that hypoglycemia is a predictor of poor outcome in people with type 2 diabetes. It is also a predictor of higher risk for premature death [4–6]. The important implication however is on clinical side. It is the frequent elevation of blood glucose pre or post dinner. These glucose readings are rarely taken by the patients. As a result adequate insulin doses are not delivered pre-dinner, giving rise to high post-dinner glucose. Thus the fasting hyperglycemia continues and can be confused with the growth hormone release mentioned above.

10.3 Few Other Aspects of Fuel Metabolism

10.3.1 Ketone Metabolism

We have seen the clinical significance of development of ketone bodies in the circulation in the discussion of DKA. Any person who is involved in the treatment of diabetes must have a grip on the ketone issue. Highly inadequate circulating insulin and high levels of glucagon are the primary reasons (which may arise from any cause) for the development of ketosis. However the body has evolutionarily adapted to this also. In such situations even when hyperglycemia is preponderant, the brain utilizes as much as 40% of the energy requirement by using ketones. Ketones in its turn stimulate insulin secretion.

In some startling discoveries since 2015 is the improvement of the cardiac function in heart failure in diabetes. This condition has so far been resistant to treatment. The promise has come from the serendipitous discovery on administration of a class of drugs called SGLT2i which was developed to block the glucose filtered in the proximal tubules of the kidney as a measure to control diabetes by wasting glucose and cause weight loss. This results in glucosuria and a state of decline in the available fuels for energy needs. This state leads to a low-grade production of ketones, which the cardiac muscle utilizes for its fuel requirement. In the trials conducted on these drugs, within a week it has shown significant improvement in the action of cardiac muscle over the conventional treatments in vogue for long. The improvement in the cardiac muscle function continues to do so in greater measures over several weeks as shown in the trials. It is also suggested that the change in the substrate utilization of the cardiac muscle arises out of a mildly hypoxic state the failing heart faces in which the ketones serve as a useful fuel for the energy supply needed.

10.3.2 Other Hormones, Fuel, and Enzymatic Interplay

There are many other fuels, hormones, and nervous controls which finally contribute to the secretion of insulin. Together they help to synchronize the secretion of insulin ([1], p. 44). This helps in finer regulation of glucose absorbed as it travels through the gastric, duodenal, splenic, and mesenteric veins to form the portal vein.

Free fatty acids (FFAs) are an important fuel substrate that is consumed everyday by the body. A person with a body weight of 70 kg consumes as fuel, only 160 g of carbohydrate that calculates as 640 kcal/day. The total body requirement would be anywhere up to 2000 calories in a sedentary individual. Most of these remaining calories come from FFAs.

10.3.3 The Normal and Abnormal Fatty Acid Glycerol Metabolism

Normal insulin levels cause lipogenesis to which the adipose tissues are sensitive. When the insulin levels are low, hormone-sensitive lipase (HSL) acts upon the adipose tissues and causes lipolysis releasing triglycerides in the circulation. Up to 50%

of fuel requirement in the body is by the utilization of FFAs. In resting conditions 90% of the muscle metabolism is from FFAs. In activity/exercise it shifts initially to glucose uptake but later consumes FFAs for its fuel requirement (see later). Under normal insulin levels, glucose metabolism is the preferred pathway for skeletal-cardiac muscle fibers and adipose tissues. In insulinopenic states also, brought out best in prolonged starvation, there is a switch in metabolism to free fatty acids and ketones. When insulin level is normalized or increased due to administered insulin, hormone-sensitive lipases will be inhibited, and triglyceride release will be cut off. Full oxidation of FFAs under normal insulin levels especially if potassium is also supplemented with glucose may keep intracellular milieu of myocardium optimal, not collect acid products of FFA metabolism, and cause less dysrhythmias.

As the fasting prolongs, the muscle metabolism shifts from glucose consumption to FFAs consumption, to spare glucose for the brain (discussed below further). The constantly working cardiac muscle also depends mainly on FFAs in addition to normal glucose consumption. Further actions of increased FFAs will be discussed under the beta cell defects.

10.3.4 Postabsorptive Phase

As soon as the postabsorptive phase starts and the insulin levels decline, the FFAs are released from the adipose tissues. Seventy-four percent of these FFAs and glycerol are mobilized from the visceral fat tissue under the effects of glucagon and norepinephrine and to a lesser extent by growth hormone ([1], p. 269). Cortisol may cause lipolysis in low insulin level conditions and in more prolonged fasting. This visceral fat release has the advantage of getting absorbed in the portal venous circulation and passes through the liver. The 3 carbon glycerol can be readily converted in 6 carbon glucose under the gluconeogenic process to maintain the glucose levels in blood and prevent hypoglycemia ([1], p. 67). FFAs released under low insulin conditions also impair the insulin-induced lipogenesis and gluconeogenesis ([1], p. 270).

Box 10.1 Skeletal-Cardiac Muscle Metabolism

Preferred metabolite—glucose

Insulinopenia—switch to FFA and ketones

Further starvation—only FFA

Lipoprotein lipases of skeletal and cardiac muscle increase use of FFA

Box 10.2 Adipose Tissue Abnormality

Insulinopenia—lipolysis

FFA used by cardiac/skeletal muscle

Spare glucose for the brain

Ketones—muscle use is proportional to the concentration of ketones

Sparing ketones for the brain

Lactates and pyruvate amino acids are the secondary sources of gluconeogenic substances also discussed below.

10.4 Exercise Physiology in Normal and Diabetic State

Although this topic does not concern us with the main focus of this volume, for the benefit of the residents in particular, a few facts may be worth mentioning. Exercise undoubtedly increases insulin sensitivity which persists after long hours. Targeted exercises can reduce the central obesity which is detrimental to the individual as a harbinger of cardiovascular disease in type 2 diabetes. Exercise has many other benefits like losing weight, lifting depression, and improving the cognitive functions especially in the older individuals. Rigorous exercise can lead to decreased insulin resistance to as long as 36 h. Overall it leads to better control of glucose.

Type 2 diabetes exercise, especially the strenuous ones, is likely to lead to retinal problems and can uncover a cardiovascular disease. Hence prior assessment of it is necessary, and avoiding strenuous exercises may be a better strategy. In type 1 diabetes, it is mainly the supply of calories during and after exercise, and appropriate adjustment of doses is necessary.

As much as exercise, it is the physical activity overall in the day that must also be kept in mind. The chief investigator of Indian Diabetes Prevention Program done on the lines of the Finnish DPP in personal communication to the first author said that huge decrease in the physical activity stands out as the single most important factor leading to early development of diabetes, which can be postponed by its introduction.

At this stage we will quickly take a brief look at how and where exogenously administered insulin differs from the portal insulin in physiologic conditions. We will discuss after that the physiological actions of insulin on different tissues, proteins, and fuels for energy production and maintenance of the organism.

10.5 Circulatory Physiology of Exogenously Administered Insulin

One may particularly note that exogenous administration of insulin, whether intravenous or subcutaneous, results in high levels of it in venous-arterial blood. This being part of systemic circulation does not, as the first-phase pass, go through portal venous circulation. The high arterial insulin levels will cause deposition of circulating glucose in muscles and lipid deposition in the adipose tissues. But the small arteries supplying the beta cells also have higher insulin levels which now effectively suppress the beta cell secretion of insulin as well as glucagon.[3] It causes low

[3] In the initial stages of newly detected diabetes with high levels of glucose, fasting generally above 250 mg, it is a recommended practice to start the patient on insulin for a few weeks. This gives beta cells rest and replenishes its contents and can respond to glucose challenges of the newly detected diabetes better, offsetting the need for insulin. The results of this intervention could be remarkable.

levels of both portal venous insulin and glucagon. During the feeding and the postabsorptive phase in diabetes, the glucose tends to be higher since it does not have the advantage of high levels of portal venous insulin and native insulin resistance to deposit the absorbed nutrients directly in the liver.

Such high levels of arterial exogenously administered insulin effectively suppress glucagon and effect lipogenesis as well. This is often seen as the initial weight gain in patients treated with insulin. At this level insulin also carries out other functions of insulin at lesser levels of concentration, detailed below. Many other non-metabolic actions of insulin are described in Chap. 12. But there are other important mechanisms for this anabolism which will be described below.

Unless insulin deficiency is concomitantly associated with high levels of glucagon, ketosis does not develop. Thus ketosis is prevented, in patients treated with insulin until some overwhelming cause results in insulin resistance at which the available insulin in plasma becomes ineffective. Increased insulin resistance under very low plasma insulin levels lead to DKA or HHNS as discussed earlier. In long standing, particularly in type 1 diabetes, there is degeneration and also the death or decline of alpha cells that produce glucagon. Hence these patients become less prone to ketosis and very severe hyperglycemia.

The exogenous insulin in circulation is mainly degraded in the kidneys by various insulinases, since little of it goes to the liver through its 30% of arterial supply (the remaining 70% coming from the portal vein). This has important implications on insulin administration in diabetic end-stage or significant nephropathy (ESRD). In ESRD the functional kidney mass declines. Hence less insulin is degraded and the circulating pool of insulin will be higher. This rise, it was supposed for long, will be compounded in using longer-acting insulins and hypoglycemia more frequent. The excess of circulating insulin in ESRD frequently comes to light if a patient is admitted with severe hypoglycemia, under insulin administration, or often with oral hypoglycemic drugs. This equally often is the stage at which the significant kidney disease is diagnosed for the first time.

In clinical practice the apprehension associated with use of intermediate-acting insulins in ESRD has long disappeared and is routinely used. If the ESRD gets complicated by sepsis or any other major illness, the insulin requirements could go substantially up. In the author's opinion, this is a result of high native insulin resistance in Indians compounded by the additional destabilizing illnesses.

10.6 Insulin Levels, Its Actions with or Without Exogenous Insulin Administration

The myopic view that insulin controls only glucose must first be abandoned since the potential of insulin in normalcy of body is enormous and outside the function of glucose control. The second understanding is about the correlation of insulin with its action as dependent on its plasma levels, whether due to exogenously administered insulin or usage of secretagogues. The latter gets released in the portal venous circulation but not the first one. The third understanding required for optimal or aggressive usage of insulin is in connection with the resistance it faces at the tissue level. It happens in the garden variety of type 2 diabetes or in additional pathological situations imposed on the existing diabetic state as discussed below. The fourth is the clear knowledge of the insulin pharmacokinetics and insulin pharmacodynamics in which the next chapter will discuss. It includes an understanding of the half maximal duration and life of insulin in plasma. This knowledge is necessary about each and every kind of insulin available today. The understanding also needs to extend to other drugs, injectable or oral which work especially on the minimization of insulin resistance as well as maintaining beta cell mass and optimal functions to the extent possible.

Glucose homeostasis is a complex interplay of a large number of hormones, enzymes and transcription factors, mRNA formations, epigenetic changes on the DNA, and so on. The information given below does not cover all these aspects but only those which are clinically relevant. Multiple mechanisms work for the glucose homeostasis, with positive feedback and feed forward reactions as well as negative feedback mechanisms. There is a redundancy of such mechanisms which enhances preservation of the species in hostile situations internally as well externally. The importance of this information lies in the fact that many of these molecules are directly dependent on adequate insulin levels and its optimal cellular actions. The point to be further emphasized is that insulin acts beyond maintaining its own enzymatic and protein synthesis mechanisms for glucose control. It influences so many processes beyond that. It also turns out to have a role in tissue and cellular preservations. In the sections to follow, all these matters will be explained.

10.6.1 Different Levels and Different Actions of Insulin

Supraphysiological insulin levels and hyperinsulinemia are two different entities. In the progress from impaired fasting glucose (IFG) to impaired glucose tolerance (IGT) to frank diabetes to insulin requiring type 2 diabetes, the insulin profile changes. In the first two phases the hyperinsulinemic response begin and then peak. This response arises in the beta cells of the pancreas. Hence it is endogenous. Even when it is higher than the insulin responses found in normal individuals to fasting as well as post-prandial states, it is not sufficient to control the glucose levels to optimal. The hyperinsulinemic response arises out of the resistance it faces in the abovementioned stages one after another. Thus clinically insulin resistance can be defined in a simple manner as higher insulin levels with higher glucose levels in different stages. Frank diabetes develops once the hyperinsulinemic response results in beta cell failure to secrete adequate insulin to control glucose. This is considered to occur as a result of both beta cell exhaustion and reduced beta cell mass.

More than 100 μU/mL could be considered supraphysiological. As explained above, it cannot arise on account of hyperinsulinemic response. These levels will be reached only on administration of exogenous insulin. Hence supraphysiological level of insulin is an exogenous phenomenon. It results in many biological effects. In supraphysiological levels of insulin with adequate/liberal presence of amino acids in plasma, the process of protein synthesis starts. From energy point of view, each nitrogen bond to build amino acids and protein requires four ATP molecules. At the same time, lesser but physiological levels of plasma insulin can stop the proteolysis. This may be seen in frankly hyperinsulinemic patients who do not lose weight or their muscle mass either. The loss of muscle mass is early to start in any catabolic process or prolonged fasting or starvation. Thus insulin has two more actions outside the glucose control—anti-catabolic and protein synthesizing—both important for physiological maintenance of tissue.

The plasma level of insulin required causing glycogenesis effectively in the liver and muscle is higher than the other actions like preventing lipolysis which occurs at a much lower insulin level. It is considered to be around 100μU/mL. These levels can effectively produce glycogenesis in the liver and muscle mass. Muscle mass contains 300–500 g of glucose in the form of muscle glycogen under the influence of insulin in steady state ([1], p. 128). The actions in these two organs are most fundamental to blood glucose homeostasis.

The fourth, i.e., antilipolytic, action that prevents excessive fatty acid accumulation in blood occurs at even lower insulin levels. Adipose tissue is exquisitely sensitive to this action of insulin which can be affected at 6–60 picomols/L of insulin ([1], p. 265). It also suppresses glucagon at such concentration avoiding all effects of glucagon, like lipolysis. When level of insulin falls below that critical level, high amounts of free fatty acids (FFAs) appear in blood; they inhibit insulin secretion as well as produce defects in insulin actions ([1], p. 265). It also increases the hepatic gluconeogenesis due to enhanced supply of glycerol with FFAs. Both these effects, together, lead to hyperglycemia. Hyperglycemia in turn increases insulin resistance by downregulating the GLUT 4 transporters in the cells and tissues increasing insulin resistance. Continuation of this state will spiral the rise in glucose in blood.

Adequate levels of insulin as found during the fed state switch off the gluconeogenic process quite effectively. During starvation or in more prolonged fasting state or under stress or catabolic states, the insulin levels decline. The glucagon, norepinephrine and epinephrine, growth hormones, and corticosteroids increase. The intertwined mechanisms of these actions of various substances and their activator/suppressor hormones can be seen more clearly under these circumstances. With it, the intricate intracellular signaling molecules also get activated or suppressed, but these details are not necessary for clinically appreciating the hormone interplay. Hence they are not discussed. The sum total of the resultant actions are the acceleration of the process of gluconeogenesis.

Gluconeogenesis is the enzymatically synthesized glucose using three carbon moieties like amino acids, glycerol, lactates, and pyruvates into glucose. Lactates and pyruvates are products of anaerobic glycolysis of glucose in the muscles. They are carried to the liver by circulation and are converted to glucose. Lactates are produced in any state of hypoperfusion under reduced perfusion pressure and hypoxemia of tissues. Adequate levels of plasma insulin and correction of hypoperfusion under reduced perfusion pressure thus facilitate the conversion of lactates to pyruvates and its entry into Kreb's cycle for full aerobic consumption to produce 38 molecules of the energy storage molecules of ATP. Amino acids come from diet or from muscle breakdown as in insulin-deficient states. The amino acid lost maximally from the muscle is alanine which by a single step can be converted into pyruvates which is a useful molecule for energy production. In all these states, the initial substantial loss of alanine later decreases. Glycerol comes from the hydrolysis of triglycerides where three free fatty acid molecules attached to glycerol. They are hydrolyzed, and free fatty acids and glycerol are liberated in the circulation. Ten percent of all gluconeogenic substances come from glycerol ([1], p. 132).

All gluconeogenesis processes are not indicative of catabolic state. They occur predominantly in normal physiological states it operates. For example, the muscle activity results in the production of lactate and pyruvates since muscle metabolize glucose only in the anaerobic way. These products are carried to the liver to be converted in glucose and recirculated for the muscles and other tissues like kidneys to be taken up. In low insulin states, the FFAs and glycerol are also released in the circulation. FFAs enter the aerobic glycolysis by complex enzymatic regulation in mitochondria and are oxidized. Glycerol goes in formation of new glucose. In addition to the glucose consumption, many tissues including muscles and heart use FFAs as their fuel.

10.7 Insulin and Protein Metabolism

Preservation of an organism, its cells and tissues is intimately connected with intracellular protein synthesis and ATP production for energy to achieve this. It is in this area insulin seems to achieve the singular distinction of being a purely anabolic hormone and regulator of cellular function. A considerable body of intensive research exists on the basis of the inferences drawn and the clinical experience of insulin usage. This information will be used to illustrate the role insulin plays here.

Protein metabolism broadly will fall into two categories. One is synthesis, and the other is breakdown of the proteins as per the functional requirements of cells. Excessive breakdown of proteins in any hyper-catabolic state has grave significances. Impaired protein synthesis is a grave danger to cell preservation. The balance between the two determines the total body protein and of the individual tissues, as well as the concentration of the specific proteins. Protein turnover is important to increase and maintain the cell size but is also important for tissue repair, adaptation, and remodeling ([1], p. 275–6). Specific proteins are synthesized and catabolized for specific functional demand by the cells. Proteins serve the functions of differentiation, cell growth, gene repair, and energy production. There is an intrinsic balance between the production and catabolic destruction between different proteins in the normal state. Any minor disturbance in this balance can lead to severe dysfunction within the cells.

Logically one may surmise that disturbances in the content, function, and integrity of these proteins could be the cause of chronic diabetes complications. Studying this regulation with respect to insulin is complicated by many other hormones contributing to these processes. The other confounding factors are the age, old age in particular, activity levels, diet issues, pregnancy, and other illnesses. With advances in molecular biology, tracer technology has helped in this search. Human genome project has identified new genes, and the knowledge has advanced ([1], p. 277).

10.7.1 Protein Synthesis and Insulin in Normal Physiology

Summarizing the various research findings, it could be safely stated that insulin adequacy or hyperinsulinemia needs to be supplemented by liberal, i.e., more than physiologic availability of the amino acids for protein synthesis. Experimentally the evidence for protein synthesis is less concurrent in humans. It has however come to be known that different protein structures in the cells like mitochondria, nuclei, ribosomal proteins, contractile structures like myosin heavy chains, and stability of the actin filaments, which constitute the cytoskeleton, respond to insulin to be preserved. Integrity of the nerve fibers is to an extent dependent on insulin adequacy and effects. (For more details about the effects on nerves, see the monograph of the first author Diabetic Neuropathy in Clinical Practice.) It is likely that development of diabetes may chronically cause alterations to these responses.

One significant finding is that of the insulin response elements within the DNA, that too in the gene promoter regions. Transmission of the insulin signal would upregulate the formation of different proteins, preexisting enzymes, or other processes. In summary the net results are that insulin increases the mRNA production for several genes and growth factors and it stabilizes the mRNA and initiates and maintains the mRNA transcription. This is an important reaction in protein formation. Elongation of mRNA, needed for protein synthesis, is distal to the initiator tRNA sequence in the process, but insulin seems to have considerable effect at these later stages also. Insulin selectively upregulates the translation of mRNA. This facilitation is recycling based and the mRNA contents do not have to change.

After a detailed appraisal of animal models, it is fair to assume that insulin also influences the formation of ribosome proteins and upregulates the rRNA (ribosomal RNA) synthesis. It appears to be quite possible that the intracellular insulin after its dissociation from the receptor influences the insulin response elements in nuclear DNA either directly or through the second messenger system or by phosphorylation of its substrates. There are many short sequence DNA insulin response elements (IREs) which code for different proteins, hormones, etc. These actions are massively important for cell preservation and functions ([1], p. 275–89). It also stimulates growth-related proteins. Insulin also helps in the uptake of branched-chain amino acids in muscles which the liver is unable to metabolize which offer an additional source of fuel to muscles in acute catabolic states as well as in normal conditions.

In insulin-deficient state, there is formation of vacuoles in the cytoplasm in which the lysosomes, polysomes, and endoplasmic reticular structures are found in which changes are reversed (unless autophagy supervenes) by insulin sufficiency. Insulin influences the collagen formation, thereby helping tissue repair. The effects can be summarized in a table given below.

10.7.2 Protein Breakdown in Standardized and Catabolic Conditions

280 g of protein is synthesized and broken down in the body under standard conditions much of it inside the cells. Among the numerous intracellular proteins there in cells, both these rates are continuous but vastly different. For example, basic proteins have a different pathway for protein breakdown and can be prevented by insulin sufficiency. Many others have a lysosomal pathway. In normal conditions these rates are tightly regulated maintaining the homeostasis. Disruptions in these rates will affect the cellular as well as organism's functions and its regulation greatly, in both normal and catabolic states. The proteins fall into acidic, basic, and neutral proteins. Then there are long-life proteins, enzymatic proteins, and structural proteins. The acidic, basic, and neutral proteins in insulin-insufficient cells are degraded uniformly in time. This is detrimental to the availability of these proteins for cell functions, but there is another aspect to it. Synthesis of these proteins at rates required for the cell functioning has a balance with degradation. Protein destruction becomes uniform but the rate of synthesis of the same proteins being different the required rate corresponding to destruction is not achieved. Then there will be a mismatch of function to be carried out due to inadequacy of some proteins at that point of time. It is easy to see how it will affect the coordinated cell functions.

Box 10.3 Intracellular Actions of Insulin

- Insulin stimulates transcription of ribosomal RNA
- Stimulates or inhibits transcription of specific mRNAs
- Preferentially recruits ribosomes in polysomes
- Increases ternary complex formation and peptide chain initiation
- Stimulates preferentially, translation of specific mRNA
- Increases the stability of specific mRNAs
- Inhibits protein degradation and regularizes normal degradative process
- Inhibits ribosomal degradation
- Inhibits lysosomal degradation of macromolecules

As noted elsewhere the enzymatic turnover of proteins that is both breakdown and synthesis is rapid. Long-life proteins take more time to be formed. Fibrinogen is synthesized faster than albumin. This is clinically important. Since the rate of albumin synthesis is slower, the deprivation of amino acids in the catabolic process for long will lead to hypoalbuminemia and profound circulatory abnormalities and is a marker for death. Amino acids with severe insulin deprivation, glucagon, and beta agonists increase the lysosomal breakdown of longer-living proteins which are 90% of all the hepatic protein and 10–20% of all muscle protein breakdown. Insulin adequacy is a key factor in interorgan transfer of amino acids to maintain the milieu.

In general terms breakdown of proteins is essential process to eliminate potentially lethal accumulation of abnormal, damaged, or foreign proteins. Formation of normal proteins will on the other hand help in cell repair, tissue remodeling, and facilitating numerous metabolic pathways.

There cannot be a more striking example of insulin anabolism of muscle tissue than the newly diagnosed type 1 diabetes patients put on insulin. The wasting of muscles is stopped, the muscle mass increases rapidly in weeks to months. Given that, between the insulin-induced protein synthesis and insulin prevention of protein breakdown, the latter seems to be the more important effect of insulin. The observation of hypertrophy of the kidneys in type 1 diabetes could be due to either heightened protein synthesis or greater inhibition of protein breakdown or both. The evidence is contradictory on this, but hypertrophy is a consistent finding in this situation.

In type 2 diabetes once insulin sufficiency is restored, the prevention of protein breakdown may be the predominant mechanism. Even in hypoinsulinemic states in type 2 diabetes, muscle breakdown is not that prominent a feature ([1], p. 275–89).

10.8 Nonmetabolic Actions of Insulin

Insulin has widely spread receptor population on a variety of different tissues/cells which on signaling address different nonmetabolic functions. Few of these are described below:

1. On ovarian granulose cells, signaling is coupled with estrogen/progesterone balance. Insulin administration alters gonadal steroid metabolism. This alteration is independent of changes in gonadotropin secretion in insulin-resistant women with the polycystic ovarian syndrome.
2. Insulin has an intrinsic property for vasodilation. Insulin also mediates skeletal muscle vasodilation. This contributes both to insulin sensitivity and responsiveness in lean humans [7].
3. Insulin, especially when administered at higher doses, exerts a variety of nonmetabolic effects; it has a vasodilatory [8], anti-inflammatory, and antioxidative effect. It also has antiaggregatory effects on platelets in particular. It affects coagulopathies through its actions of fibrinolytic and thrombolytic effects.
4. Endothelial cell has insulin receptor which helps transcytosis of the insulin molecule from the intravascular space to the interstitial space from where it can reach its target tissues for further action [9].
5. Intensive insulin therapy for critically ill patients protects the endothelium [10]. There are positive inotropic and cardioprotective effects of insulin.
6. These are of particular benefits for patients who have cardiovascular disease [11–16].

10.8.1 Human Growth and Insulin

Insulin signals through phosphoinositol 3-kinase and Ras MAP kinase with normal IGF 1 activity cause cell growth (mitogenic) and differentiation ([1], p. 148–9). In

Table 10.1 Insulin actions of gene products

Glycolytic enzymes	– Glucokinase, pyruvate kinase	Stimulated
Lipogenic enzymes	– Fatty acid synthetase	Stimulated
Formation of glucose transporters (muscle)	– GLUT 4	Stimulated
Gluconeogenic gene	– PEPCK	Inhibited
Secretory proteins	– Albumin, amylase, GH	
	Alpha 2 microglobulin	Helped
Reproductive proteins	– Ovalbumin, casein formation	Helped
Lens protein	– Delta crystalline formation	Helped
Axons and dendrites	– Tubulin	Stabilized

mutated insulin receptor individuals, there is insulin resistance which may lead to additional diabetes mellitus in such individuals along with growth retardation. Individuals with hypoinsulinemia due to any cause like pancreatic agenesis or glucokinase defect lead to severe growth retardation indicating that insulin has a major role in the normal growth of the human fetuses ([1], p. 174). Insulin also acts on the cytoskeletal actin and polymerizes it to facilitate GLUT 4 membrane translocation ([1], p. 174). Insulin and IGF 1 has neurotrophic effects on sensory, motor, and sympathetic neurons. Insulin and IGF 1 deficiency causes apoptosis of neural tissue; Schwann cells undergo apoptosis which can be reversed by IGF 1 through activation of PI 3 kinase. Insulin deficiency causes inhibition of neuritic growth and leads to apoptosis of autonomic neurons ([1], p. 174).

10.8.2 Other Gene Products and Insulin

Some genes, of which the products are listed below, are more sensitive to insulin and respond in a disproportionate way. Many of them have important implications in the anabolic or anti-catabolic way of insulin action (Table 10.1).

10.9 Beta Cell Defects in Type 2 Diabetes Leading to Insulin Secretion Impairment

The foremost is the loss of first-phase insulin release. It starts within a few minutes after food is ingested, reaches a high peak, and tapers initially sharply and then more slowly. This is under the enteroinsular axis and rise in systemic glucose. In type 2 diabetes, this phase is lost with profound effects on glycogen synthesis and adequacy of systemic glucose as well as insulin levels. This phase does not occur in intravenous administration of glucose since there is no gastric stimulation after meal ([1], p. 150–1).

In prandial states there is a second phase of peak insulin release a couple of hours after the food is ingested. It has the same shape as the first phase but the height of the peak is less. In type 2 diabetes, this phasic release of insulin is delayed further and is decreased in the quantum of insulin release. There is a marked flattening of the glucose-induced insulin release [17]. This secretory defect of beta cells persists even after control of diabetes.

Insulin secretion occurs in an oscillatory manner in small bursts every 8–16 min and is quite regular in nondiabetic state. The normal maintenance of glucose and FFAs levels may correspond to these oscillations which are lost. The oscillations become shorter in peak and are irregular ([1], p. 257). These defects are apparent even in IGT states ([1], p. 265–7). The unrestrained hepatic glucose output added by the increased gluconeogenic process thus is an important pathophysiological feature in type 2 diabetes ([1], p. 265–7).

References

1. Joslin EP. Joslin's textbook of diabetes mellitus. 14th ed. Lippincott, Williams and Wilkins, USA 2005, Indian Edition
2. UKPDS. The Lancet. 2000.
3. Pickup, Williams. Textbook of diabetes. Oxford: Blackwell Publication; 1992.
4. Zoungas S, Patel A, Chalmers J, et al. Severe hypoglycemia and risks of vascular events and death. N Engl J Med. 2010;363:1410–8. https://doi.org/10.1056/NEJMoa1003795.
5. Hsu P-F, Sung S-H, Cheng H-M, et al. Association of clinical symptomatic hypoglycemia with cardiovascular events and total mortality in type 2 diabetes: a nationwide population based study. Diabetes Care. 2013;36:894–900. https://doi.org/10.2337/dc12-0916.
6. Gitt AK, Bramlage P, Binz C, et al. Hypoglycaemia is more frequent in type 2 diabetic patients with co-morbid vascular disease: an analysis of the DiaRegis registry. Eur J Prev Cardiol. 2012;19:765–72. https://doi.org/10.1177/1741826711411104.
7. Dunaif A, Graf M. Insulin administration alters gonadal steroid metabolism independent of changes in gonadotropin secretion in insulin-resistant women with the polycystic ovary syndrome. J Clin Investig. 1989;83(1):23–9. https://doi.org/10.1172/JCI113864.
8. Baron AD, Steinberg HO, Chaker H, Leaming R, Johnson A, Brechtel G. Insulin-mediated skeletal muscle vasodilation contributes to both insulin sensitivity and responsiveness in lean humans. J Clin Invest. 1995;96:786–92. https://doi.org/10.1172/JCI118124.
9. King GL, Johnson SM. Receptor-mediated transport of insulin across endothelial cells. Science. 1985;227:1583–6.
10. Langouche L, Vanhorebeek I, Vlasselaers D, et al. Intensive insulin therapy protects the endothelium of critically ill patients. J Clin Invest. 2005;115:2277–86.
11. Groeneveld ABJ, Beishuizen A, Visser FC. Insulin: a wonder drug in the critically ill? Crit Care. 2002;6:102–5.
12. McNulty PH, Pfau S, Deckelbaum LI. Effect of plasma insulin level on myocardial blood flow and its mechanism of action. Am J Cardiol. 2000;85:161–5.
13. Dandona P, Aljada A, Mohanty P, et al. Insulin inhibits intranuclear nuclear factor kappaB and stimulates IkappaB in mononuclear cells in obese subjects: evidence for an anti-inflammatory effect. J Clin Endocrinol Metab. 2001;86:3257–65.
14. Ferrannini E, Galvan AQ, Gastaldelli S, et al. Insulin: new roles for an ancient hormone. Eur J Clin Investig. 1999;29:842–52.
15. Das UN. Is insulin an endogenous cardioprotector? Crit Care. 2002;6:389–93.
16. Parsonage WA, Hetmanski D, Cowley AJ. Beneficial haemodynamic effects of insulin in chronic heart failure. Heart. 2001;85:508–13.
17. Levy J, Malaisse WJ. The stimulus-secretion coupling of glucose induced insulin release. XVII. Effects of sulfonylurea and diazoxide on insular biosynthetic activity. Biochem Pharmacol. 1975;24:235–9.

Insulin Pharmacodynamics, Pharmacokinetics, and Insulin Regimens

11

Contents

11.1 Introduction

Pharmacodynamics is the action the drug has on the body. The main elements connected with it are the plasma concentration, protein binding, and the receptor affinity. Half-life in plasma is the duration in which the drug level falls to 50%.

S. Kelkar et al., *Towards Optimal Management of Diabetes in Surgery*,
https://doi.org/10.1007/978-981-13-7705-1_11

Pharmacokinetics is how the drug travels in the body over time and their variations in concentration across time in blood. So far we have dealt with considerable details both these aspects of insulin in the body tissues and cells. Here these functions will be more fully understood against the backdrop of pharmacotherapy of insulin and its pharmacokinetics from a different perspective in all kinds of situations in diabetes.

This chapter however will have to be substantially dissociated from the postoperative management of patients since usage of insulin in all kinds of situations, mainly in type 2 diabetes, has a wider applicability. This discussion will help in treatment of patients who have recovered from the acute or routine surgical/medical situations, are stable, and are in continuing need of insulin at the time of discharge. In the chapter on Commonly Asked Questions, many more insulin-related aspects have been covered.

The detailed description below is based on the PKPD properties of the regular as well as the short-acting insulins, intermediate insulin of both human and analogue type, as well as the long-acting varieties. The discussion will also cover the pluses and minuses of all insulin varieties and the limits as well as comparability of actions and side effects between these types of insulin. Then it will be easier to understand the varied insulin regimens.

While the gross distinction of regular, short-acting and longer- or intermediate-acting insulin is well known to medical fraternity, a few more details could be helpful, especially for surgical fraternity, residents, nurses, and anesthetists. This is more relevant today because newer, finer, and more elegant varieties of insulin within these two categories are available. They work more predictably, almost with mathematical quantification. The understanding of insulin pharmacokinetics vis-à-vis the rate of calorie infusion, calorie consumption, and insulin effects has been detailed in the various chapters.

11.2 Types of Insulin Available Today

India adapted the human insulin over a decade beginning from the mid-1980s to early 1990s. First the modified pig insulin enzymatically converted to human insulin with all the properties of it as a highly purified and monocomponent insulin was prepared. Soon the recombinant human insulin was manufactured by using the yeast *Saccharomyces cerevisiae* or by the *E. coli* route by genetic manipulation of insulin gene. This has made insulin of the highest purity and effectivity available all over the world in any quantities for over 25 years now.

Two types of crystalline insulin have existed. Regular one is from the pig or beef or the human variety; the second the modified loosely crystalline short acting analogues of human insulins. In the discussion below, human crystalline insulin variety will be represented by the word regular variety. The other varieties are the regular human insulin mixed with protamine giving NPH insulin or with zinc giving the lente insulin, by converting regular human insulin to intermediate-acting one. Both NPH and lente insulin have duration of action lasting for about 16–22 h which is much longer than the rapid-acting insulin which has 6–8 h of action. The third variety in human insulin is that of premixed insulin where NPH and regular human insulin are mixed in certain proportions.

Similarly, there are three varieties of insulin analogues—fast- or short-acting insulins—lispro, aspart, and glulisine. Lispro and aspart are also available as the intermediate-acting variety, premixed with the fast- or short-acting variety.

11.2.1 The Regular Human Insulin: Structure and Changes After Subcutaneous Injection

The manufactured rapid-acting insulin exists as a hexamer, i.e., it has six insulin molecules crystallized with a zinc molecule. It is water soluble. Injected in the subcutaneous fat, it undergoes dissociation which results in the formation of three dimers, i.e., two insulin molecule structures which later are converted in the tissues into a monomer and a single insulin molecule. The monomer is then absorbed in the bloodstream. This process takes some time; hence this insulin starts acting in 30 min. Rapid-acting insulin peaks in concentration at about 2 h, which starts declining in 4 h the effective activity lasts for 6 hours from time of injection [1]. At least one third of the insulin is locally degraded and is not available for action. This insulin is therefore well suited to control the prandial excursions of glucose.

The important clinical implication and limitation of this pharmacokinetics are that the administration of rapid-acting insulin over the longest fasting period overnight will not act beyond 3 PM since the plasma levels decline and little or no trace of it will be found in blood in the morning. This leaves a minimum of 5 h gap before breakfast time and the next regular human insulin administration with low levels of insulin in the plasma. That will lead to increased fasting glucose levels through increased hepatic out of glucose at 10 g/h compared to 1 g/h in people without diabetes. The intermediate- and long-acting insulin varieties are useful to control this situation. The different ways to combine these two will be discussed below. The fasting being high, the subsequent control of the post-breakfast and other prandial blood glucose levels will be more difficult to control. The clinical reality of usage of regular human insulin is different. Three times use of rapid-acting insulin without the backing of intermediate- or long-acting variety is not at all uncommon even today. These patients will hardly ever come under control, the insulin doses will continue to increase, and the weight gain will continue.

When a patient has stable circulation, the 6–8 h of action of regular human insulin remains uniform for that duration. Fever, tachycardia, flushing, and thyrotoxicosis, i.e., all causes of hyperdynamic circulation, may have opposite effect; insulin absorption may be faster (see below also). In hypotension, cutaneous vasoconstriction or shock subcutaneous insulin route should not be resorted to since insulin absorption will be delayed and erratic and may fail to produce appropriate concentration at the right time which makes it unreliable in these situations.

The second implication of this delayed time to start its action results in the advice of injecting the short-acting insulin at least 30 min before the meal time. This is inconvenient and worrisome for the patient if he cannot adhere to it. If she manages to do that, the next 30 min of waiting before breakfast can begin will be spent under the apprehension as to when hypoglycemia will supervene. Fast-acting analogues seem to be a good alternative for this, discussed below. In addition the insulin action is highly variable in the same patient as well as in different patients injected with same dose of insulin under similar conditions. The intraindividual variation for regular human insulin is up to 25%. The same is found to be about 50% for longer-acting insulin [1].

The rapid or the short-acting insulins are also given by the intravenous route. We have discussed the numerous details connected with it in the chapters gone by. The intermediate-/long-acting insulins are used *only by subcutaneous route* and never by intravenous route. Intravenous insulin has a short half-life in blood. When insulin infusion is discontinued, no detectable insulin will remain in blood in about 60 min. The half-life of insulin is about 7 min by this route. The liver and kidneys will degrade insulin presented to them.

11.2.2 Intermediate-Acting Insulin: Structure, Tissue Changes, and the Pharmacokinetics

In isophane or neutral protamine hagedorn (NPH) insulin, there is no excess of protamine. This is called stoichiometric proportions for mixing. The highly basic protein protamine forms poorly soluble crystals delaying the absorption once injected [1]. This aspect is also found to be useful in mixing the regular human insulin with it without the possibility of conversion of the latter to the intermediate variety. This excess conversion takes place when rapid-acting insulin is mixed with lente insulin preparation. The NPH has a delayed peak and long duration of action of this insulin. It peaks at 5–7 h after injection and has duration of action from 12 to 15 h. It is therefore usually administered twice daily to provide a 24-h uniform basal insulin supply once with evening meal and once with breakfast. There is a contrast between the mealtime in India and in Western European countries. In India it is much later in the evening. Injection of NPH at the time of an especially early evening meal may result in much lower level of insulin before breakfast of the next day. This can lead to higher fasting levels. Therefore it is easier and convenient to administer NPH at bedtime in Western societies. Since the evening meal in India is delayed, there is no particular advantage in taking regular human insulin with dinner and NPH at bedtime as practiced in the west. The duel injection therapy thus becomes cumbersome. Pharmacokinetically speaking, it may be contended that it does not have any advantage, although this has not been studied.

The other intermediate-acting lente insulin has excess of zinc in acetate buffer mixed with the regular human insulin resulting in insoluble insulin-zinc complex lengthening the period of action. Hence its degradation to insulin monomers takes longer time. On an average, the action starts by 2 h, reaches its peak between 4 and 7 h, and continues to act at that level till about 14–16 h from the time of injection. The extent of delayed action will depend on the size and type of insulin crystal. Semilente insulin preparation is the amorphous form. Ultralente insulin preparation has larger crystals hence longer duration of action. A 30% of semilente and 70% ultralente are mixed to prepare the lente formulation. Human ultralente and lente have a similar duration of action to that of isophane insulin. There is a disadvantage of mixing lente with regular human insulin in the same syringe. There is excess of zinc ions in lente which will convert some of the regular human insulin to long-acting insulin. This does not happen in premixing with NPH [1]. The case with premixed insulins is a little different which will be discussed separately in Sect. 11.3.1.

11.3 Pharmacodynamics of Different Insulins and Combinations of Insulin

The intermediate-acting insulin provides *continuous and uniform basal levels* of insulin for 24 h to maintain the basal glucose disposal, round the clock. Since the concentrations start declining by 12–16 h, it has to be administered twice a day—usually with breakfast and bedtime or dinner as discussed above. The intermediate-acting insulins thus will provide effective basal levels throughout the night and day. However, NPH cannot always control the postprandial glucose elevations which make it essential to combine it with rapid- or short-acting insulin with each meal which can achieve this.[1]

Insulin glargine covers 24 h with a constant basal level. To cover the prandial glucose rise, it has to be combined with three mealtime injections of either the rapid-acting or short-acting insulin. Glargine cannot be mixed with either of them and hence has to be given as the fourth injection. It is generally administered at bedtime. It however eliminates the need for two injections of NPH. But it does not reduce the number of injections. NPH use has been associated with somewhat more frequent and somewhat unpredictable hypoglycemic episodes. The advent of long-acting insulin glargine and much later insulin detemir discussed below emerged as having superior advantage in this respect.

A combination of regular NPH and regular rapid-acting insulin or analogue of NPH and analogue short-acting insulin can be used. Both these varieties of NPH insulin can be mixed in a single syringe with rapid-/short-acting insulin (see below). This cannot be done with glargine as shown above. It is also available as a fixed dose of NPH and rapid-acting premixed variety. Two concentrations which are maximally used are 30:70 and 50:50 where the first number indicates the concentration of the rapid acting and the second number depicts the concentration of intermediate variety. The analogue premixed insulin is routinely used in a concentration of 30:70 as above. In these varieties, the individual concentrations and the pharmacodynamic properties do not change since there is no excess protamine. In other words, the time-action profiles of premixed insulins are as if both the components have been injected separately. The aim of such mixtures is to provide a time-action profile that is characterized by a rapid onset of action to cover the prandial insulin requirements,

[1] In attempts to minimize the fears associated with insulin administration for the first time, a regime called BIDS is sometimes used. It spells out as bedtime (intermediate) insulin daytime sulfonylurea. Single NPH rarely is effective and lasts for a short time if at all. It is better to start with two injections of intermediate-acting variety 12 h apart if insulin regime becomes necessary. Such regimes of insulin combined with OHAs are not discussed here.

followed by a second phase with a longer ongoing action to cover the basal insulin requirements called the "biphasic" profiles.

11.3.1 Premixed Insulin Regimen

Several premixed insulin preparations are commercially available with a variety of fixed ratios of regular and analogue insulin and regular or analogue NPH insulin from 10/90 to 50/50, 25% lispro with 75% isophane (Humalog Mix 25), or 50% lispro with 50% isophane (Humalog Mix 50), or 30% aspart with 70% isophane like analogue (Novomix 30/70). Here the first number always depicts the rapid-acting component and the second the intermediate variety [1].

Most frequently the premixed insulin of a chosen concentration is given before breakfast and before dinner. The rapid-acting variety controls the prandial glucose excursions at breakfast and after dinner. The basal levels of insulin are maintained by NPH through 24 h. There is a small interval of overlap between them each time it gets injected. This will in most situations control the fasting and post-dinner glucose as well but may not at times control the post-lunch glucose rise. If the regular premixed insulin is changed to analogue NPH premixed insulin, the doses in terms of units are just the same, that is, unit-to-unit exchange in a switch from one to other [1].

1. Lunch in India can be the bigger meal. In this simple regime, it may not be always possible to control post-lunch blood glucose since there is no rapid-acting insulin at lunch. There are two alternatives to control the situation.
   (a) A small dose of 6–10 U of rapid-acting insulin injection before lunch can be given. If regular-/rapid-acting insulin is used, it may be given 30 min prior to time for lunch. If short-acting insulin is used, it has to be given just before the lunch starts. The disadvantage of this regimen is that it requires the use of two different varieties of insulin with different properties. It could also give rise to confusion about which one to use and they may get switched.
   (b) Instead of using two varieties, the premixed insulin can also be used before lunch. The dose could be determined by the pre- or post-lunch glucose level. The disadvantage of using two different insulins will be eliminated. Using three premixed doses has been suggested for a long time, but there are no trials to show that this is as safe or more effective. This commonsense approach suggests that such administration will at most increase the basal insulin which may not be particularly risky, but the post-lunch will be controlled. In practice it usually works well under good monitoring and dose adjustments.
2. A situation may develop where both fasting and the post-lunch glucose are higher than acceptable. Such a situation points to the possibility that both the premixed doses are likely to be lower than needed. There are many ways of controlling the situation.
   (a) The golden rule is to Fix the Fasting First by increasing substantially the night dose first, achieve normal fasting levels, and wait for the post-lunch to decline on its own.

(b) If that does not happen in full measure and the post-lunch continues to be high, the morning premixed dose can then be increased. Many professionals believe that 50:50 combinations for this purpose are better which makes sense. Logically 50:50 have a greater component of short-acting insulin to control prandial excursions. The evidence in trials at least, conducted many years ago, did not show much difference, but the trials could be biased towards 30:70 being the most used hence the best brand.

These two strengths are also available as a ready-made prefilled NovoPen 3 which gives higher convenience and accuracy of dosage compared to syringes for many reasons. If a patient is already on these pen injections prior to surgery, the same can be used postoperatively in situations above. However, if the patient is not on these pens and if the patient is expected to return to oral hypoglycemic drugs after a few weeks, this costly device need not be imposed on them.

(c) The clue to the quantities of night insulin to be increased to control fasting lies in doing pre-dinner or post-dinner blood glucose. The wide use of self-monitoring of blood glucose makes it easy for the patient to test these glucose levels. The need to run to the laboratories at odd hours is eliminated. If this level is also high, the doses can be raised with more confidence. The night insulin of intermediate variety is considered with reservation by many practitioners for fear of hypoglycemia. It is necessary to remember that given in appropriate doses, it can balance the excess hepatic glucose output in the postabsorptive phase of food cycle, which starts 5 h after the ingestion of food as discussed earlier. However it must be said that longer-acting insulins now available are a better replacement for intermediate-acting ones.

(d) There is a distinct possibility of hypoglycemic episodes developing in these attempts. They can be attributed to either excessive dose administration due to inexperience or the drug-diet activity mismatch leading to the derailment of the entire process of glucose control, causing fear in the patient. In such situations, it may be better to refer such brittle diabetes to an expert and get the doses stabilized. Clearly the experience to manage this situation is vital here.

3. In case of brittle diabetes especially in wards, this insulin regimen should be shifted first to what is called the basal-bolus regimen. In fact this could be the best regime as the patient starts shifting towards normal food intake as he recovers from his illness. When the patient waits for discharge, the basal-bolus could be shifted to one of the premixed twice daily insulin regimens.

11.3.2 The Basal-Bolus Insulin Regime

The basal-bolus regimen or the multiple subcutaneous insulin injections (MSII) are given as three regular-/short-acting insulins at three major meals and a corresponding NPH at bedtime. In postoperative situation when the patient is in the wards, this regime is particularly useful for the following reasons. Firstly, it is easier to monitor the blood glucose at specified intervals even with minimum monitoring. Secondly, all four insulin injections are administered by the staff, and the patient does not have to worry about it. Thirdly, it is easier to discharge the patient by converting the MSII doses to two premixed insulin doses.

It can be initiated by giving regular human insulin three times with intermediate-acting insulin at night or three short-acting analogue insulin injections with meals with long-acting analogues like glargine.

Intermediate-acting human insulin used at bedtime is much less expensive than long-acting analogues. Regular human insulin however is more prone to irregular hypoglycemic episodes or is less effective in controlling postprandial excursions without some hypoglycemia since it stacks up in the plasma. Short-acting analogue insulins do not stack up in plasma. Cost however will be the major constraint in most situations if analogue insulins are used.

11.3.3 More Complex Regimen: Split Mix and CSII

The two regimens given below are somewhat complex and need experience and hence may be sparingly used. In the split mix variety, the ratio of the intermediate-acting NPH to the rapid-acting insulin can be changed as per the glucose values. Here we are not confined by the fixed ratios of the premixed varieties. In this regime the injections are drawn from these two separate vials in a single syringe on the basis of units decided and given twice daily in the morning and night with usual monitoring practice.

CSII or continuous subcutaneous insulin infusion and mechanisms around it have many levels of complexities. It is probably of best use in extremely brittle diabetes. It involves more than multiple glucose monitoring, by self or by sophisticated devises implanted in the abdomen. The insulin quanta and the rate are either programmed in algorithmical manner or by self-adjustment. It probably has no place in the daily surgical arena. The disadvantages CSII has are high complexity of management, high need for backup services, burdensome patient education, and high costs. It also can suffer from pump failures leading to hyperglycemia, run away pump discharge leading to hypoglycemia, or wide swings. It is mentioned here for completing the subject at hand.

11.4 Molecular Structure, Pharmacokinetics, and Pharmacodynamics of Analogue Insulins

The pharmacokinetics and pharmacodynamics of rapid-acting insulin analogues and their clinical consequences have been reviewed in detail from which the important observations are derived [2]. In the later discussions, more specific references have also been quoted. We are deeply indebted and grateful for this review to Dr. PD Home.

Lispro, aspart, and glulisine are the short-acting insulins in vogue. Intramolecular comparison between these three analogue molecules suggests that they are equally efficacious and safe [2]. All types of insulins have to dissociate from hexamer to monomers before being absorbed in blood. The speed of action and the duration both depend upon the molecular structure. As the name suggests, the short-acting insulins act in less than 30 min or even earlier after subcutaneous injection. These insulins exist in a destabilized hexameric form. That is the reason for their quicker conversion to dimeric and monomeric forms as compared to regular human insulin. The latter is a stable hexamer and hence takes more time to dissociate in a monomer.

These changes come from the modification of the protein structure of human insulin. It is achieved by either substituting or exchanging two terminal amino acids. These are located at the end of peptide chain B of the human insulin molecule in lispro and glulisine. Only one amino acid change leads to the formation of aspart. Since all these substitutions are carried outside the receptor combining insulin surface/site, these remain identical to human insulin with respect to receptor binding, receptor affinity, and actions and are safe [1].

In lispro and aspart, a zinc molecule is present, whereas in glulisine it is a substance called polysorbate 20. It ensures the stability of glulisine while in vial formulation in the absence of zinc found in the other two. The pharmacologic action of all three starts within minutes, peaks in 30 min, and tapers off in 3–4 h. This profile, unlike that of rapid-acting insulin described above, reduces the possibility of delayed postprandial hypoglycemia considerably.

The issue is whether there are substantial reasons for using them in hospitalized patients to start with. The issue can be settled on the evidence shown under trials regarding the severity and frequency of hypoglycemia as well as glucose control by these molecules. The causes for hypoglycemia especially in the hospitalized patients who have been on human insulin administration are many. The patient may develop hypoglycemia if delivery of meal is considerably delayed, and/or the patient eats less than expected, an unpredictable element, or other medical conditions, including liver and kidney disease. One frequent factor is the fasting that starts at unusual time for imaging procedures, disruptions due to shifting for various investigations. In addition there are several other mechanisms discussed in Chap. 6 as well as Chap. 5 of this volume that predispose to hypoglycemia in a hospitalized patient.

Use of short-acting insulin analogues reduces the frequency and risk of hypoglycemia in the outpatient setting. It may hence be a better choice than regular human insulin for the treatment of hyperglycemia in hospitalized patients who are not critically ill [3]. Meyer et al. also demonstrated that in hospitalized noncritical patients, glulisine gave a much better control. The frequency of hypoglycemia was a little higher within a short period of 4 days, but the level of it was not significantly low as compared to hypoglycemia occurring if regular human insulin is used [4].

Tested in people with type 1 diabetes, the peak plasma concentration of the short-acting analogue insulin roughly doubles that of human insulin. The time to reach maximum concentration is also lesser than half of human insulin. The time of fall to less than 20% concentrations is about 4 h. In these 4 h, the human insulin absorption continues for a couple of more hours and higher levels last longer. This is the reason for higher frequency of hypoglycemia with human insulin.

Short-acting analogue, glulisine, was administered at the same time immediately before meal with human insulin. It showed a much lower postprandial maximal glucose excursion, much less time to reach that level and smaller area under the curve for glucose excursion over 0–4 or 0–2 h. The possible reason for the quicker onset of action is the zinc-free formulation of insulin glulisine compared with insulin lispro and aspart. However, when human insulin is administered 30 min before a meal, these differences are partly obliterated and narrowed (see below).

11.5 Hypoglycemia and HbA1c Levels: Comparing Regular Human to Analogue Insulins

The frequency of major hypoglycemia requiring the assisting of some other person decreases with short-acting analogues. Major nocturnal hypoglycemia in particular is more dangerous. When compared with human insulin, short-acting analogues reduce it substantially. The time for which the short-acting analogues remain in the subcutaneous tissues as is expected is the reason for such decreases. HbA1c reduction was maximally seen when patients previously on all-human insulin regimen were switched to all-analogue regimen. After shifting, there was significant reduction in hypoglycemic episodes, 42.4–20.3 per patient year. The nocturnal hypoglycemic events were also reduced from 11.8 to 2.1 episodes per patient year. Both these observations were highly significant [2].

11.6 Studies of Analogues as Biphasic Insulin in Comparison with Human Biphasic Insulins

Biphasic analogue insulins result in a more physiological insulin profile when compared with human biphasic insulin as expected. The postprandial glucose excursions also were much reduced than biphasic human insulin. It also significantly lowers rates for nocturnal hypoglycemia and major hypoglycemic events.

Treatment satisfaction score is an important consideration. People were more comfortable with rapid-acting analogues than human insulin. One of the reasons for satisfaction could be due to the abolition of the waiting time of 30 min when human premixed insulins are to be used. The all-analogue premixed insulins are used immediately before food.

Insulin aspart also is as safe as regular human insulin given intravenously in patients who have undergone cardiac surgery [5]. If the transition to subcutaneous insulin is planned during the postoperative recovery phase, aspart could be a better choice. In India the liberal or ubiquitous use of insulin analogues has a limitation of cost.

11.6.1 Long-Acting Insulin Glargine

The pH of the subcutaneous tissues is 7.3. Glargine has an acidic pH of 5.5. Glargine therefore precipitates and forms a depot after the injection. It is then absorbed rather slowly which gives a relatively uniform concentration without peaks, over approximately 20–24 h after administration. It also follows the pattern of basal endogenous insulin secretion [6].

The uniform basal levels continue to dispose of glucose at a basal rate. It therefore needs a supplementation of some agent to cover and lower the prandial peaks. Glargine can thus be combined with OHAs as well. In this combination, the possibility of reaching the desired level of HbA1c level without hypoglycemia is quite good. This is in contrast to NPH combined with OADs where such a level may not be reached. Compared to the regime of premixed insulin use with OHAs, insulin glargine and OHA gave the same results without severe hypoglycemia. Insulin glargine and OHA use compared to insulin detemir with OHAs resulted in similar outcomes of better control and less frequent severe hypoglycemia. It also best serves for bolus insulins at prandial times. With respect to the fear of hypoglycemia, Glargine fairs better than some other regimens used [7].

The risk of severe hypoglycemia was lower in IGlar than in NPH, when the data was analyzed solely for the risk of hypoglycemia. IGlar compared to premixed insulins with this consideration did not show any differences. The case was similar when insulin detemir was used in place of glargine. Less number of patients discontinued the treatment in glargine compared to those who discontinued treatment in NPH arm. The number of premature withdrawals due to adverse events was significantly lower in insulin glargine with bolus insulin than insulin detemir with basal insulin added in addition to OAD therapy [5].

11.6.2 Insulin Detemir

As a new molecule claiming, the long-acting insulin status detemir had to first demonstrate the non-inferiority to NPH insulin and to demonstrate that outside the glucose control and HbA1c lowering, it had additional features that would prove its superiority over NPH. The following are the results of systematic reviews on this comparison.

Majority of RCTs which compared insulin detemir versus NPH in patients with type 1 diabetes indicate that both the regimens with respect to HbA1c lowering give a similar level of glycemic control. But the effect of insulin detemir in lowering fasting plasma glucose was greater than NPH [8–13]. A distinct feature of detemir is that it does not get stored in the subcutaneous tissues like NPH or glargine but is bound to albumin. That makes it virtually a depot carried by blood, and the release of detemir will be governed by the physicochemical concentration gradient. This is one of the reasons why one of the trials listed below has shown that it does not accumulate, produces less intra subject variability, and produces less frequent hypoglycemia including nocturnal due to its steady state compared to NPH. But with respect to glargine, this effect is the same for both the molecules.

There is a definite and large reduction in the risk of developing major hypoglycemia with insulin detemir versus NPH insulin. It was found to be 69% lower in a long duration trial of 24 months which enrolled 495 patients. Similarly the risk of nocturnal hypoglycemia was lower by 46% in that study with an additional substantial lowering of HbA1c with insulin detemir [14]. In couple of other trials, frequency of nocturnal hypoglycemia was consistently lower with insulin detemir—26% and 50% [15].

Frequency of hypoglycemic events with insulin detemir compared with NPH insulin was different in different trials involving type 2 diabetes. In one 26-week basal-bolus RCT, the rates of overall and nocturnal hypoglycemia were 38% in insulin detemir group against 47% in NPH group [16, 17]. Major hypoglycemia was not reported with the use of insulin detemir. The NPH group had three such episodes [17].

Detemir with OHAs combined compared with NPH with OHAs also found the detemir arm with significantly lower hypoglycemic events, including nocturnal hypoglycemia. If both insulin detemir and NPH insulin were given in the evening, the hypoglycemic episodes still were lower with detemir [18, 19]. In a basal-oral combination therapy with both these insulins, insulin detemir similarly showed lower event rate of overall and nocturnal hypoglycemia [19]. In addition, insulin detemir has consistently shown less weight gain compared to NPH insulin.

NPH insulin is unpredictable in its absorption and action. This extends to within-subject variability—a common issue with NPH [20–22]. Variability in absorption produces peaks and troughs of plasma insulin concentrations resulting in unpredictable hypoglycemia and unwanted hyperglycemia. Insulin detemir has a less variable time-action profile than NPH insulin. This avoids wide swings in plasma insulin levels and also lowers day-to-day (within-subject) variability [12, 14].

11.7 The Subcutaneous Route: Steps of Injection Method for All Types of Insulins in Vials

All the steps detailed below must be followed meticulously to ensure that dully mixed appropriate dose of insulin are delivered.

11.7.1 Insulin Syringes and Vials: Points to Be Noted

Insulin syringes and vials both come as 40 U of insulin per mL or 100 U/mL. In 10 mL vials, the total units of insulin would thus be 400 or 1000. The vial strength and the insulin injection capacity should be the same. Otherwise highly inappropriate doses will be delivered with disastrous consequences. The insulin needles come in numbers as high 31. They have a protective coating. Hence the needles should not be cleaned with spirit or any other material. These fine needles hardly cause any pain. Strictly speaking they should be used only once. In a resource-poor country and by clinical experience, it may be safely stated that they could be easily used many times over. They should be changed if the insertion is found difficult or painful. Safely they may be changed every 5–7 days depending upon the number of usage.

11.7.2 The Preparation for Injection: Method

1. The appropriate vial of insulin to be injected along with the appropriate corresponding syringe strength should be brought out to the room temperature at least half an hour before but not more.
2. At the time of injection, the vial must be tilted up and down 15–20 times, but not shaken vigorously as it creates fibrils of insulin. Alternatively it could be rolled between the palms.
3. The piston of the insulin syringe of corresponding strength should be withdrawn to the level of insulin units to be injected. These unit levels are marked on the insulin syringe.
4. The vial should then be held upright, and the air-filled insulin syringe needle should be inserted through the rubber, and the air is pushed in. The air may also get sucked on its own. The rubber top also need not be cleaned with spirit.
5. The insulin then should be drawn slowly holding the syringe at eye level to avoid inaccurate withdrawal. Slow withdrawal avoids air bubbles to come in the syringe.
6. The syringe should then be withdrawn without pressing the piston. If there are any air bubbles, they should be removed by gentle flicking of the syringe or by pushing the piston a little.

11.7.3 The Method of Injection

1. Any skin over the surfaces mentioned below which if ordinarily clean does not need to be sterilized by spirit.
2. The insulin syringe then must be held like a pen and brought to the surface of injection perpendicular to it.
3. A thick fold of the surface should be raised by using the other hand, and the needle is inserted perpendicular to the surface in a single swift manner.
4. Raising the fold and giving the injection perpendicularly ensures that the short needles go in to the subcutaneous fat to form a depot and not intramuscularly where the absorption is very fast.
5. Care should be taken *not to press the piston* before inserting the needle.
6. Once in situ the piston should be pressed slowly and fully till all the contents of the syringe are delivered.
7. The injection should be held in position for a count of five and should then be withdrawn quickly and unhesitatingly.
8. Any insulin vial and its syringe after its use should be returned to the door compartment of the refrigerator after capping.

The injectable surfaces are the infraumbilical portion of the abdomen and lateral and the anterior aspects of the thighs. Insulin as a rule should not be injected on the deltoid, but the posterior surface of the arms may be used. However it is cumbersome to use it since it requires someone else to properly inject hence must not be used.

Any person with diabetes will be involved in day-to-day activity or exercise. Insulin injected in the thighs is prone to get absorbed faster than the time of its desired stay, leading to a decrease in the steady levels, usually over 6 or 16 h, respectively, depending upon whether it is short-acting or intermediate-acting insulin. This may raise the level of blood glucose inappropriately.

The abdomen is a relatively undisturbed surface even during activity or exercise. Hence the insulin absorption would be uniform and will maintain the insulin levels to the desired length of time. This is likely to lead to more appropriate control. Injecting on the arms will also create the same situation as on the thighs and is even more undesirable for reasons stated above.

References

1. Insulin pharmacology Lutz Heinemann, 2002.
2. Home PD. The pharmacokinetics and pharmacodynamics of rapid-acting insulin analogues and their clinical consequences. Diabetes Obes Metab. 2012;14:780–8.
3. Dailey G, Rosenstock J, Moses RG, Ways K. Insulin glulisine provides improved glycemic control in patients with type 2 diabetes. Diabetes Care. 2004;27:2363–8.
4. Meyer C, Boron A, Plummer E, Voltchenok M, Vedda R. Glulisine versus human regular insulin in combination with glargine in noncritically ill hospitalized patients with type 2 diabetes: a randomized double-blind study. Diabetes Care. 2010;33:2496–501; http://care.diabetesjournals.org on 30 Aug 2010.
5. Chawla M, Malve H, Shah H, Shinde S, Bhoraskar A. Safety of intravenous insulin Aspart compared to regular human insulin in patients undergoing ICU monitoring post cardiac surgery: an Indian experience. J Diabetes Metab Disord. 2015;14:20.
6. Lepore M, Pampanelli S, Fanelli C, et al. Pharmacokinetics and pharmacodynamics of subcutaneous injection of long-acting human insulin analog glargine, NPH insulin, and ultralente human insulin and continuous subcutaneous infusion of insulin lispro. Diabetes. 2000;49:2142–8.
7. Rys P, Wojciechowski P, Rogoz-Sitek A, Niesyczyński G, Lis J, Syta A, Malecki MT. Systematic review and meta-analysis of randomized clinical trials comparing efficacy and safety outcomes of insulin glargine with NPH insulin, premixed insulin preparations or with insulin detemir in type 2 diabetes mellitus. Acta Diabetol. 2015;52(4):649–62, Published online: 14 Jan 2015.
8. Home P, Bartley P, Russell-Jones D, et al. Study to evaluate the administration of detemir insulin efficacy, safety and suitability (STEADINESS) study group. Insulin detemir offers improved glycemic control compared with NPH insulin in people with type 1 diabetes: a randomized clinical trial. Diabetes Care. 2004;27:1081–7.
9. Russell-Jones D, Simpson R, Hylleberg B, Draeger E, Bolinder J. Effects of QD insulin detemir or neutral protamine Hagedorn on blood glucose control in patients with type I diabetes mellitus using a basal-bolus regimen. Clin Ther. 2004;26:724–36.
10. Pieber TR, Draeger E, Kristensen A, Grill V. Comparison of three multiple injection regimens for type 1 diabetes: morning plus dinner or bedtime administration of insulin detemir vs. morning plus bedtime NPH insulin. Diabet Med. 2005;22:850–7.
11. Vague P, Selam JL, Skeie S, et al. Insulin detemir is associated with more predictable glycemic control and reduced risk of hypoglycemia than NPH insulin in patients with type 1 diabetes on a basal-bolus regimen with premeal insulin aspart. Diabetes Care. 2003;26:590–6.
12. De Leeuw I, Vague P, Selam JL, et al. Insulin detemir used in basal-bolus therapy in people with type 1 diabetes is associated with a lower risk of nocturnal hypoglycaemia and less weight gain over 12 months in comparison to NPH insulin. Diabetes Obes Metab. 2005;7:73–82.

13. Standl E, Lang H, Roberts A. The 12-month efficacy and safety of insulin detemir and NPH insulin in basal-bolus therapy for the treatment of type 1 diabetes. Diabetes Technol Ther. 2004;6:579–88.
14. Bott S, Tusek C, Jacobsen LV, et al. Insulin detemir under steady-state conditions: no accumulation and constant metabolic effect over time with twice daily administration in subjects with type 1 diabetes. Diabet Med. 2006;23:522–8.
15. Kølendorf K, Ross GP, Pavlic-Renar I, et al. Insulin detemir lowers the risk of hypoglycaemia and provides more consistent plasma glucose levels compared with NPH insulin in type 1 diabetes. Diabet Med. 2006;23:729–35.
16. Hermansen K, Fontaine P, Kukolja KK, Peterkova V, Leth G, Gall MA. Insulin analogues (insulin detemir and insulin aspart) versus traditional human insulins (NPH insulin and regular human insulin) in basal-bolus therapy for patients with type 1 diabetes. Diabetologia. 2004;47:622–9.
17. Fajardo Montañana C, Hernández Herrero C, Rivas Fernández M. Less weight gain and hypoglycaemia with once-daily insulin detemir than NPH insulin in intensification of insulin therapy in overweight type 2 diabetes patients: the PREDICTIVE BMI clinical trial. Diabet Med. 2008;25:916–23.
18. Hermansen K, Davies M, Derezinski T, Martinez Ravn G, Clauson P, Home P. A 26-week, randomized, parallel, treat-to-target trial comparing insulin detemir with NPH insulin as add-on therapy to oral glucose lowering drugs in insulin-naive people with type 2 diabetes. Diabetes Care. 2006;29:1269–74.
19. Philis-Tsimikas A, Charpentier G, Clauson P, Ravn GM, Roberts VL, Thorsteinsson B. Comparison of once-daily insulin detemir with NPH insulin added to a regimen of oral antidiabetic drugs in poorly controlled type 2 diabetes. Clin Ther. 2006;28:1569–81.
20. Scholtz HE, Pretorius SG, Wessels DH, Becker RH. Pharmacokinetic and glucodynamic variability: assessment of insulin glargine, NPH insulin and insulin ultralente in healthy volunteers using a euglycaemic clamp technique. Diabetologia. 2005;48:1988–95.
21. Heise T, Nosek L, Rønn BB, et al. Lower within-subject variability of insulin detemir in comparison to NPH insulin and insulin glargine in people with type 1 diabetes. Diabetes. 2004;53:1614–20.
22. Becker RH, Frick AD, Teichert L, et al. Fluctuation and reproducibility of exposure and effect of insulin glargine in healthy subjects. Diabetes Obes Metab. 2008;10:1105–13.

Metabolic Havoc of Uncontrolled Diabetes

12

Contents

12.1 The Altered Physiology of Tissues

The metabolic havoc arising out of altered physiology of tissues leads to a continuously existing diabetic state. Basic defects have already occurred, and whether the glucose control is excellent or poor, the balance of actions between

S. Kelkar et al., *Towards Optimal Management of Diabetes in Surgery*,
https://doi.org/10.1007/978-981-13-7705-1_12

various organs, hormones, and fuels is always precarious as it can destabilize at the slightest provocation. Over a period of years, diabetes does initially cause functional as well as structural alterations later in organs and tissues. Thus there are the cumulative effects of years of being in diabetic state. These changes reach a stage of such deterioration that managing life becomes difficult. It must also be understood that diabetic state begins years before the actual diagnosis of diabetes is or can be made. IGT is a precursor of diabetes and exemplifies the diabetic state in organs, tissues, hormones, and fuel statuses. It is also widely believed that diabetic state on an average starts about 5–7 years in type 2 diabetes before diagnosis.

As shown in earlier pages, before any of these four elements are affected, it is at the cellular level that the effects of insulinopenia and insulin resistance are most profound. Thus the consequent alterations change the cellular integrity and cause cell loss. To believe that the grosser-level parametric understanding of diabetes and basing solutions on that will anyhow mitigate the problem is not true. The myriad effects of diabetes where no cell, tissue, or organ is spared are of a much finer level as shown below. Alert continuous background awareness of it will go a long way in intelligently and not mechanically managing diabetes. This pathophysiological knowledge is also necessary since it helps in explaining various situations to the patients and relatives satisfactorily without resorting to facetious replies.

Needless to say it will thus lead to decision-making with application of a critical, clinical reasoning and not leaving that process to machines to give an answer. More often than not, after a few years of graduation, the physiology of the organ systems is forgotten. One may believe otherwise, but the knowledge of any specialty is formed on the understanding of physiology, anatomy, and biochemistry. In today's world, medicine has graduated from cytoplasm to nucleus, and molecular biology has come to fore. It has fundamentally affected the content of our understanding of tissues. A fair acquaintance to this new knowledge should be a legitimate expectation. *A sound understanding of physiology and biochemistry on the other hand is necessary for surgeons and anesthetists as well.* A lot of iatrogenic problems are on account of lack of good understanding of physiology, hence starting at the basic level only.

Diabetes can serve as the central paradigm for noncommunicable diseases. Truly, it can signify, amplify, and illuminate physiological and biochemical mechanisms. It affects, more than any other disease, the most central process of life, i.e., developing utilizable energy for the body. While dealing with this somewhat odd topic, we have to make certain basic premises clear. The affected person is able to live without any external help in his day-to-day functioning. She may or may not have an end-organ disease and may or may not have optimal body as well as laboratory parameters. She may be controlled or uncontrolled. The range of these alterations varies from mild to the most severe, viz., as in diabetic ketoacidosis and in hyperosmolar coma, even when it is not necessarily complicated by end-organ disease. We will discuss the alterations essentially in the steady state and not in the severely complicated forms mentioned just above.

12.2 The Bases of Diabetic State

The diabetic state on one hand is the result of, inadequate secretion or inadequate action of insulin, due to paucity or defects of beta cells or both and insulin resistance on the other. The resistance most notable in the liver, muscle, and adipose tissue is putative to the development of type 2 diabetic state and may increase further in an obese diabetic. Among other things the efficient regulation of a normal physiological process of glucose control, gluconeogenesis, and other fuels is disturbed. Glucagon is the main player in this process, and cortisol, epinephrine, norepinephrine, and growth hormone, its allies, who synergize in greater or lesser measure with it. This is a disequilibrating/equilibrating process as insulin is secreted during postprandial and switched off during fasting state. Despite this constant disequilibrium, the abundant resources and reservoirs in our body try to reequilibrate this state and contain as much as it can the likely strain on cells, tissues, or body functions. It is high time to realize that proper care of these resources and reservoirs must be taken by us clinicians, for our patients, especially with diabetes.

Box 12.1 Bases of Diabetic State 1
Inadequate plasma insulin
Insufficient secretion
Resistance to action
Failure of β-cell function
Decline in β-cell number
Insulin resistance in liver, muscle, and adipose tissue

Box 12.2 Bases of Diabetic State 2
Gluconeogenesis: ↑ fasting
Hepatic glucose output
Counter-regulatory hormones
Epinephrine, cortisol, glucagon Growth hormone and norepinephrine under positive and negative feedback

All in all, an unstable state of hyperglycemia remains that may roughly correspond to a diabetic state, but it certainly is not coextensive with it.

12.3 The Components of Diabetic State

The component physiology of tissues in diabetic state can be subdivided in many parts. The most basic level would be the biochemical abnormalities described in brief in the tables above. These changes result in alteration of blood composition which has its own transgressive effects on physiological checks and balances. This process once chronic enough affects vessels and capillaries, all of which are not only cells but basement membranes and in the vascular system, the endothelium, and the medial compartment with its thin layers of muscle cell. From there on, it will finally affect organs and make them functionally less efficient by forcing them to cope with, one, the vascular changes and, two, an altered metabolism, the heart being a prime example.

The component bases of diabetic state:

1. Biochemical abnormalities and altered plasma concentration.
2. Alteration in physiological coagulation process.
3. Alteration in immune responses in a diabetic.
4. Effects of insulinopenia related to protein metabolism.
5. Altered organ metabolism under abnormal tissue lipases and hyperglycemia.
6. Pathological basis of diabetes complications: glycosylation, oxidant stress, essential fatty acid abnormalities, and sorbitol/myoinositol abnormalities.

Box 12.3 Components of Diabetic State 1

Biochemical alterations
Altered plasma composition
Altered protein metabolism
Altered organ metabolism
Dehydration

Box 12.4 Components of Diabetic State 2

Alterations in immune function
Glycosylation
Altered sorbitol/myoinositol metabolism, omega fatty acids
Hypercoagulable state

12.3.1 Biochemical Alterations and Its Effects

An insulinopenic state is also a hyperglucagonemic state. Both produce ultimately through glucagon action, an uninhibited high fasting hepatic glucose output through glycogenolysis. Glucagon also causes release of free fatty acids and glycerol. Insulinopenia leads to incomplete combustion of free fatty acids and results in progressively increasing ketone formation. Glycerol is used for increased gluconeogenesis. Insulinopenia also leads to the loss of anti-catabolic actions which normally preserve muscle protein. The result is the loss of alanine and glutamine from the muscles. Excessive accumulation of free fatty acids and glycosuria-induced dehydration increases the viscosity of blood which makes the passage of blood through arterioles and venules slower. This may predispose to intravascular thrombosis.

If the uncontrolled state of diabetes is complicated by any other stress factor(s), it will give rise to a few more biochemical abnormalities. The release of CRH or counter-regulatory hormones occurs as the first reaction to a stress. Cortisol, growth hormone, or epinephrine and norepinephrine fully and effectively demonstrate their effects in the presence of glucagon. This enhances or accelerates the gluconeogenic process. These hormones also increase insulin resistance, thereby decreasing influx of glucose into the tissues resulting in hyperglycemia. Catecholamines stimulate calcium-dependent adrenergic activity by blockage of insulin secretion by alpha 2 inhibition. Catecholamines initiate lipolysis and glycogenolysis from the muscle and liver with an effect similar to glucagon and prevent insulin-stimulated glucose disposal.

Cortisol in particular mobilizes amino acids from muscles, which causes proteolysis. Through aminoacidemia it produces glucagon stimulation and facilitates glucagon effect on gluconeogenesis. It acts in synergy with catecholamines. Growth hormone also produces lipolysis, increases insulin resistance, and causes hyperglycemia.

Box 12.5 Insulinopenia: Low Insulin Levels

Hyperglucagonemia reduces insulin-dependent glucose disposal
Glycogenolysis
Lipolysis-ketogenesis
Proteolysis ↑ losses of amino acids, hepatic protein breakdown, +ve nitrogen balance not easy, to restore

Box 12.6 High Levels of Counter-regulatory Hormones (CRH)

Catecholamines
Lipolysis
Inhibit insulin secretion
Cortisol: decreases insulin receptor affinity
Proteolysis aminoacidemia

12.3.2 Altered Physiology of the Coagulation Process

Diabetes is associated with a hypercoagulable state. The primary abnormality is that of hyperactive platelets as assessed by standard platelet aggregation assays. Lipid abnormalities like familial hypercholesterolemia or as found in diabetes may increase platelet membrane cholesterol content, decrease fluidity, and enhance platelet reactivity to agonists in vitro. The factors implicated in diabetes in the production of hypercoagulable state are as follows:

- Increase in prothrombin fragments 1 + 2 leading to greater thrombin production.
- Increase in fibropeptide A, thromboxane A2, and adhesion molecules.
- Increased activity of procoagulant protein factors VII X and von Willebrand factor.
- Increase in platelet factor 4 and platelet-derived growth factor.
- Increased Lp(a) lipoprotein lipase, competing with plasminogen and resulting in less available plasmin and less fibrinolysis.
- Increased plasminogen activator inhibitor (PAI) results in decreased availability of plasmin for fibrinolysis.
- Cytokine release leading to monocyte chemotactic factor, macrophage recruitment through growth factors, formation of foam cells and macrophage-derived growth factor.
- Hyperproinsulinemia, increased insulin level, increased growth factors.
- Hyperlipidemia, low HDL cholesterol.
- Dehydration or raised hematocrit in the presence of diabetic hypercoagulable state.

The seriousness of platelet activation and endothelial dysfunction in diabetic state should be emphasized and understood. It does not take very long for these effects to materialize. In patients with type 2 diabetes, as little as 4 h of acute hyperglycemia is accompanied by these effects. It also results in leakage from endothelial cells. In diabetic hyperglycemic patients after myocardial infarction, there is no reflow phenomenon. All these factors may explain the increased incidence of the same [1–3].

One of the important factors to set the coagulation cascade in motion is dehydration. That can alter the rheology, i.e., the resistance faced by the blood in capillary traversing time, slowing it down in the microcirculation. Slower passage could become a nidus for starting the coagulopathy cascade. Dehydration assumes great significance as severely uncontrolled diabetics are more likely to be dehydrated due to osmotic diuresis. Diabetes thus increases predisposition to thrombosis (see below also).

12.3.3 Infection, Inflammation, and Vascular Damage in Diabetes

It is a commonsense relationship. One paves the way for the other and must be treated simultaneously. Hyperglycemic infections particularly associated with diabetes are malignant otitis externa, emphysematous cholecystitis, pyelonephritis, cystitis, and necrotizing fasciitis. Tuberculosis is far more common in diabetes and is more difficult to diagnose and treat. AIDS has a more unbridled course in persons with diabetes.

Components of the infective inflammatory process, more virulent, are endotoxemia in gram-negative bacteria. Endotoxins are the lipopolysaccharides (LPS). Then there are staphylococcal superantigens. Each is accompanied by massive release of cytokines. LPS leads to increased secretion of interleukin-1 which in turn leads to

IL-6/IL-8 and tumor necrosis factor-alpha (TNF alpha) production. Sympathetic stimulation and increased ACTH and steroid, angiotensin II, and other acute phase reactants lead to vascular wall damage. Polymorphonuclear (PMN) superoxide bursts on adhered endothelium further increase the vascular damage. IL-1, IL-6, IL-8, and TNF alpha induce adhesion molecules leading to increased platelet aggregation and activation of clotting cascade leading to disseminated intravascular coagulopathy.

12.3.4 Intravascular Coagulation and Multiorgan Failure

Increased vascular wall damage leads to loss of plasma in inflamed tissues, hypovolemia, hypotension, splanchnic vasodilatation, mucosal and tissue hypoxia, increased anaerobic glycolysis, reduced pH, reduced vasomotor response, and decreased myocardial contractility. This facilitates the bacterial entry from the gut. TNF-α is central to infection and affects post-receptor signaling pathways by affecting the phosphorylation. Increased sympathetic amines lead to β_2 stimulation and reduction in insulin secretion. Angiotensin II affects intracellular signaling.

12.3.5 Alterations of Immune Functions: Ineffective Containment of Infection

12.3.5.1 Hyperglycemia and Neutrophil Function

Neutrophil function studies have been undertaken in type 1 diabetic patients mostly. Hyperglycemia seems to affect the variable degree of the two important immune functions, phagocytosis or intracellular killing of bacteria. The summary of these studies also seems to suggest that these functions are significantly improved with tightening of glycemic control [4–7].

There are other factors independent of glycemic status affecting the neutrophil function. To put it otherwise, these factors will continue to affect the functions even after euglycemia has been restored completely [4–7]. Further to it, diabetes seems to hasten earlier apoptosis of leukocyte when compared with their nondiabetic relatives. It suggests a possibility of a potential underlying genetic defect which may play a role [8–10].

Hyperglycemia in the range of 12 mmol/L or 216 mg/dL makes a patient with diabetes more prone to develop infections as shown in the Australian guidelines, mentioned elsewhere in this volume. The limit of 250 mg/dL held by the Australian guidelines earlier was changed to 210 mg/dL for infection proneness. This lowered range corresponds more closely with the abovementioned limit. In the chapter on Special Situations in Surgery in Diabetes Part 1, we have cited many studies where the optimum levels of diabetes control, least likely to lead to systemic or surgical site infection without hypoglycemia and/or mortality, were between 140 and 170 mg/dL. Within the cardiac surgery varieties, this lower limit is far more desirable. Obviously a variety of changes in the immune function are induced by hyperglycemia.

12.3.6 Wound Healing and Hyperglycemia

It may be argued that by achieving good blood glucose control before, admission costs can be brought down. There are three issues: One - as tight postoperative blood glucose as possible should be achieved. Second – is insulin the best method for it or other non insulin methods if it can be achieved. Of the two ways which method of glucose control has a higher chance of laying proper collagen adequately for wound healing, scar strength postoperatively? Both viewpoints however agree that adequate blood glucose control will produce better healing.

In type 1 diabetics, decreased capillary volume, fibroblast numbers, collagen synthesis, tensile wound strength, increased edema, leukocyte migration, and overall cellularity of the inflammatory response at the surgical site are reduced compared with nondiabetic controls. Among studies done with human forearm abrasion, only one studied the leukocyte migration under blood glucose level of 160–240 mg/dL. It could not show that hyperglycemia played a primary role in these defects mentioned above. However these effects were reversible to some degree with insulin therapy.

Ulcers are much uglier in leprotic patients compared to diabetic ulcers. But leprotic ulcers remain localized and hardly ever produce septicemia which is common to diabetes. Metabolically speaking, the absence of diabetes is the only difference in these two ulcerative processes, which may lead to an easier spread of infection.

Bacterial endotoxemia in hyperglycemic state causes slower response in number and speed of polymorphonuclear cells or the neutrophil migration. Decreased diapedesis, that is, formation of foot processes for bacteriophagy at the site of infection and inflammation, decreased chemotaxis and lowered cell-to-cell adherence which occurs in hyperglycemia. Hyperglycemia also decreases the function of the natural killer cells due to reduction in the superoxide bursts which kill bacteria. The cytokine synthesis, that is, the inflammatory response and decreased complement activity, combines to exacerbate inflammation and increase the risk of infection in hyperglycemic conditions. As Langouche argues intensive treatment with insulin will prevent these effects [11].

Monocytes and macrophages are known to have insulin receptors. It is also observed that various functions of these white cells are deficient in an environment of hyperglycemia and normalize in euglycemic surroundings. The phagocytosis especially in diabetic ketoacidosis is distinctly poor if blood glucose is above 250 mg/dL. Killing after phagocytosis is also poor; lymphocyte responses are also slower. This capacity is restored with normoglycemia. CD4+ lymphocytes decrease. Antibody-dependent cellular cytotoxicity is also decreased. A defect in opsonization has been suggested to account for this. The monocytes have decreased lectin-like receptors with decreased affinity. The adhesive molecular action also shows some delay.

The proneness to infection and failure of an infection to localize at a place are familiar phenomena in diabetes. This is best illustrated in case of diabetic foot. These two processes can be traced to the altered physiologic mechanisms described above. A person with diabetes who is well controlled does not show increased susceptibility to get newer infections even during surgery (see Chap. 7).

12.3.7 Alterations in Protein Metabolism in Insulinopenia

In the chapter on insulin physiology, this topic has been extensively dealt with. Here we will elaborate a couple of more points. The insulin effects on protein metabolism are so salutary that they justify the title of the only truly anabolic hormone in the body, conferred on insulin. Inhibiting excessive unregulated proteolysis is achieved by basal insulin levels. It keeps normalcy of the protein catabolism. Regulation of proteolysis and prevention of excessive proteolysis seem to be a more useful and stronger action of insulin than new protein synthesis.

12.3.8 Protein Metabolism and Insulin: The Experimental Backdrop

Protein metabolism with or without insulin has been studied with both in vivo and in vitro techniques. Initial methods consisted of determining synthesis rate and quantitative machinery of protein synthesis, i.e., rates of production or turnover time of mRNA, tRNA, eukaryotic factors, enzymes, and ribosomes. Amino acids, glucose, and insulin form the raw materials for them. Several discrete reactions occur in protein synthesis of insulin with the above molecules. In metabolic energy terms, protein synthesis is a costly process, and the presence of insulin becomes important. The various levels at which insulin affects protein synthesis are gene transcription level, mRNA level, translational level on ribosomal proteins, elongation level on ribosomal proteins, nonstructural cellular proteins, and effects on cellular organelles, enzymes, polysomes, and structural or long-lasting proteins. These effects are operative in "all cells" of the body.

The simplest investigation in protein metabolism is to see nitrogen balance in a steady state. It was a crude method, telling nothing about what changes occur in the individual body tissue. Accumulation of radiolabeled amino acids in tissues forms a major step in newer, more refined studies. The radiolabel usually used is C^{13} or N^{15}, in human studies. Only essential amino acids are labeled. These techniques in vitro are adopted to treat small pieces of tissues—liver slices, atrial strips, diaphragm, skeletal muscle, etc. Elaborate perfusion systems have been developed, like in isolated heart. Cell cultures of primary hepatocytes, fibroblasts, and cardiac and skeletal myocytes give uniformity of cell types but not tissue atmosphere. Techniques of molecular biology have tried to locate insulin-responsive genes recently.

12.3.9 Insulinopenia and Cellular Changes

Intracellular protein degradation under insulinopenic conditions is different from normal protein degradation. In insulinopenia, large intracellular vacuoles appear in which the mitochondria, rough and smooth endoplasmic reticulum, and glycogen collapse. The changes are detectable. Insulin and amino acid infusion reverse these changes. At normal level of concentration, it requires the help of insulin to reverse these changes. In protein degradation, regulated events can take place only in the presence of adequate insulin by increasing the stability of lysosomal enzymes. Insulinopenia causes increased fragility of lysosomes and thereby self-destruction of cells by the lysosomes.

12.3.10 Type 2 Diabetes and Gene Expression Profile in Muscle

Studies conducted on insulin-insufficient and insulin-sufficient tissue atmosphere in vivo and studied through microarray technique, analyzing thousands of genes expressed in muscles, have underlined the importance of insulin on normal muscle maintenance. As many as 85 gene transcripts were affected in type 2 diabetes and insulinopenia. Out of these 85 gene transcripts, 74 gene transcripts were found to improve in insulin-sufficient state.

Supposedly these transcripts represent the genes responsible for prevention of chronic complications of diabetes. The remaining 11 transcripts that did not improve in insulin-sufficient state may be responsible for pathogenesis of muscle insulin resistance. Another 29 gene transcripts for growth factors, structural as well as contractile proteins like myosin heavy chain and troponin T and in energy metabolism like UCP3, ATP synthase, cytochrome c oxidase, glycogen synthase, myosin light chain, alpha actin, etc., genes involved in protein metabolism, signal transduction, fatty acid metabolism, and tissue development are altered (improved) under insulin-treated type 2 diabetic patients. This research is mentioned more to underline the profound actions of insulin on such a large scale and how insulinopenia affects each and every aspect of structure and function of muscles diabetic state. These gene functions are not related to glucose metabolism under insulin [12].

It is not only insulin supplementation in patients with type 2 diabetes. The quantum of insulin administered is more important. In type 2 diabetes, majority of mitochondrial transcripts were expressed at a lower level when they were infused with low-level insulin glucose infusions of 0.25 mU/kg of lean body weight. The expression of these mitochondrial transcripts got corrected with high-dose glucose infusion, 1.5 mU/kg of lean body weight. This study also is mentioned for the above purpose to underline the deep influence insulin has on muscles which has an abundance of mitochondria [13]. As emphasized elsewhere, supraphysiologic levels of insulin with amino acid abundance are needed for protein anabolism.

12.3.11 Tissue and Organ Alterations Under Insulinopenic Conditions

Endothelium is a large organ recognized for its local vasodilatory actions as per the needs of the tissues through the production of nitric oxide. In hyperglycemia nitric oxide production is reduced leading to a more likely vasoconstrictor action in the blood vessels [11]. Insulin administration increases the NO production. High loss of capillary endothelium is found in the retina, heart, and kidneys.

The discussion below is largely based on Joslin's *Textbook of Diabetes Mellitus* 14th (special Indian) edition 2005, pp. 809–17 [14, p. 809–7].

Loss of pericytes around the capillaries, in the retina, leads to the development of various abnormalities of diabetic retinopathy like protein leak and microaneurysms. Increased expression of vascular endothelial growth factors in diabetes is partly responsible for retinal and renal changes.

Death of cardiomyocytes that increased severalfold occurs through the activated apoptotic pathways. Failure of development of new vessels during ischemia leads to higher cardiac muscle loss and affects remodeling. Intramural fibrosis is increased. All these changes together lead to congestive heart failure, reinfarction of the myocardium, heart failure during infarcts as well as the diastolic dysfunction of cardiac muscle. Hypertension also affects the microvasculature.

Generalized thickening of vascular and nonvascular basement membrane occurs due to excess production of various collagen-type fiber and reduction in the normal degradation which disturbs the balance and alters its properties like electrical charge sites in kidney, losing albumin.

12.3.12 Few Specific Effects of Hyperglycemia or the Pathological Basis of Diabetic Complications

Hyperglycemia gives rise to a cascade of biochemical reactions leading to excess glycosylation of proteins, excessive oxidant stress, essential fatty acid availability, or otherwise, and altered sorbitol-myoinositol metabolism forms the basis of many microvascular abnormalities. These are briefly discussed below.

12.3.13 Glycosylation

The higher the glucose and longer the duration of hyperglycemia, the greater is the covalent attachment of glucose to the N-terminal of proteins. Long-lasting stable proteins undergo this reaction and reach a level of glycosylation which is measurable (like in hemoglobin over several weeks). This covalent bond results in an unstable Schiff's base, and with a series of rearrangements they undergo, a brown fluorescent advanced glycosylation end product (AGE) is obtained. It is also accelerated by the excess production of reactive oxygen species that are elevated in hyperglycemia. It also has profound effects on the normal collagen turnover. It reduces the endothelial NO production, increases the expression of endothelin 1, and activates growth factors.

Glycosylation can result in a change in the electrical character of basement membranes and the impedance it causes normally to the exudation or leaking of proteins, like albumin, which is lost in urine. Proteins that can be glycated are numerous such as albumin and hemoglobin, and coagulation proteins are also glycosylated. The last ones add to the altered coagulation states. Due to these inflammatory changes produced by the AGE and its attachment to the receptor for AGE (RAGE), TNF alpha,

IL-1, and other cytokines are released, effects of nitric oxide are quenched, and all these changes will result in a more inflammatory, vasoconstrictive, and proaggregatory atmosphere in tissues. Collagen, basement membrane proteins, and DNA are particularly disposed to the formation of AGE, like the vascular and neural tissue. Effects of glycosylation on DNA could be lasting. Single-strand breaks and impaired DNA repair are reported in endothelial cell cultures with severe hyperglycemia. It can take place in quite a ubiquitous manner.

12.3.14 Free Radicals and Tissue Damage in Diabetic State

The discussion below is largely based on Joslin's *Textbook of Diabetes Mellitus* 14th (special Indian) edition 2005, pp. 840–52 [14, p. 843].

Generation of free radicals or the reactive oxygen species (ROS) and the cellular mechanisms to quench excess ROS production is a normal body process. It arises mainly in the leucocytes and mitochondria. The respiratory chain of mitochondria is an electron transport system which forms exchangeable electrons. Oxygen is the final acceptor of electrons. When it accepts one extra electron, it becomes a superoxide radical O_2^{-e}. This is a hyperactive element. H_2O_2 is among the many others like lipid peroxides that are produced. These cause lipid peroxidation in the brain and nerves unless quenched. Advanced glycation end products (AGE), combined with their receptor RAGE, increase the production of these ROSs, which in turn cause increase in AGEs which then quench the endothelial NO affecting the vasodilatory activity. Smoking, ionizing radiation, X-ray exposures, and long periods of uncontrolled hyperglycemia are the frequent causes of excess radicals which the body find difficult to quench.

There are more than 12 antioxidant molecules in normal milieu which will neutralize these peroxides. These molecules decrease in hyperglycemic states. Hyperglycemia with its increased flux of glucose through tissues is a source, cause, and catalyst for the production of increased supraphysiological levels of free radicals and decrease in the defensive cellular mechanisms [14, p. 840–52]. Excess free radical release could also be responsible for DNA strand breaking and stress-activated pathways leading to apoptosis. The ROS also decreases the cellular defenses like superoxide dismutase and glutathione and causes destruction of the cells.

12.3.15 The Polyol/Sorbitol Pathway

Hyperglycemia activates this pathway. In the simplest schema, it diverts the glucose to other non-glycolytic pathways and products like sorbitol increase. This overwhelms the capacity of sorbitol dehydrogenase to form from accumulated sorbitol fructose to be metabolized. Aldose reductase also reduces the intracellular antioxidants. Sorbitol does not diffuse, draws water, breaks lens fibers, and can cause cataract much earlier.

An activated polyol pathway reduces the myoinositol and taurine in the nerves which are potent antioxidants. Sorbitol and hyperglycemia decrease myoinositol uptake and myoinositol incorporation in the nerve fibers. This may cause further nerve dysfunction. While it is known that neural tissue does not need insulin to transport glucose in the cells, the protein formation in nerves is a consideration. Tubulin that forms the building blocks of microtubules of all cells as well as neuronal axons and dendrites is more stable in the presence of insulin.

Box 12.7 Glycosylation Causes

Covalent attachment of glucose to N-terminals of proteins
Long-life proteins, coagulation proteins undergo the reaction—collagen, hemoglobin, etc.
DNA proteins susceptible, DNA breakages, protein defragmentation
Bonding proportional to average blood glucose, time of this average
Inflammatory changes in tissues

Box 12.8 Glycosylation Effects

Basement membrane thickening in muscle, capillary bed
Decreased vascular bed
Decreased muscle blood flow
Decreased insulin-induced glucose disposal, hyperglycemia, and reduced muscular energy
Increased oxidative state and tissue damage, quenching nitric oxide

12.3.16 Omega-6 (W6)/Omega-3 (W3) Fatty Acids and Milieu Interior

These two essential fatty acids can be obtained only through diet. Fish is the richest source of W3. They are unsaturated. 3 and 6 indicate number of unsaturated double bonds. It is believed that they should be consumed in a ratio of 5:1. Modern agriculture and food and cooking methods are supposed to have caused a marked decline in W3 fatty acid content. The biological changes produced by them are subtle. W6 acts through the arachidonic acid pathway which gives rise to prostaglandins with potential to a proinflammatory, vasoconstrictive, proaggregatory, and procoagulant atmosphere in diabetes. W3 activates the production of prostcyclins which are antithrombotic, antiaggregatory, vasodilatory, and anti-inflammatory. It is also supposed that W3 replaces W6 fatty acid in membranes of endothelial cells improving their physicochemical stability and functional integrity.

12.3.17 Alterations in Metabolism of Some Important Organs

Under adequate insulin levels, glucose metabolism is the preferred pathway for cardiac and skeletal muscle fibers and adipose tissues. In insulinopenic state, brought out best in prolonged starvation, there is at first an increase in glucose metabolism of the muscles from 10% in resting conditions. Later the FFAs and ketones are used from 50% to 90%, and there is a switch in metabolism. Hormonal lipases release triglycerides, and the tissue lipases hydrolyze the FFAs to be consumed by these two organs. That increases the level of VLDL and glycerol in the plasma. This spares glucose for the brain which does not utilize any other substance normally for metabolism.

As starvation proceeds and ketones are produced by the liver, the skeletal muscles reduce FFA utilization and switch to ketones which muscles utilize almost proportional to the ketone concentration in plasma. In still more prolonged starvation or in ketoacidosis, skeletal muscles switch back to FFAs. This transition serves two purposes. As starvation proceeds gluconeogenic process alone may not be sufficient for the brain. High levels of ketones are then utilized by various organs along with glucose. As much as 40% of all brain energy requirements can then be met by ketones. When insulin is readministered, the proper utilization of FFAs and glucose takes place in cardiac and skeletal muscles. Full oxidation of FFAs under insulin may keep intracellular milieu of myocardium optimal, not collect acid products of FFA metabolism and cause less dysrhythmias especially if potassium is also supplemented with glucose. When insulin concentration is adequate, lipogenesis takes place.

Box 12.9 Skeletal-Cardiac Muscle Metabolism

Preferred metabolite glucose
Insulinopenia—switch to FFA, ketones
Further starvation-only FFA
Lipoprotein lipases of skeletal and cardiac muscle ↑ use of FFA

Box 12.10 Adipose Tissue Abnormalities

Insulinopenia, lipolysis
FFA used by cardiac-skeletal muscle
Spare glucose for the brain
Ketones and muscle use are proportional to the concentration of ketones
Sparing ketones for the brain

In summary we have detailed the profound physiological alterations in insulinopenia. Large numbers of persons with type 2 diabetes are insulinopenic, and insulin happens to be the most important single nonsurgical element that needs to be used adequately to produce its singular effects and avoid the problems of insulinopenia, in the perioperative that is essentially a catabolic state.

References

1. Gresele P, Guglielmini G, De Angelis M, et al. Acute, short term hyperglycemia enhances shear stress-induced platelet activation in patients with type II diabetes mellitus. J Am Coll Cardiol. 2003;41:1013–20.
2. Williams SB, Goldfine AB, Timimi FK, et al. Acute hyperglycemia attenuates endothelium-dependent vasodilation in humans in vivo. Circulation. 1998;97:1695–701.
3. Iwakura K, Ito H, Ikushima M, et al. Association between hyperglycemia and the no-reflow phenomenon in patients with acute myocardial infarction. J Am Coll Cardiol. 2003;41:1–7.
4. Dziatkowiak H, Kowalska M, Denys A. Phagocytic and bactericidal activity of granulocytes in diabetic children. Diabetes. 1982;31:1041–3.
5. Gin H, Brottier E, Aubertin J. Influence of glyceaemic normalization by an artificial pancreas on phagocytic and bactericidal functions of granulocytes in insulin dependent diabetic patients. J Clin Pathol. 1984;37:1029–31.
6. Kjersem H, Hilsted J, Madsbad S, et al. Polymorphonuclear leucocyte dysfunction during short term metabolic changes from normo- to hyperglycemia in type 1 (insulin dependent) diabetic patients. Infection. 1988;16:215–21.
7. Repine JE, Clawson CC, Goetz FC. Bactericidal function of neutrophils from patients with acute bacterial infections and from diabetics. J Infect Dis. 1980;142:869–75.
8. Molenaar DM, Palumbo PJ, Wilson WR, et al. Leukocyte chemotaxis in diabetic patients and their nondiabetic first-degree relatives. Diabetes. 1976;25(Suppl 2):880–3.
9. Tennenberg SD, Finkenauer R, Dwivedi A. Absence of lipopolysaccharide-induced inhibition of neutrophil apoptosis in patients with diabetes. Arch Surg. 1999;134:1229–33.
10. Glister BC, Vigersky RA. Perioperative management of type 1 diabetes mellitus. Endocrinol Metab Clin North Am. 2003;32:411–36.
11. Langouche L, Vanhorebeek I, Vlasselaers D, Perre SV, Wouters PJ, Skogstrand K, Hansen TK, Van den Berghe G. Intensive insulin therapy protects the endothelium of critically ill patients. J Clin Invest. 2005;115(8):2277–86, http://www.jci.org.
12. Sreekumar R, Halvatsiotis P, Schimke JC, Nair S. Gene expression profile in skeletal muscle of type 2 diabetes and the effects of insulin treatment. Diabetes. 2002;51:1913–20.
13. Asmann YW, Stump CS, Short KR, Conen-schimke J, Guo Z, Bigelow M, Nair KS. Skeletal muscle mitochondrial functions, mitochondrial DNA copy numbers, and gene transcript profiles in type 2 diabetic and nondiabetic subjects at equal levels of low or high insulin and euglycemia. Diabetes. 2006;55:3309–19.
14. Joslin EP. Joslin's textbook of diabetes mellitus. 14th ed. Boston, MA: Lippincott, Williams & Wilkins; 2005, Indian edition.

Commonly Asked Questions

13

Content

Q1: What are the abnormalities/mechanisms which result in type 2 diabetes?

Over a period the beta cell secretion of insulin increases in those prone to develop diabetes or those who have lifestyle issues as in impaired glucose tolerance. It later declines as this hyperinsulinemic response leads to beta cell exhaustion and apoptosis and insulin insufficiency start, leading to initially postprandial but later progressive hyperglycemia. Portal venous insulin levels decrease, and hepatic glucose output increases due to it and increased glucagon secretion. The persons prone to develop diabetes have insulin resistance in the three primary tissues which results in the declining quantity of insulin ineffective for the adequate glucose disposal.

In type 2 diabetes, one of the earliest abnormalities is the dampening as well as the irregularities of the intervals at which small insulin bursts regularly occur. This essentially leads to irregularity in the basal insulin-induced glucose disposal. This beta cell defect is considered to be one of the pathogenetic factors in type 2 diabetes. In addition the immediate or early peak insulin secretion response to food intake as found in people without diabetes is also lost in people with diabetes. The normally occurring second physiological surge postprandially is lower and delayed causing postprandial hyperglycemia. This issue is discussed in greater detail in the earlier chapters of the volume. This is a simplified version of the same.

Q2: Emphasis on intensive monitoring and therapy like blood gases, central lines have been made. Do you think it can be generally affordable?

It is high time we realize that diabetes is one of the few diseases which damage most body systems. Due care has got to be taken, and therefore sophistication of equipment and higher expenditure are inevitable for better results. In modern

S. Kelkar et al., *Towards Optimal Management of Diabetes in Surgery*,
https://doi.org/10.1007/978-981-13-7705-1_13

medicine where serious disorders are treated, unmonitored intervention is a disaster. Therefore costs will go up.

Judicious use of monitoring and optimal treatment modalities based on solid evidence does bring the costs down considerably. To achieve that, the treating team should be sensitive to cost issue and strive to achieve it without diluting the mandatory actions. Medical fraternity today does not really attend to this aspect and has been accused of doing interventions neither necessary nor should be done too frequently as are done to increase the revenue. The consideration to lower the "total burden" of a patient wherever possible with and some "give and take" on costs of doing something and not doing certain thing can solve the problem.

Spending on central lines, for example, is a good way of simplifying management. The quality of management is better, pain to the patient is less, and veins are preserved. It brings in a lot of precision and avoids dehydration and fluid overload. Thrombophlebitis in a diabetic when peripheral veins are used can be troublesome. In central lines properly put and removed the moment they are not required, thrombophlebitis is much less.

Judicious monitoring generally reduces costs. It is however a rarity in acute clinical medicine, which we have discussed elsewhere in the volume. Judicious monitoring is an "attitude," and the least that can be emphasized is that cultivating it is advisable.

Q3: A frequent reliance on blood gas has been mentioned which is costly. Moreover, it is a facility available only at a few places. How do we solve this problem?

Emphasis is on the judicious use of ABG and not frequent use. Investigative modalities like arterial blood gas analysis when available may be more frequently used, while the clinicians are on the learning curve. It helps clinicians to precisely make a diagnosis of abnormalities. The search for causes of abnormalities becomes easier. Once the familiarity with these techniques is achieved and ability to correlate its data clinically is developed, the reliance on blood gas will decline saving costs.

Once an initial blood gas is done, there is generally little necessity to repeat it in most cases since the other simpler clinical bedside parameters can guide us to intensify or de-escalate the treatments. Identifying it as redundant or costly will not be proper. Mixed acidosis, for example, is a condition identified on arterial blood gas only. Translating it to clinical picture and treating it are important. In the absence of arterial blood gas, the simpler lab parameters aided by clinical judgment are the final answer. Finally, it is the development of heightened clinical acumen, precise observation, and sharp judgment within that is the "last word." Sophisticated monitoring helps develop that.

Q4: You have mentioned the Leuven studies. Their results are not confirming but often contradictory. How do you explain that?

The many studies conducted under the leadership of Greet Van den Berghe are sometimes referred to as the Leuven studies. All of them have been conducted on critically ill patients of different types. This will partly explain the variances, but these should not be understood as contradictory results among the many trials.

First such study to appear was in 2001 conducted at a single center. The cohort was of only critical surgical cases. It was a nurse-driven protocol and was not blinded. The spectacular success of this study in reducing the mortality by 42% could be because of the one-to-one nurse-to-patient ratio. It was higher than the nurse-to-patient ratio in most ICUs. Additional support was made available with a study physician for narrow range glucose maintenance. The physician was not involved in clinical care. This level of supportive staffs could have helped maintain the glucose levels and reduced incidence and magnitude of hypoglycemic events as well as other adverse outcomes.

A similar instance can be cited of the secondary trial analysis of DCCT. DCCT also was spectacularly successful and also had high level of support of every kind to the trial population, which was not available in day-to-day management of the control group of type 1 diabetes. This was considered to be one of the major reasons for the success of DCCT. It is unclear if the results of this study can be generalized to other surgical ICUs, much less medical ICUs, or operating rooms in normal situations where so much support cannot be offered.

63% of these patients were recovering from cardiac surgery. Blood glucose level more than 110 mg/dL was used as the criterion to put these patients on intravenous insulin on arrival to the ICU. All of them were not having diabetes [1].

A significant percentage of them received calories by the route of total parenteral nutrition (TPN) of which the details are given in this chapter below. TPN causes hyperglycemia and through additional mechanisms causes insulin resistance. To control that aggressive insulin infusion rates would be required to maintain a narrow range of blood glucose.

The control group of this study was treated conventionally—that is to say that the target blood glucose was more lax in this group, whereas both groups were treated in identical methods. The value of this study was a single variant and what effects it could cause on the outcome. The mortality in the control group was quite high. Quite a few argued that intensive insulin therapy significantly reduced high relative risks. The 42% reduction in mortality otherwise could not be expected otherwise [1].

The second study from Van den Berghe was published in 2006. Here the cohort was completely different. It was conducted on 1200 medical ICU patients, again with a single variant between the two groups tight control and conventionally treated ones with intensive insulin therapy (IIT) and conventional therapy [2]. It did not show any mortality benefit with IIT against the control group. This is the most critical difference between the 2001 and the 2006 studies. This has been considered contradictory by some. Following remarks may be considered to decide if it is really so.

These two cohorts were completely different to begin with. Medical illnesses have a higher prevalence of death in general. Such severe illnesses are more likely to occur in the elderly and with long-standing diabetes. Hence failure to reduce mortality should not be held against in the 2006 study. More importantly tight control of glucose should also not be characterized as a detrimental or a useless method of treatment. The treatment group did receive other benefits over the conventional group like reduced adverse effects on the kidneys and reduced number of days on ventilation and reduced critical care neuropathy.

If we look at the ACCORD study, the mainstay was tight control of blood glucose and the blood pressure as well. The blood pressure control level was considered to be the factor for so many deaths in elderly patients [3]. Tight control of glucose has at least not resulted in mortality in excess of the conventional group even if there was no reduction.

An important factor however emerged when both studies were pooled for multivariate analysis. It concluded that hypoglycemia could be an independent predictor of death [4]. It suggested maintaining blood glucose levels at 8.3 mmol (150 mg/dL) to be the most important factor in reducing mortality. This is the most significant lesson of blood glucose control in critical medical illnesses. In addition, it appears that to protect the kidneys and the nervous system, blood glucose had to be kept at 6.1 mmol (110 mg/dL). This tight level of control did provide additional survival benefit. The pooled data reaffirm the higher risk of hypoglycemic events, 11.3% against 1.8% in the IIT group in medical acute illnesses but not in surgical critical illnesses [4].

Q5: Emphasis on monitoring may look excessive to a care provider. Your comments on this!

The one thing we have tried to emphasize is judicious, even minimal monitoring. The latter can give as precise a control as any, under certain conditions as explained elsewhere. We have also given in great detail as to what to do for many different clinical situations practically without too much monitoring, with mid drip monitoring as an example. Another emphasis laid in these pages is that monitoring without action needed and action without monitoring are unacceptable. If these two principles are borne in mind, the issue of frequent/excessive monitoring becomes hypothetical.

Q6: What antidiabetic treatment may be required postoperatively if a patient has had preoperative uncontrolled diabetic status on substantial OHA dose?

The general prevalence of many type 2 diabetes patients who should have been on insulin preoperatively but were not was uncontrolled due to OHA failure and had an uncontrolled preoperative that is pre-admission status, all point to the following possibilities that can coexist singly or multiply in one patient for which all of them would require insulin in postoperative early and later as well.

The surgical condition for which the patient is admitted can be the cause for pushing the earlier "controlled" diabetes on OHA, in an uncontrolled state. These patients may go back on tablets after the resolution of the surgical condition.

Primary OHA failure is by definition failed control after due modifications in diet, exercise, and complimentary use of OHAs within 3 months of starting the treatment. To clarify further, such a patient should not have active infection, tuberculosis, stress, unacceptable obesity, unregulated diet, absence of exercise, and so on. These patients will have lost weight in recent times acutely or subacutely and will *tend towards* a lean diabetic status. These patients will usually continue to need insulin postoperatively.

It is necessary to understand this category of lean type 2 diabetes or the latent autoimmune diabetes in adults (LADA). These are known to have diabetes and have less than optimal weight for their height and age, and they have been losing weight for a long time. They may be on OHAs but are not controlled, although they are not ketotic. The body mass index is likely to be less than 19 kg/m^2 of their height in males and 17 kg/m^2 in women. It is supposed that in India, a large number of people with diabetes are lean or bordering on that status. Secondly, many of these lean patients are treated like type 2 diabetes. In actuality however they are supposed to be type 1 diabetes in evolution. These patients in all likelihood will continue to need insulin.

Tubercular infection in perioperative period, many times diagnosed on table, is a definite indication for continuing insulin. Urinary infection at times can be troublesome, and such patients if uncontrolled on OHAs will need insulin for variable time.

In type 1 diabetes, the question of substituting insulin does not arise. During gestational diabetes mellitus, the question of OHA does not arise. There are a number of studies with OHAs in pregnancy, but we are firmly inclined to use of insulin in GDM. In postdelivery or post caesarean, if the diabetic status persists and if the mother is breastfeeding the child, she will be in need of insulin. The reason is that the OHAs may get secreted in the milk and cause hypoglycemia in the child due to neonatal pancreatic insulin secretion.

If a woman has diabetes and becomes pregnant, she will require insulin during the antenatal period, during and after delivery and lactation. Maturity-onset diabetes of the young (MODY) who become diabetic before 25 or 30 years of age and may have OHA failure in about 5 years after diagnosis needs insulin. They will continue to do so postoperatively. Older persons with diabetes and with secondary OHA failure have what is called as insulin-requiring diabetes mellitus (IRDM). Postoperatively, in convalescence they will continue to need insulin. Therefore there are many varieties of diabetics who will continue to need insulin postoperatively.

Q7: Are there any differences in the hypoglycemic potential of various drugs used to lower/control blood glucose?

All drugs in a particular class do not have the same hypoglycemic potential. It depends primarily on the duration of action of these drugs and the dissociation constant between them and the SUR receptors in case of different sulfonylureas. The higher it is and dissociation occurs at lower glycemic rise, the less is the potential for developing hypoglycemia from the use of such a drug. Many of the oral drugs should be discontinued before surgery to avoid hypos. The detailed answer will be found in Chap. 5.

Q8: Type 2 diabetes needs many drugs to achieve normoglycemia and many more to control other parameters and complications. Are there any significant drug interactions?

Yes there are. These interactions can either potentiate or diminish the action of any drug when two or more drugs are used. This can happen even if these drugs are from across the different classes of drugs that have to be used simultaneously. Hypertension, dyslipidemia, cardiovascular risk factors, acute infections, or chronic ones like tuberculosis, recurrent urinary tract infections, boils, and carbuncles are among the comorbidities encountered in diabetes far more frequently than the population without diabetes. The outcomes also are more grave and management more difficult. Multiple drugs are used for diabetes control, control of other comorbidities arising from it, and also for new abnormalities arising over a period in substantial number. Many are capable of some potentization or reduction of action of its own or of the other drugs.

Most of these actions will occur on account of the drugs being common substrates to a variety of cytochrome P450 isoforms of its enzyme. HIV AIDS if present greatly complicates the entire picture and has grave prognosis.

We have described below those interactions which are clinically significant. We are indebted to a well-structured detailed review by Scheen L, mentioned below, for this information [5]. In addition there is a tendency to use multiple drugs in one capsule or tablet, a polypill which reduces the number of different drugs to be consumed everyday and supposedly produce equal benefits. We do not favor the polypill idea to the extent that we do not recommend combination of even two drugs of different classes unless it has some extraordinarily compelling logic. Our principle objections arise from the differences of drugs in combination with functions, different times of administration, and the number of doses recommended based on their pharmacodynamics and pharmacokinetics. Last but not the least, for several years that these combinations are in the market, we are unable to be convinced that they are as or more effective. In fact the parameter controls are far from being in proper ranges in either direction, be it glucose or blood pressure. These drug classes include not only oral hypoglycemic drugs but all the other categories of comorbidities mentioned above.

Within the diabetes field scores of trials have been conducted comparing different combinations against a placebo or *against a single component* to show that they are more effective. At its best these trials may show safety and demonstrate that the pharmacokinetics and the pharmacodynamics remain unchanged and there are no intermolecular interactions within them. Considered otherwise these are dubious explanations to justify combining the drugs. The avenue that the combinations open is to create many more brands that can be sold at higher MRP and would be called by some as market-oriented profit motives.

Drug interactions between different classes of drugs

UKPDS and three more trials have shown a positive association when the sulfonylureas and metformin are both given as separate drugs, not combined in one pill, for cardiovascular mortality. It still remains the classic, basic, and mainstay combination which vary the other drug introductions [6]. As of now the issue of interaction between them is not at all settled in a definite conclusion.

Among the drugs that induce disturbance of metabolic that is glucose control are the antiretroviral and the second-generation or atypical antipsychotic drugs. Lipid-lowering agent simvastatin coadministered with repaglinide has shown increased incidence of adverse reactions. Those on atorvastatin and thiazolidinediones (TZD) showed that the adverse reactions of the former like myalgia and raised hepatic enzyme levels were three times more likely to be among those who were taking the latter drugs as well. Gemfibrozil, the triglyceride-lowering agent coadministered with repaglinide, not only enhances but also considerably prolongs the glucose-lowering effect of repaglinide. Repaglinide administered with other lipid-lowering drug class of bezafibrate of fenofibrate does not produce these reactions. Gemfibrozil with rosiglitazone potentiates all the actions of the latter. In addition concern has been expressed that this combination also increases the concentration of rosiglitazone which may result in increase in the risk of adverse reactions.

Among the non-OHA drugs, high doses of diuretic thiazide and nonselective beta-blockers may increase blood glucose by increasing insulin resistance. Nonselective beta-blockers also inhibit to some extent insulin secretion. Beta-blockers also block the early adrenergic reaction if a hypoglycemic episode is to occur. It may take the patient directly to a neuroglycopenic state and coma without realizing the onset of hypoglycemia. It also blocks the counter-regulatory hormones.

ACE inhibitors increase insulin sensitivity and insulin secretion, an effect known for a long time. ACE inhibitors have cardioprotective and renal protective effects and hence are essential drugs in diabetes. It is supposed to have an odds ratio of 4.3, and patients may present with severe hypoglycemia among hospital admissions. But clinically as is well known, this event is negligible.

Tuberculosis is many times commoner in people with diabetes. Rifampicin is the principle weapon to fight it. It however increases the metabolism of gliclazide measured as area under the curve method by as much as 70%, glimepiride by 34%, repaglinide by 57%, rosiglitazone by 65%, and glibenclamide to choose a few [7]. What it means is that the glycemic control worsens considerably with the use of rifampicin. However in any significant and extensive tuberculosis, the patient as a rule should be on insulin therapy. Hence these interactions may not occur that frequently unless OHAs are used and insulin omitted.

On the other hand, many commonly used antifungal agents increase the area under the curve by 138% for glimepiride, which is bound to lower the glucose significantly to cause hypoglycemic episodes. The use of glibenclamide with doxycycline and quinolones like ciprofloxacin and gatifloxacin has the potential to induce hypoglycemia. It should be kept in mind by clinicians. Cyclosporin A used in renal transplant patients with glibenclamide increases the cyclosporine A concentration in steady state by 57% which necessitates more frequent assessment of cyclosporine levels, identifying the cause and appropriate reduction in doses of the former. Metformin has almost no clinically important interactions with any drug classes normally used in diabetic patients.

Q9: What are the indications, contraindications, advantages, disadvantages, and side effects of total parenteral nutrition (TPN)? How is glycemic control affected and how is it managed?

The issues leading to the need for TPN

Theoretically it is recommended *that at least 180 (Alberti) to 200 g of dextrose should be infused per day* in the immediate postoperative period in ICUs under insulin to control or reverse hypercatabolic state. It comes to 8 U of 5% intravenous glucose or 4 U of 10% intravenous glucose in 24 h, i.e., 4000 or 2000 mils. This translates to the use of 5% or 10% glucose at 200 or 100 mils of glucose, respectively, round the clock, for a few days. In practice it is extremely difficult to reach this level of supplementation for many other limitations of the diabetic state. Five percent dextrose is available with saline and can be constituted with potassium, but 10% dextrose does not have a saline component which additionally makes it less desirable. Ten percent glucose concentration is injurious to the veins and more difficult to control than 5% dextrose; it cannot be managed by simply doubling of IV insulin dose [8].

Nonglucose-containing fluids are the fluids of choice when the need is to infuse large volumes at fast rates for rehydration. Glucose infusion has to be per force a constant rate infusion as shown repeatedly in this volume. Balancing these needs of both fluids and glucose supplementation is difficult when the clinical situation demands administration of many other fluids like blood or blood products. It may affect the supply of the caloric needs.

The solution to the situation where the supply the calories is required to be stepped up enteral feeding should be begun as soon as patient's condition permits. Five percent dextrose normal saline easily available in India is used till then, with potassium supplements as needed till the patient settles down. The degree of catabolism would be less, and the anti-catabolic insulin action still does its work in this period also. If normal oral intake is restored in a few days after the surgery or the acute illness, role of dietician is encouraged in this regard. In this aspect of management, doctors should know more about diet and dietician about catabolism and its prevention. The maximum possible, gradually increasing intake of proteins, within the limits of diabetic nephropathy which will be found in large number of these cases, cannot be adequately emphasized. There is no need to consider TPN in these early recovering cases.

As stated repeatedly these calories have to be spread uniformly over 24 h. This is absolutely essential because people with diabetes in surgical situations need high doses of insulin for burning even the seemingly minor elevations in the rat of calorie supplementation. Maintaining the quasi-uniformity of calories in 4 hourly oral/nasogastric feeding and issues related to it has been discussed in postoperative management earlier. A staged and incremental planning of nutrition is essential.

When this smooth transition from IV dextrose for a few days to full oral intake is not possible, in relatively small number of cases, in the postoperative period, TPN emerges as the option. These would typically be hypercatabolic states with one or many causes. At the cost of repetition, one may emphasize that low-volume high-calorie nutrition, qualitatively similar in composition, is recommended, even if it is high in lipids. TPN has this advantage [1, 2].

TPN is the best option of nutrition supplements in surgery with or without diabetes, particularly in critically ill patients who do not show adequate improvement over weeks of treatment and may have other medical problems. TPN requirement is emphasized by the accentuated catabolic nature of major or emergency surgical situations in diabetes and its necessary correction. TPN may look costly to start with but is now agreed to be a cost-effective in the long run. It also improves clinical outcomes in critically ill patients like severe burns, prolonged ileus, after transplantation, trauma, abdominal surgery, pancreatitis, and long-term ventilation [9].

The maximum caloric needs depending on degree of illness are just about 25–35 calories/kg/day. Some malnourished critically ill patients may require only 15–25 calories/kg/day [10–12]. Patients with or without diabetes do not show any difference in adverse reactions to the administered TPN due to hyperglycemia [13, 14].

In the first paper published by Greet Van den Berghe in 2001, the calorie supplementation methods are described. All patients requiring intensive care were started with only intravenous glucose 8–12 g/h. From the next day onwards, the nutrition was to administer total protein-derived calories required for 24 h. It was calculated on the basis of balanced composition of 0.13–0.26 g nitrogen/kg/24 h. It was to deliver 20–30% total calorie requirement. Additional 20–40% calories were given as lipids or nonprotein calories. The mode of giving the calories was either total parenteral nutrition or it could be a combination of parenteral and/or enteral nutrition or could be full enteral feeding. Whether to start enteral feeding on the next day on or as early as possible was decided on the judgment of the physician looking after these patients [15]. Wherever enteral feeding was not possible, TPN would be the most logical as well as the only option.

Total intravenous or parenteral nutrition substantially bypasses the first-pass hepatic circulation of nutrients that would come via the stomach. The insulin therefore is not released appropriately by the pancreas by activating the neuroendocrine axis. Hence, we need to have higher circulating insulin levels. One must be aware of it while loading the plasma with nutrients and make adjustment to give higher doses of subcutaneous or intravenous insulin to keep the blood glucose levels normal.

Parenteral amino acids are a good source of protein and may not cause immediate rise of glucose. However some of them may be used up in gluconeogenesis.

The American Association of Clinical Endocrinologists and American Diabetes Association (AACE/ADA) have issued certain recommendations with respect to glycemic levels to be attained in critically ill patients with any forms of nutrition supplementation as above. It is a consensus statement. It says that a blood glucose level between 140 and 180 mg/dL in critically ill patients is the preferred one [16]. As has been shown repeatedly in this volume, it matches perfectly with the recommendations the authors have been making much before 2008.

A glucose load sufficient to meet the demands of the brain and basic cellular functions is the main consideration in deciding how much glucose per day should be administered within the TPN supplementation. The recommended dose for glucose is 4 mg/kg/min in nondiabetic critically ill patients. However the same rate in patients with established diabetes will undoubtedly need higher insulin use in those who need intensive care in particular. It would be desirable to reduce the hyperglycemic excursions during TPN. The total dextrose infusion was limited to 150 g/day to avoid hyperglycemia [12, 17–19]. Very high quanta of intravenously administered glucose during TPN will also need higher rates of insulin infusions and high insulin plasma levels. Together these two factors will have some adverse effects. It accelerates lipogenesis in the liver and fat tissue and more heat is generated. It also leads to a higher CO_2 production due to full oxidation of glucose. It will lead to higher work of breathing [20, 21].

Indications for TPN

In postoperative or any critical illness, patients are not able to consume for the next few or several days all the calories needed for recovery either in ICUs or in general wards. Hence some criterion is necessary to decide when to start special nutritional methods like TPN. If a patient cannot take in more than or equal to 60% of his nutritional needs for at least 5 days in the ICU, or 7–14 days in the general ward, the patient should be given special nutrition support. This is supported by evidence to be a better approach than early initiation of TPN as shown below.

Very early initiation is started with infusion of 20% glucose on day 1 followed by enteral/parenteral nutrition on day 2 to meet the calorie requirement. However if the total parenteral nutrition is withheld until day 8, it has been shown to result in much reduced ICU infections, early recovery of organ dysfunction, reduced ICU stay, and lowered health-care costs. One way of doing it is to supplement approximately 30% of the nutrition needs by oral route. The remaining is supplemented by total parenteral route. This significantly lowers the high tissue concentration of glucose and reduces insulin resistance, and significantly less insulin is needed to be infused. This maneuver can still achieve a glucose level of 100 mg/dL [22, 23].

The macronutrient composition modifications of TPN

The macronutrients are glucose, proteins, and fats. The recommendations are at least 2 g/kg/day of glucose as the only carbohydrate in parenteral nutrition formulations, 0.7–1.5 g/kg/day of lipid emulsions, and 1.3–1.5 g/kg/day of amino acids calculated according to the ideal body weight [8, 12, 24, 25]. Many professional societies and experts have recommended this. Lipid supplementation is to be carried out by using soybean oil-based lipid emulsion. This is the only approved formulation in the USA. It has a high content of linoleic acid and ω-6 polyunsaturated fatty acids (PUFA.) With it there is a likelihood of excessive inflammatory response during stress and trauma. Soybean oil is likely to generate higher levels of arachidonic acid which in turn may lead to the generation of eicosanoids causing more inflammation [26–28]. Infusion of ω-6 PUFA can have other contrary effects also. These effects are immunosuppressive and decrease endothelial function of generating nitric oxide. It may also decrease autonomic nervous system activity. This has led to the development of lipids with lower linoleic acid content. This can be done by adding olive oil (ClinOleic; Baxter, Chicago, IL, USA), deceasing soybean oil content. This has improved the safety of TPN [26, 29–31]. However soybean vs. olive oil-based lipid emulsion has not shown any difference in the frequency of infectious or noninfectious complications in hospital or ICU stay. Similarly it has not shown any difference in glycemic control or inflammatory plus oxidative stress markers in medical and surgical ICU patients [32]. This is the only trial that compared clinical outcomes between ICU patients receiving these two lipid-based parenteral nutrition.

Disadvantages of TPN

Prolonged TPN bypasses the gastric route of nutrition supplements. It leads to gut mucosal atrophy, overfeeding, and hyperglycemia. The risk of infectious complications, deaths, and hospital complications in critically ill patients increases. TPN-induced hyperglycemia is more likely for the patients to be admitted to the

ICU. They also require a more protracted administration of parenteral nutrition when patients without hyperglycemia are compared with this [8, 33, 34].

Maintaining infusion rate properly and using a separate intravenous line can keep the parameters of controls within limits better. Intravascular thrombosis and lipemia during parenteral lipid infusion can be avoided if the rate of supplementation is adequately matched with disposal of the nutrients. Intermittent testing for lipid levels may also be desirable.

Thrombophlebitis due to intravenous injections can be very troublesome and is highly undesirable in people with diabetes. Hypertonic glucose boluses cause it maximally. We have suggested gentler speeds and other methods of administering the same in problems relating to hypoglycemia. Also in femoral central lines, lower limb infusions should be avoided. Some of the worst phlebothrombosis and abscesses can be seen with people with diabetes.

Insulin therapy during total parenteral nutrition

Hyperglycemia should be corrected, and normoglycemia should be maintained at all costs. One way is to change the nutrient contents. Or insulin infusion should be appropriately changed during TPN [35]. The use of subcutaneous as well as intravenous insulin is quite effective in maintaining normoglycemia in patients on TPN [10, 18]. As has been repeatedly stated earlier, critical illness or hemodynamically unstable patients must be treated by intravenous continuous insulin infusion and not subcutaneous insulin. Separate insulin infusion is more effective over long intervals of TPN also for reasons like flexibility of doses rapidly and frequently. It will be cost-effective as it will reduce all consequences of intermittent or prolonged hyperglycemia. Adding insulin to the TPN bag loses these advantages as one gets bound by the fixed doses which cannot be varied for excellent control. The fact that insulin added to TPN mixture is clinically safe does not make it the choice [36].

When glucose is used alone with insulin, there are two recommendations of how much each should/could be infused. For every 11 g of dextrose, 1 U of insulin in patients with diabetes is effective. TPN containing as much as 150–300 g of carbohydrates per day can thus be effectively controlled for hyperglycemia. 1 U of regular insulin for every 10 g of dextrose can be started as a baseline ratio. If hyperglycemia results, the insulin should be upscaled or glucose infusion quantum can be reduced [10, 37]. If high insulin resistance is suspected, the insulin-glucose ratio of 1 U to 4 g of dextrose during TPN in subjects with diabetes achieved normoglycemia [38]. Needless to say that these formulae may work or may have to be upscaled or lowered, the quantum of which will be determined by the level of insulin resistance hence will have to be individualized (Ref. Chap. 1).

Insulin use in patients without diabetes on TPN

Glucose infusion could be higher in patients without diabetes who are on TPN at 20 g of glucose with 12 U of insulin. If blood glucose is above 140 mg/dL, the glucose can be reduced to 15 g without changing insulin at 1 U/h in ICU. Nondiabetic hyperglycemia was managed also by daily insulin dose of 0.3 ± 0.2 U/kg/day [39, 40].

This note on TPN has been developed on the basis of a fine review by Gosmanov Aidar R and Umpierrez Guillermo E [26] for which we gratefully acknowledge our debt to both the authors.

Q10: How has the Alberti regime evolved over years? Its transition to the insulin infusion through to the Syringe pump needs more clarification

The most important change Alberti regimen brought about was the shift from very high levels of insulin hourly to low-dose insulin infusion starting with 5–7 U/h. This has not changed as the base rate. The Alberti regimen recommends 180 g of glucose, i.e., 7.5 g of glucose per hour IV. This has changed marginally between 150 and 200 g of glucose IV in different situations. However with the Alberti regimen, the glucose-to-insulin ratio is fixed. It cannot be varied independent of each other if the blood glucose level is unsatisfactory. The alternative was to prepare several dextrose infusions with different insulin concentrations. The insulin concentrations could start from 1 to several units of insulin for every 100 mil of dextrose and a fixed dose of and potassium. If blood glucose was not adequately controlled, the bag of IV fluid had to be discarded or at least kept aside for a possible reuse. This was clumsy. A new bag of glucose with the possible appropriately higher quantum of insulin had to be started. There were some basic algorithm for glucose levels and likely required insulin infusion rate, something like sliding scale. Frequent changes of infusion made this regimen labor intensive which contributed to inadequate glycemic control but a lot of wastage of IV fluids. What it did achieve was to virtually eliminate the dangers of both severe frequent hypoglycemia and hypokalemia [41]. A 10% dextrose also did not come with the normal saline component which has been shown to be a disadvantage at many places in the preceding chapters in detail.

Two developments established the variable rate insulin regimens as the best. Reliable but large volume infusion pumps and rapid glucose monitoring meters became available. Over the 1990s, the availability of rapid glucose assessing meters became quite widespread though greater accuracy took its time to occur. The small-volume insulin pumps of great accuracy were available in the new millennium. Insulin and glucose administered separately had become common practice in the Oxford region by 1993. More than 70% of anesthetists used variable rate insulin infusions by then to achieve good control of glucose levels during major surgery [42]. What was overlooked was to use a dextrose concentration which also had a normal saline component. This mechanical adoption of the Alberti regimen inevitably exposed diabetic patients to the development of hyponatremia with it dangerous complication over short run. Hyponatremia, even if it was a laboratory parameter in many symptoms of cerebral edema with lethargy and headache, seizures, coma, and even death, was the danger always lurking in the background [43].

To avoid hyponatremia as a complication, additional infusion of 0.9% sodium chloride in the event of hyponatremia was suggested, but the rate of glucose infusion remained unchanged at 100 ml/h [44]. The obvious risk of fluid overload was always there. The simple solution was to use DNS to avoid this. We have discussed this issue in connection with the usage of Ringer's lactate also in an earlier chapter which may be worth referring to. We have also commented on the sliding scales at a few places. Both Alberti and the separate infusion methods or regimens depended on low to moderate hourly doses of insulin as the precursors, but it was difficult to upscale insulin rapidly especially in stress and high insulin resistance we have harked upon. Thus today it is dextrose normal saline at a fixed rate of 100–125 mils/h and a separate variable insulin infusion as the norm.

Q11: Between the analogues and human insulins, which are the preferred insulins?

This question has been substantially answered in the section on Pharmacokinetics and Pharmacodynamics of Insulin in this volume. We may still add that rapid-acting human insulins are more predictable in action and more dependable especially by intravenous route and have a cost advantage as well. This is further accentuated if the insulin usage is going to be short in perioperative period. If the cost consideration is not there, analogue insulin is better for subcutaneous use for various reasons discussed in the abovementioned chapter.

Q12: What is the difference between multiple monitoring and glucose profiling?

Glucose profiling is a technique used to decide the adequacy or otherwise of any antidiabetic treatment regime, generally in ambulatory diabetics. It can be applied to adjust doses in preoperative stage as well. Six to seven blood glucose readings are taken as described earlier. As regards multiple monitoring, we have used these words essentially in the perioperative context. Here the next glucose estimation is directed by the preceding reading or to calculate the insulin quanta to be administered in the upcoming insulin infusions, which unlike glucose profiling would be more random in time sequence.

Q13: How are deficits of sodium, potassium, and bicarbonates calculated on the basis of serum levels and ABG readings?

The calculations can be done by the following formulae:

- Total deficit of Na^+ = (140 − S. Na) × 0.6 × kg body weight.
- Total deficit of K^+ = (4 − S. K) × 0.3 kg body weight.
- Total deficit of bicarbonate = (ABE) × 0.3 × kg body weight.

In pH below 7, 100 ml sodium bicarbonate is diluted with 400 ml of distilled water and given at 200 ml/h and venous pH checked after 30 min and repeated if necessary.

The formulae to be used for calculating osmolarity and correction of sodium in hyperosmolar states are given in the corresponding topic.

Q14: In how many days can the patient be put on oral hypoglycemic agents again and insulin withdrawn after surgery?

It is relevant only in Type 2 diabetes and Gestational Diabetes. Patients with type 2 diabetes, well controlled preoperatively, can go back to OHAs again. In minimalistic surgeries like cataract, laparoscopic or orthopedic clean surgeries this can happen by the next day. In case of infected surgical conditions, especially with long scars it is wise to continue insulin till the infection completely disappears and the scar heals firmly. The strong anabolic actions of insulin come helpful in such situations. Procedures like sternotomy site or any other surgery in which infections occur more frequently insulin coverage is probably more desirable even if the preoperative control on OHAs was good. If diabetes persists after delivery in GDM and if the woman is lactating she should be controlled with insulin since OHAs likely to cross placenta will have deleterious effects on the fetus through pancreatic stimulation leading to hypoglycemia. This has been contested and OHAs have been shown to be as effective in controlling GDM as insulin in many cases without fetal affection. But we *do not* subscribe to it and use only insulin, regular or analogue during GDM.

Infection and scar healing are the two major considerations to continue as long as one can with insulin postoperatively.

Q15: Does substitution within various sulfonylureas help?

No. It does not help if the patient is well controlled and does not have hypoglycemic episodes under a particular SU. If such episodes are frequent, substituting SUs with lower hypoglycemic potential may work. Otherwise there is no place for substitution. One must ascertain that such people do not have any renal or hepatic impairment. Many of them may not even need OHAs if they normalize weight and diet and do exercises. The relative potential of various OHAs is answered in a separate question in this chapter. Some SUs have been converted to longer-acting forms. There are no studies to support substituting normally acting SU by extended-release SUs. Repaglinide is a good substitute for replacement of SUs in early renal failure.

This class concept is applicable to all the other oral drugs used to treat diabetes and its comorbidities. In the classes of gliptines, ACE inhibitors and ARBs, cholesterol-lowering agents, and antibiotics, several molecules have been marketed, each having some extra advantage over others or a limitation. It stands to reason to get familiar with a couple of molecules from each class and get the experience with close observation than prescribing them by random substitution with the other.

Q16: Does 5% dextrose with 5% fructose solutions have any disadvantages or advantages?

Oral fructose from low-calorie fruits produces less glycemic swings as compared to oral glucose, especially when mixed with meals. In susceptible type 1 patients with diabetes, it can cause exacerbation of hypertriglyceridemia if it is given IV; hence caution is needed. Fructose directly enters glycolytic pathway for which it may not need insulin. But the total glucose load from that point can be considered as glucose plus glucose load or fructose plus fructose load. To this extent additional insulin requirement could be assumed for supplementation, while insulin dose is decided. Secondly fructose cannot be given as 10% solution IV since the brain cannot utilize fructose which has to be complimented as 5% dextrose with 5% fructose IV.

Q17: Are there formulae to calculate insulin doses while converting a patient on IV insulin to subcutaneous insulin?

In general the total dose consumed by the patient in 24 h IV to remain normoglycemic is the basis for SC doses. There may however be need for supplemental doses of insulin since 30% of SC insulin is degraded reducing available insulin quantum. If hyperglycemia prevails, these doses have to be up scaled. In clinical practice the calculations, if they serve well, are helpful. The formulae do not usually achieve normal glucose values only a nearby value. Further control should be by using common sense and not using another formula. Glucose control is an art; the best way is to stop chasing glucose levels but rein it in by aggressive increase in the insulin doses.

Those patients on insulin and under control prior to need for any surgery could possibly go back to their previous dose. If a patient postoperatively is considered as insulin-requiring type 2 diabetic, the dose can be calculated as 0.5–0.7 per kg body weight per day to start with. But in many cases, it may have to be upscaled to 1.2 U of insulin.

The total daily dose is calculated by different formulae for SC switch.

1. The last stable hourly insulin infusion rate multiplied by 24 can be considered as the insulin dose for 24 h [45].
2. When the patient is nil per oral and is not receiving IV dextrose but is receiving insulin infusion at a particular rate over 6–8 h interval, the average of all such dose intervals can be considered as the hourly dose for subcutaneous insulin injections.
3. The average dose of the (last) 6 h should be multiplied by 4. If the average is taken from 8 h, it should be multiplied by 3 to arrive at the possible total dose for 24 h [46]. An additional calculation attached to it is to multiply the above dose by 0.7 or 0.8 again. The product is considered as dose reduction for safety. To complete the understanding, the figures 0.7 and 0.8 when multiplied by body weight represent the possible need for insulin in a day in stable nonstress conditions. It may go as high as 2.2 or more in stable as well as stressed conditions [47].
4. If the patient is taking full nutrition, average hourly drip rate of previous 6 h be multiplied by 20 for total daily dose.
5. Minimal nutrition is defined as the patient taking only 50% of the calories needed or if the patient is nil per oral. The average hourly drip rate over prior 6 h needed for glucose control may then be multiplied by 40 to decide total SC insulin dose [48].
6. Patients in hospital could be on basal and prandial insulin supplementation. The total dose requirements can be considered as the average mean hourly rate of insulin infusion in last 12 h, multiplied by 24 as the daily insulin requirement [49].
7. The 24-h basal requirement can be calculated as patient's hourly insulin infusion rate during stress and while nil per oral. It is multiplied by 24. This will undoubtedly need additions of short- or rapid-acting insulin for glycemic excursions—authors [50].

Q18: What is the status of high-protein diets in perioperative situation?

The question implies whether in diabetes, protein supplementation higher than the recommended one has any value. It does not. The issue in India is different. Many Indian patients with diabetes on diet may not be able to meet the recommended protein intake, particularly the vegetarians. The normal recommendation is 1–1.2 g of protein/kg ideal body weight. If there is renal involvement, then depending upon the degree of renal insufficiency, it has to be reduced to 0.8 or 0.6 g/kg ideal body weight, both normally or during surgical situations. High-protein diets are particularly contraindicated in even incipient nephropathy as it worsens the renal injury. In patients with diabetes undergoing any type of major surgery, where oral intake is going to be deferred for, a few days or more attention to adequate protein supplementation are mandatory. The details are given on the question of TPN above. In highly catabolic states, higher supplementation is given. Adequacy of insulin administration with it is important.

Only protein diet, high-fiber diets, and recently for weight loss and diabetes a high-fat high-protein with low or no carbohydrate keto diet are under practice. While prescribing any diet, the prescriber must take into account various comorbidities of diabetes but *most importantly the feasibility* of carrying out the same for long periods.

Q19: At what dose of insulin an OHA be considered for substitution?

Any person, whose diabetic status can be managed with less than 20 U of insulin per day, in the absence of significant renal disease, can be considered for substitution of OHAs postoperatively. They should be started on low doses of SUs with low hypoglycemic potential and then gradually increased over a few weeks. Addition of other OHAs will have to be considered simultaneously for control. If they do not achieve euglycemia, then they should be quickly shifted back to insulin.

Q20: How high can insulin doses go?

Theoretically there is no limit to it. Patients on high doses of glucocorticoids preoperatively or in gestational diabetes or hyperosmolar hyperglycemic states are some examples where as high as 200 U or more per day may be needed. Careful multiple monitoring and dose fixation are required in these conditions.

Q21: What are "sick day rules"?

Sick day rules mean the modified ways of food and fluid intake as well as insulin administration schedule and doses. These are generally far more important for type 1 patients with diabetes. In a person with type 1 diabetes, any illness will cause the blood glucose to rise even if such a person is not eating well. As a result the patient, relatives, or even the treating physician tends to reduce insulin or temporarily withhold insulin. Actually the insulin doses need to be either increased, or small doses have to be given with every small food intake; the glucose monitored and insulin doses increased more boldly.

The sick day rule is that the calorie supplementation should continue as small portions as solids if tolerated or liquids frequently, with as liberal hydration as possible. A cup of 250 mL or more of sugar-free fluid every hour is recommended. Water, weak tea or herbal tea, or many such beverages that can be prepared in India like thin buttermilk with a little salt and many more can be considered useful to maintain hydration and prevent dehydration. This has to be coupled with continuing the same doses of insulin or an arbitrary increase of insulin doses by 20%. The presence of sickness despite increased insulin doses will not result in hypoglycemia but may bring the glucose levels to a more acceptable level and prevent the onset of acidosis, vomiting, and nausea, making way for better and more easily tolerated food and liquid intake while the therapy instituted for its new destabilizing disease progresses. The insulin dose can be divided in smaller but increased number of doses under monitoring at short intervals till a substantial reduction in glucose level is obtained. Moreover, patients should be given instructions on how to initiate additional subcutaneous insulin supplementation in the event of continued hyperglycemia.

In acute surgical situations, the sick day rules do not apply. In type 2 diabetes, the OHAs should not be discontinued, and the food and fluid intake as mentioned above should continue. If these measures are not sufficient or nausea is severe, such patients with medical conditions will need hospitalization.

References

References on Q4: You have mentioned the Leuven studies. Their results are not confirming but often contradictory. How do you explain that?

1. Berghe G, Dodek P. Intravenous insulin nomogram improves blood glucose control in the critically ill. Crit Care Med. 2001;29:1714–9.
2. Van den Berghe G, et al. Intensive insulin therapy in the medical ICU. N Engl J Med. 2006;354:449–61.
3. The ACCORD Study Group. Effects of intensive blood-pressure control in type 2 diabetes mellitus. N Engl J Med. 2010;362(17):1575–85, nejm.org. 29 Apr 2010.
4. Van den Berghe, et al. Intensive insulin therapy in mixed medical/surgical intensive care units: benefit versus harm. Diabetes. 2006;55:3151–9.

References on Q8: Type 2 diabetes needs many drugs for normoglycemia and many more to control other complications. Are there any significant drug interactions?

5. Scheen Andre J. Drug interactions of clinical importance with antihyperglycemic agents an update. Drug Saf. 2005;28(7):601–31.
6. UK Prospective Diabetes Study (UKPDS) Group. Intensive blood-glucose control with sulphonylureas or insulin compared with conventional treatment and risk of complications in patients with type 2 diabetes (UKPDS 33). Lancet. 1998;352:837–53.
7. Surekha V, Peter JV, Jeyaseelan L, et al. Drug interaction: rifampicin and glibenclamide. Natl Med J India. 1997;10:11–2.

References for Q9: What are the indications, contraindications, advantages, disadvantages, and side effects of total parenteral nutrition (TPN)? How is glycemic control affected and how is it managed?

8. Alberti KG, Marshall SM. Diabetes and surgery. In: Alberti KG, Krall LP, editors. Diabetes annual/4. New York: Elsevier; 1988. p. 248–71.
9. Ziegler TR. Parenteral nutrition in the critically ill patient. N Engl J Med. 2009;361:1088–97. [PubMed: 19741230].
10. McMahon MM, Rizza RA. Nutrition support in the hospitalized patient with diabetes mellitus. Mayo Clinic Proc. 1996;71:587–94.

11. Bantle JP, Wylie-Rosett J, Albright AL, Apovian CM, Clark NG, Franz MJ, Hoogwerf BJ, Lichtenstein AH, Mayer-Davis E, Mooradian AD, Wheeler ML. Nutrition recommendations and interventions for diabetes: a position statement of the American Diabetes Association. Diabetes Care. 2008;31(Suppl 1):S61–78. https://doi.org/10.2337/dc08-S061.2008.
12. McClave SA, Martindale RG, Vanek VW, et al. Guidelines for the provision and assessment of nutrition support therapy in the adult critically ill patient: Society of Critical Care Medicine (SCCM) and American Society for Parenteral and Enteral Nutrition (A.S.P.E.N.). JPEN J Parenter Enteral Nutr. 2009;33:277–316.
13. Mesotten D, Gielen M, Wouters PJ, Desmet L, Vlasselaers D, Vanhorebeek I, Langouche L, Van den Berghe G. Effect of tight glucose control with insulin on the thyroid axis of critically ill children and its relation with outcome. J Clin Endocrinol Metab. 2012;97(10):3569–76. https://doi.org/10.1210/jc.2012-2240. Epub 2012 Aug 7.
14. Van den Berghe G, et al. Intensive insulin therapy in mixed medical/surgical intensive care units: benefit versus harm. Diabetes. 2006;55:3151–9.
15. van Den Berghe G, et al. Outcome benefit of intensive insulin therapy in the critically ill: Insulin dose versus glycemic control. Crit Care Med. 2003;31(2):359–66.
16. Moghissi ES, Korytkowski MT, DiNardo M, et al. American Association of Clinical Endocrinologists and American Diabetes Association consensus statement on inpatient glycemic control. Endocr Pract. 2009;15:353–69. [PubMed: 19454396].
17. Rosmarin DK, Wardlaw GM, Mirtallo J. Hyperglycemia associated with high, continuous infusion rates of total parenteral nutrition dextrose. Nutr Clin Pract. 1996;11:151–6. [PubMed: 9070016].
18. McCowen KC, Bistrian BR. Hyperglycemia and nutrition support: theory and practice. Nutr Clin Pract. 2004;19:235–44. [PubMed: 16215111].
19. Ahrens CL, Barletta JF, Kanji S, et al. Effect of low-calorie parenteral nutrition on the incidence and severity of hyperglycemia in surgical patients: a randomized, controlled trial. Crit Care Med. 2005;33:2507–12. [PubMed: 16276174].
20. Schutz Y, Thiebaud D, Acheson KJ, et al. Thermogenesis induced by five different intravenous glucose/insulin infusions in healthy young men. Clin Nutr. 1983;2:93–6. [PubMed: 16829417].
21. Askanazi J, Weissman C, Rosenbaum SH, et al. Nutrition and the respiratory system. Crit Care Med. 1982;10:163–72. [PubMed: 6800701].
22. Casaer MP, Mesotten D, Hermans G, et al. Early vs late parenteral nutrition in critically ill adults. N Engl J Med. 2011;365:506–17. [PubMed: 21714640].
23. Lidder P, Flanagan D, Fleming S, et al. Combining enteral with parenteral nutrition to improve postoperative glucose control. Br J Nutr. 2010;103:1635–41. [PubMed: 20211036].
24. Singer P, Berger MM, Van den Berghe G, et al. ESPEN Guidelines on Parenteral Nutrition: intensive care. Clin Nutr. 2009;28:387–400. [PubMed: 19505748].
25. Via MA, Mechanick JI. Inpatient enteral and parental nutrition for patients with diabetes. Curr Diab Rep. 2011;11:99–105. [PubMed: 21170688].
26. Gosmanov AR, Umpierrez GE. Medical nutrition therapy in hospitalized patients with diabetes. Curr Diab Rep. 2012;12:93–100. [PubMed: 21997598].
27. Yaqoob P. Lipids and the immune response. Curr Opin Clin Nutr Metab Care. 1998;1:153–61. [PubMed: 10565342].
28. Yaqoob P. Monounsaturated fatty acids in parenteral nutrition; evaluation of risks and benefits. Br J Nutr. 2005;94:867–8. [PubMed: 16351759].
29. Buenestado A, Cortijo J, Sanz MJ, et al. Olive oil-based lipid emulsion's neutral effects on neutrophil functions and leukocyte-endothelial cell interactions. JPEN J Parenter Enteral Nutr. 2006;30:286–96.
30. Garcia-de-Lorenzo A, Denia R, Atlan P, et al. Parenteral nutrition providing a restricted amount of linoleic acid in severely burned patients: a randomized double-blind study of an olive oil-based lipid emulsion vs medium/long-chain triacylglycerols. Br J Nutr. 2005;94:221–30. [PubMed: 16115356].

31. Siqueira J, Smiley D, Newton C, et al. Substitution of standard soybean oil with olive oil-based lipid emulsion in parenteral nutrition: comparison of vascular, metabolic, and inflammatory effects. J Clin Endocrinol Metab. 2011;96:3207–16. [PubMed: 21832112].
32. Umpierrez GE, Spiegelman R, Zhao V, et al. A double-blind, randomized clinical trial comparing soybean oil-based vs olive oil-based lipid emulsions in adult medical-surgical intensive care unit patients requiring parenteral nutrition. Crit Care Med. 2012;40:1792–8. [PubMed: 22488002].
33. Cheung NW, Napier B, Zaccaria C, Fletcher JP. Hyperglycemia is associated with adverse outcomes in patients receiving total parenteral nutrition. Diabetes Care. 2005;28:2367–71. [PubMed: 16186264].
34. Pasquel FJ, Spiegelman R, McCauley M, et al. Hyperglycemia during total parenteral nutrition: an important marker of poor outcome and mortality in hospitalized patients. Diabetes Care. 2010;33:739–41. [PubMed: 20040658].
35. Quigley EM, Marsh MN, Shaffer JL, Markin RS. Hepatobiliary complications of total parenteral nutrition. Gastroenterology. 1993;104:286–301. [PubMed: 8419252].
36. Sajbel TA, Dutro MP, Radway PR. Use of separate insulin infusions with total parenteral nutrition. JPEN J Parenter Enteral Nutr. 1987;11:97–9.
37. Hongsermeier T, Bistrian BR. Evaluation of a practical technique for determining insulin requirements in diabetic patients receiving total parenteral nutrition. JPEN J Parenter Enteral Nutr. 1993;17:16–9.
38. Valero MA, Leon-Sanz M, Escobar I, et al. Evaluation of non-glucose carbohydrates in parenteral nutrition for diabetic patients. Eur J Clin Nutr. 2001;55:1111–6. [PubMed: 11781679].
39. Jakoby MG, Nannapaneni N. An insulin protocol for management of hyperglycemia in patients receiving parenteral nutrition is superior to ad hoc management. JPEN J Parenter Enteral Nutr. 2012;36:183–8.
40. Sarkisian S, Fenton TR, Shaheen AARaman M, Raman M. Parenteral nutrition-associated hyperglycemia in noncritically ill inpatients is associated with higher mortality. Canadian journal of gastroenterology. J Can Gastroenterol. 2010;24:453–7. [PubMed: 20652162].

References for Q10: How has the Alberti regime evolved over years? Its transition to the insulin infusion through to the Syringe pump needs more clarification

41. Milaskiewicz RM, Hall GM. Diabetes and anaesthesia: the past decade. Br J Anaesth. 1992;68(2):198–206.
42. Eldridge AJ, Sear JW. Peri-operative management of diabetic patients. Any changes for the better since 1985? Anaesthesia. 1996;51:45–51.
43. Achinger SG, Ayus JC, Moritz ML. Dysnatremias: why are patients still dying? South Med J. 2006;4:353–62.
44. Grant IS, Nimmo GR, Nimmo S. Intercurrent disease and anaesthesia. In: Aitkenhead AR, Smith G, Rowbotham DJ, editors. Textbook of anaesthesia. Oxford: Churchill Livingstone Elsevier; 2007. p. 466–8.

References for Q17: Are there formulae to calculate insulin doses while converting a patient on IV insulin to subcutaneous insulin?

45. Donaldson S, Villanuueva G, Rondinelli L, Baldwin D. Rush University guidelines and protocols for the management of hyperglycemia in hospitalized patients: elimination of the sliding scale and improvement of glycemic control throughout the hospital. Diabetes Educ. 2006;32:954–62.

46. Furnary AP, Braithwaite SS. Effects of outcome on in-hospital transition from intravenous insulin infusion to subcutaneous therapy. Am J Cardiol. 2006;98:557–64.
47. O'Malley CW, Emanuele M, Halasyamani L, Amin AN. Bridge over troubled waters: safe and effective transitions of the inpatient with hyperglycemia. J Hosp Med. 2008;3:55–65.
48. Ramos P, Childers D, Maynard G, et al. Maintaining glycemic control when transitioning from infusion insulin: a protocol driven, multidisciplinary approach. J Hosp Med. 2010;5:446–51.
49. Avanzini F, Marelli G, Donzelli W, et al. Transition from intravenous to subcutaneous insulin: effectiveness and safety of a standardized protocol and predictors of outcome in patients with acute coronary syndrome. Diabetes Care. 2011;34:1445–50.
50. Magaji V, Johnston J. Inpatient management of hyperglycemia and diabetes. Clin Diab. 2011;29:3–9.

Additional Reading

Australian Diabetes Educators Association. Sick day management of adults with type 2 diabetes. Canberra: ADEA; 2014.

Robins M, Coles M, Smith D, Armstrong M, Bryant W, Homeming L, on behalf of the Australian Diabetes Educators Association. Clinical guiding principles for sick day management of adults with type 1 and type 2 diabetes. Technical document. Canberra: ADEA; 2014.

The manufacturer's authorised representative in the EU is Springer Nature Customer Service Centre GmbH, Europaplatz 3, 69115 Heidelberg, Germany. If you have any concerns regarding our products, please contact ProductSafety@springernature.com

Printed and bound by CPI Group (UK) Ltd, Croydon, CR0 4YY
30/07/2026
02181706-0002